Techniques in Anesthesia, Intensive Care and Emergency Medicine

Nishkarsh Gupta
Raveendra Shankaranarayana Ubaradka
Anju Gupta
Debendra Kumar Tripathy
Editors

Techniques in Anesthesia, Intensive Care and Emergency Medicine

Springer

BYWORD BOOKS™

Editors
Nishkarsh Gupta
Department Onco-Anesthesiology and
Palliative Medicine at DRBRAIRCH
All India Institute of Medical Sciences
New Delhi, Delhi, India

Anju Gupta
Anesthesiology, Pain Medicine,
Critical Care
All India Institute of Medical Sciences
New Delhi, Delhi, India

Raveendra Shankaranarayana Ubaradka
Jerudong Park Medical Centre
Brunei Muara, Brunei Darussalam

Debendra Kumar Tripathy
Professor and Head, Department of
Trauma & Emergency
AIIMS Raipur
Raipur, Chhattisgarh, India

ISBN 978-981-96-1201-7 ISBN 978-981-96-1202-4 (eBook)
https://doi.org/10.1007/978-981-96-1202-4

Jointly published with Byword Books

This Springer imprint is published by the registered company Springer Nature Singapore Pte Ltd.
The registered company address is: 152 Beach Road, #21-01/04 Gateway East, Singapore 189721, Singapore

Foreword

All the domains of learning—cognitive, affective, and psychomotor—have important roles and represent a continuum of processes that begin with the simplest and end with the most complex ones. Learning and practicing anesthesia, critical care, and emergency medicine is possibly the most stressful in terms of the altered physiology with rapid and largely unpredictable changes in the homeostasis, with the need for continuous and intense monitoring and invasive interventions, including surgery.

Within this context, the editors (Dr. Nishkarsh Gupta, Dr. Raveendra Shankaranarayana Ubaradka, Dr. Anju Gupta, and Dr. Debendra Kumar Tripathy) of this book have taken pains to create a simple yet practical list of topics related to the techniques of patient clinical management, monitoring, and anesthesia management. With the recent emphasis on the active implementation of Competency Based Medical Education (CBME) by the National Medical Commission (NMC) for undergraduates and the NMC and the National Board of Examinations (NBE) mandate for postgraduates in anesthesiology, critical care, and emergency medicine, this book serves as a ready reference guide. Its primary objectives are to highlight the utility of each technique, the procedural aspects, the practical difficulties, and how to circumvent and overcome them. The nursing trainees and operation theater/anesthesia technicians will also benefit from the simple language and helpful illustrations and tables in each of the chapters. The targeted use of medical and technical jargon would also cater to readers who are primarily interested in learning and practicing basic techniques. Post COVID-19, the importance of oxygen therapy has grown manifold and the chapters on airway management encompass its application in various situations, including anesthesia, critical care, and emergencies. The airway management chapters, covering topics from mask ventilation to supraglottic airway access, endotracheal intubation, jet ventilation, apneic oxygenation, and front-of-neck access, are very lucid and informative.

The lifeline of the medical field, particularly in critical specialities, is vascular access. Fittingly, the first chapter of this book focuses on peripheral venous cannulation. Central venous cannulation and the special indications and techniques of peripherally inserted central venous catheterization have also been rightfully included. Chapters on the point-of-care use of ultrasound for airway, trauma assessment, and cardiac assessment are truly contemporary. So too are the patient-controlled analgesia (PCA) systems and the target-controlled infusion (TCI) techniques, which cover the latest developments in analgesia and anesthesia, encompassing both techniques wise and drug-wise.

The contributors to this book are excellent academicians with sufficient hands-on experience and have incorporated the most recent evidence in the preparation of the manuscripts. Emphasis is placed on the practical aspects of various techniques, with salient theoretical background provided to the extent necessary, allowing the reader to understand the concepts without being overwhelmed by unnecessary or redundant information. It is also important to note that the authors have provided the details of the necessary devices and accessories, drugs and doses routinely used, and alternative interventions when a technique is unsuccessful or not indicated. All in all, this book is a concise resource suitable for every desk, not just for use in the operating room, intensive care unit, and emergency unit, but also in general wards.

Department of Anaesthesiology
Vijayanagar Institute of Medical Sciences
Ballari, Karnataka, India

S. Bala Bhaskar

Preface

Techniques play a major role in medical practice, both in elective and emergency clinical scenarios. They are either essential for surgery, mechanical ventilation, and the administration of anesthesia, etc. or can be lifesaving. The successful execution of techniques and procedures is crucial for patient safety and for the best outcome of treatment. Some techniques are basic, such as peripheral venous access and the use of bag-mask ventilation, while others are more advanced and require specialized training and qualified medical personnel to perform.

The success of any technique depends on understanding its use, selecting the right patient, thorough preparation, and the availability of equipment and expertise. While expertise is acquired through observation, hands-on training, and simulation, the other aspects must be learnt from reliable and authentic sources. While numerous techniques and their indications, contraindications, and steps are described in medical books specific to various specialties, few books have exclusively focused on the techniques and procedures used in medical practice. This book aims to fill this gap by providing a single-point learning resource that covers the majority of techniques, especially about the most basic ones. These basic and commonly used techniques are required to be performed on a day-to-day basis, and some of them are even carried out by nurses and paramedical staff.

The editors (Dr. Nishkarsh Gupta, Dr. Raveendra Shankaranarayana Ubaradka, Dr. Anju Gupta, and Dr. Debendra Kumar Tripathy), who are anesthesiologists with decades of clinical and academic experience, have kept the objectives of this book in mind. The primary objective of this book has been to present the techniques in a lucid and clear manner, covering various aspects in a way that is easily understandable by both basic medical practitioners and paramedical staff. More than 20 techniques have been covered, including seemingly simple yet clinically useful techniques and procedures, such as oxygen therapy and patient transfers. The material is presented in a simple and easy-to-understand manner, with illustrations.

It is expected that readers will welcome this book and make use of its contents, which have been prepared and put together with due diligence and care.

New Delhi, Delhi, India — Nishkarsh Gupta
Brunei Muara, Brunei Darussalam — Raveendra Shankaranarayana Ubaradka
New Delhi, Delhi, India — Anju Gupta
Raipur, Chhattisgarh, India — Debendra Kumar Tripathy

Preface

Techniques play a major role in medical practice, both in elective and emergency clinical scenarios. They are either essential for surgery, mechanical ventilation, and the administration of anaesthesia, etc., or can be life-saving. The successful conduct of techniques and procedures is crucial for patient safety and for the best outcome of treatment. Some techniques are basic, such as peripheral venous [illegible]

[illegible] and simulation, the other aspects must be learnt from reliable and authoritative sources. [illegible]

[illegible] seemingly simple yet clinically useful techniques and procedures, such as [illegible] The material is presented in a simple and easy-to-understand manner, with illustrations.

It is expected that readers will welcome this book and make use of its contents, which have been prepared and put together with due diligence and care.

New Delhi, Delhi, India — Nishkarsh Gupta
Brunei Muara, Brunei Darussalam — Raveendra Shankaranarayana Ubaradka
New Delhi, Delhi, India — Anju Gupta
Raipur, Chhattisgarh, India — Debendra Kumar Tripathy

Contents

Editors and Contributors

About the Editors

Nishkarsh Gupta, MBBS, MD, DNB, PGCCHM, MNAMS is working as Professor in the Department of Onco-anesthesiology and Palliative Medicine at DRBRAIRCH, All India Institute of Medical Sciences (AIIMS), New Delhi. He has been a keen researcher with more than 260 publications to his name. He has written 40 book chapters. He has been a pioneer in the field of difficult airway in head and neck oncology cases and has described new techniques for airway management in these patients. He has received many awards, including the Best Researcher Award by ISA and Best Reviewer Award by IJA. He has been an invited faculty at more than 100 conferences. He has conducted many airway workshops across India. He is the founder-secretary of the Society of Research and Education in Onco-Anesthesiology and Palliative Medicine. He is also a member of the national executive committees of IAPC, SOAPC and RSACP. He serves on the editorial board of several journals. He is the editor of the South Asian adaptation of two of the most widely popular books in anesthesia: *Clinical Anesthesia* by Barash and *Understanding Anesthesia Equipment* by Dorsch and Dorsch. He has also edited eight additional books, including three from Springer: the *Airway Manual*, *Onco-Critical Care*, and *Problem-Based Learning Discussions in Onco-Anesthesiology*.

Raveendra Shankaranarayana Ubaradka, MD, DNB is currently working as a Consultant Anesthesiologist at the Jerudong Park Medical Centre and Maxillofacial, Plastic and Reconstructive Surgery Centre in Brunei Darussalam. Formerly a Professor and Head of the Department of Anaesthesiology at K S Hegde Medical Academy, Nitte University (Deemed to be), Mangalore, Dr. Raveendra has made significant contributions to the field of airway management through clinical teaching, training programs and workshops, conferences, and simulation. He was instrumental in developing a focused and advanced training program for qualified anesthesiologists in fiber-optic guided airway management techniques. Teaching and training in airway management for residents and other medical and paramedical professionals has always been a passion of Dr. Raveendra. He, along with other eminent editors, has recently published a book on airway management, *The Airway Manual.* This book is a single-point learning resource for all aspects of airway management. He is also recognized for his contributions to maxillofacial anesthesia, where difficult airways are frequent. Dr. Raveendra was the founder-secretary of the All India Difficult Airway Association (AIDAA) and was part of the guidelines group of AIDAA, which published the first Indian guidelines on difficult airway management in 2016. He has delivered many guest lectures on airway management at various scientific meetings and conferences, including the 21st ASEAN Congress of Anaesthesiologists (ACA) held in Brunei Darussalam. Empowering young trainees in anesthesia and allied specialities and of allied subjects like nursing and OT technology, with knowledge and skills related to various anesthesia and critical care techniques has been a passion for Dr. Raveendra.

Anju Gupta, MD, DNB, MNAMS, PGCCHM, IDRA is working as an Assistant Professor in the Department of Anesthesiology, Pain Medicine, and Critical Care, All India Institute of Medical Sciences, New Delhi. She completed her MD at Lady Hardinge Medical College, New Delhi, and now has over 15 years of experience in anesthesia, having served as faculty on various national and international platforms. She is an avid researcher, with more than 150 publications in reputable national and international journals and over 35 book chapters to her credit. She has won several prestigious national and international awards. She serves as the Associate Editor of *JMCR*, *Airway*, the *International Journal of Regional Anesthesia*, and *Frontier Pediatrics* and as the Assistant Editor of *JOACP*. Additionally, she is a member of the editorial board of several other journals. She is a member of the international executive committee at ESRA. She is the Editor of the South Asian adaptation of two of the most widely popular anesthesia books: *Clinical Anesthesia* by Barash and *Understanding Anesthesia Equipment* by Dorsch and Dorsch. She was listed by the WFSA as the "Female Innovator and Leader 2023".

Debendra Kumar Tripathy, MBBS, DNB, MNAMS is a distinguished medical professional and co-inventor of the "Pranavayu Ventilator," a groundbreaking innovation in critical care and emergency medicine. Currently holding the position of Professor and Head of Trauma and Emergency at AIIMS, Raipur, Dr. Tripathy has had an illustrious career marked by various achievements. He has held prominent academic roles at esteemed institutions, including AIIMS Raipur and AIIMS Rishikesh, and has made substantial contributions to medical research, education, and innovation. His recognized expertise in critical care and emergency medicine, coupled with his co-editorship of the book *Airway Manual*, exemplifies his commitment to advancing medical knowledge and best practices. As an accomplished speaker and prolific author of numerous publications,

Dr. Tripathy continues to inspire and educate fellow professionals in the medical field. His steadfast dedication to patient care, along with his pioneering inventions and innovations, underscores his exceptional impact on the realm of medicine.

Contributors

Deepti Agarwal Anaesthesiology and Critical Care, U.C.M.S & GTBH, New Delhi, India

Anisha Department of Emergency Medicine, JPNTC, AIIMS, New Delhi, India

Vighnesh Ashok PGIMER, Chandigarh, India

Muralishankar Bhat Department of Anaesthesiology, KS Hegde Medical College, Mangalore, India

Geetanjali Chilkoti Department of Anesthesiology and Critical Care, UCMS and GTB Hospital, New Delhi, India

Mayur Rama Krishna Chillal Critical Care Medicine, Unity Health Network, St. Michaels Hospital, Toronto, ON, Canada

Ripon Choudhary Department of Anesthesia, LNJP and MAMC Delhi, New Delhi, India

Arindam Choudhury Department of Cardiac-Anaesthesia and Intensive Care, AIIMS, New Delhi, India

Devishree Das Department of Cardiac-Anaesthesia and Intensive Care, AIIMS, New Delhi, India

Rohini Dattatri Department of Anesthesiology, AIIMS, Bibinagar, Telangana, India

Surjyendu Ghosh Department of Onco-Anesthesiology and Palliative Medicine, DRBRAIRCH, All India Institute of Medical Sciences, New Delhi, India

Poonam Godhwal Department of Onco-Anesthesiology and Palliative Medicine, DRBRAIRCH, All India Institute of Medical Sciences, New Delhi, India

Anju Gupta Anesthesiology, Pain Medicine, Critical Care, All India Institute of Medical Sciences, New Delhi, Delhi, India

Nishkarsh Gupta Department Onco-Anesthesiology and Palliative Medicine at DRBRAIRCH, All India Institute of Medical Sciences, New Delhi, Delhi, India

Suruchi Hasija Department of Cardiac-Anaesthesia and Intensive Care, AIIMS, New Delhi, India

Karthik V. Iyer Department of Anesthesiology, Pain Medicine and Critical Care, All India Institute of Medical Sciences, New Delhi, Delhi, India

Sriganesh Kamath Department of ENT, KS Hegde Medical Academy, Mangalore, Karnataka, India
Department of Neuroanaesthesia and Neurocritical Care, National Institute of Mental Health and Neurosciences (NIMHANS), Bengaluru, Karnataka, India

Bhavna Kayarat Department of Anesthesiology, Pain Medicine and Critical Care, All India Institute of Medical Sciences, New Delhi, India

Anu Kewlani Department of Anaesthesia, Pain Medicine and Critical Care, All India Institute of Medical Sciences, New Delhi, India

Sachin Kumar Department of Anesthesiology, Pain Medicine and Critical Care, All India Institute of Medical Sciences, New Delhi, India

Kiran Mahendru Department of Anaesthesiology, Dayanand Medical College and Hospital, Ludhiana, Punjab, India

Priya R. Menon Department of Critical Care, Abu Dhabi, UAE

Raj Mohan Department of Cardiac-Anaesthesia and Intensive Care, AIIMS, New Delhi, India

Poonam Motiani Paediatric Anaesthesia, Post Graduate Institute of Child Health, Noida, Uttar Pradesh, India

P. S. Nagaraja Sri Jayadeva Institute of Cardiovascular Sciences and Research, Bangalore, India

M. R. Vishnu Narayanan Department of Anesthesiology, Pain Medicine and Critical Care, AIIMS, New Delhi, India

Parul Raina Department of Anesthesiology, Pain Medicine and Critical Care, All India Institute of Medical Sciences, New Delhi, Delhi, India

Rashmi Ramachandran Department of Anesthesiology, Pain Medicine and Critical Care, AIIMS, New Delhi, India

Vimi Rewari Department of Anesthesiology, Pain Medicine and Critical Care, AIIMS, New Delhi, India

Nishant Sahay Department of Anesthesiology, AIIMS, Patna, India

Indu M. Sen Department of Anesthesiology, PGIMER, Chandigarh, India

Ridhima Sharma Department of Anesthesia, AIIMS, Nagpur, India

Santosh Kumar Sharma Department of Anesthesia, BRD Medical College, Gorakhpur, Uttar Pradesh, India

Gyaninder Pal Singh Department of Neuroanaesthesiology and Critical Care, Neurosciences Centre, All India Institute of Medical Sciences, New Delhi, India

Tej Prakash Sinha Department of Emergency Medicine, JPNTC, AIIMS, New Delhi, India

Bharath Srinivasaiah Department of Neuroanaesthesia and Neurocritical Care, National Institute of Mental Health and Neurosciences (NIMHANS), Bengaluru, Karnataka, India

Ayush Srivastava Department of Emergency Medicine, JPNTC, AIIMS, Delhi, India

Debendra Kumar Tripathy Professor and Head, Department of Trauma & Emergency, AIIMS Raipur, Raipur, Chhattisgarh, India

Raveendra Shankaranarayana Ubaradka Jerudong Park Medical Centre, Brunei Muara, Brunei Darussalam

Vinayak PS Department of Anaesthesiology, MS Ramaiah Medical College, Bangalore, India

Manipal Hospital, Bangalore, India

Preeti Yadav Department of Anesthesiology, Pain Medicine and Critical Care, All India Institute of Medical Sciences, New Delhi, Delhi, India

1 Peripheral Venous Cannulation

Raveendra Shankaranarayana Ubaradka

Key Points
- Peripheral venous access is the most frequently used access to circulation.
- Ability to establish a reliable peripheral venous access is an essential skill.
- Choosing an appropriate size cannula and proper site is important.
- Venous cannulation can be difficult in many patients and requires additional expertise.
- Disconnection, dislodgement, extravasation, thrombophlebitis etc. are known complications.

1.1 Introduction

Peripheral venous access can be easy, difficult, or rarely impossible. It is one of the basic skills in medical care irrespective of the specialty, both in elective and emergency situations. In several clinical situations, it is absolutely inevitable to establish intravenous access. Importance of venous access, general principles, and techniques are described in this chapter.

1.2 Importance of Venous Access

Free flowing, easily accessible venous line (IV line) is the *life line* for patients who require anesthesia, emergency medical care, intensive care, or intravenous medications; (a) IV line is required for administration of anesthetic drugs, fluids (crystal odds and colloidal), and blood. Drugs are given as bolus or as infusion, (b) when there is severe hypotension due to acute and massive blood/fluid loss (which can sometimes take place within a matter of minutes), anaphylaxis, central neuronal blockade or transfusion mismatch, rapid administration of fluids, and blood could be life-saving. This requires one or more wide bore cannula.

Peripheral venous cannula is relatively easier to insert compared to central venous access and can be performed by nurses, paramedics, and other medical assistants with basic training.

1.3 Principles of Peripheral Venous Access

- Site of venous access should be visible and accessible during anesthesia for surgery or non-surgical procedures. For adult patients, ideally, 18 G should be the minimal standard size, irrespective of the severity of surgery. If surgery is a major one with potential for significant blood loss or fluid shift and if the vein

R. S. Ubaradka (✉)
Jerudong Park Medical Centre,
Brunei Muara, Brunei Darussalam

N. Gupta et al. (eds.), *Techniques in Anesthesia, Intensive Care and Emergency Medicine*,
https://doi.org/10.1007/978-981-96-1202-4_1

is prominent, a 16 G cannula can be chosen. The larger the inner diameter of the cannula, the faster the infusion rate. For older children, it is 20 G and smaller children 22 G. 24 G cannula are not very reliable, because of short length and are prone for dislodgement.
- Usually, non-dominant upper limb is preferred. Site should be as distal as possible (commonly on the dorsal of the hand), avoiding the joint and away from the artery. The venous segment chosen should be straight and without valves. However, a change in the site or limb may be required for specific surgical procedures or due to associated comorbid conditions.
- A second cannula, preferably a 16 or even 14 G cannula may be inserted immediately after the induction of anesthesia, before the surgical incision. In surgical patients, establishing an additional venous access becomes progressively difficult as the surgery proceeds, due to blood loss, vasoconstriction, hypothermia, inadequate lighting etc. Use of extension lines may be required.
- Avoid cannulations in the following areas: (a) areas of flexion, (b) previous catheter insertion site, (c) presence of bruise or phlebitis, (d) presence of A-V fistula, (e) previous lymph node dissection or mastectomy, (f) stroke, (g) cellulitis.

1.3.1 Sizes and Specifications

	14 G	16 G	18 G	20 G	22 G	24 G	26 G
Color	Orange	Grey	Green	Pink	Blue	Yellow	Violet
Internal diameter	2.0 mm	1.7 mm	1.3 mm	1.1 mm	0.9 mm	0.7 mm	0.6 mm
Length	45 mm	50 mm	45 mm	33 mm	25 mm	19 mm	19 mm
Max	270 mL/min	196 mL/min	96 mL/min	61 mL/min	36 mL/min	13 mL/min	14 mL/min

Flow depends on additional factors other than internal diameter: Height of the fluid source, type of fluid (blood flows slowly and the line has a filter also) and the length which the fluid has to travel

1.3.2 Steps of IV Cannulation (Fig. 1.1)

- Explain to the patient, select the limb and select the site.
- Make the vein prominent, clean the area with alcohol swab.
- Inject local anesthesia with a 26 G needle—not required in emergency or in unconscious patients.
- Insert the cannula and watch for blood in the hub.
- Push the cannula for a few millimeters and stabilize.
- Withdraw the needle few millimetres into the cannula, without pulling it out completely.
- Simultaneously push the catheter and withdraw the needle.
- Connect the appropriate intravenous fluid.
- Fix the cannula firmly and document the procedure and appropriate instructions.

1.3.3 Difficult Venous Cannulation (Fig. 1.2)

- Not infrequently, there will be patients in whom the venous access becomes extremely difficult if not impossible. These patients/clinical conditions include (a) patients for emergency surgery, (b) dehydration: prolonged fasting, fluid loss, (c) hypotension due to any cause, (d) obesity, (e) post chemotherapy and radiotherapy, (f) previous multiple cannulations as in patients who had multiple surgeries, intensive care unit or prolonged use of antibiotics, (g) children with congenital malformations, and (h) contracture and trauma.

Management of difficult venous cannulation situations include:

(a) Careful search for the veins which have not been utilized carefully. This requires patience and diligence and often successful. Look for

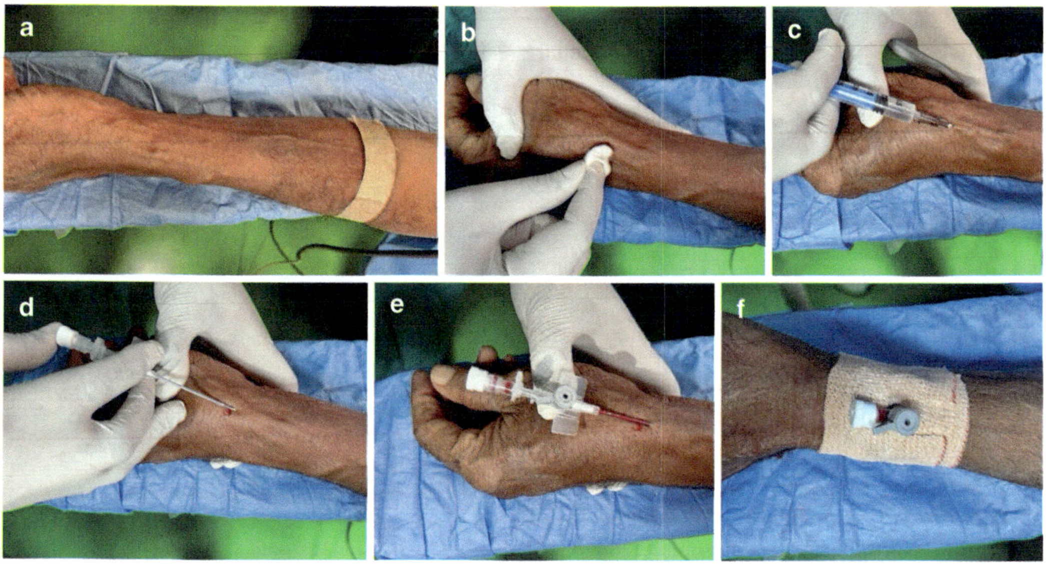

Fig. 1.1 Showing the steps of peripheral IV cannulation. (**a**) Vein is made prominent by applying tourniquet proximally. (**b**) Site is cleaned with alcohol swab. (**c**) Injecting local anesthetic. (**d**) inserting the cannula. (**e**) Needle withdrawn once cannula is inside the vein. (**f**) Cannula fixed firmly

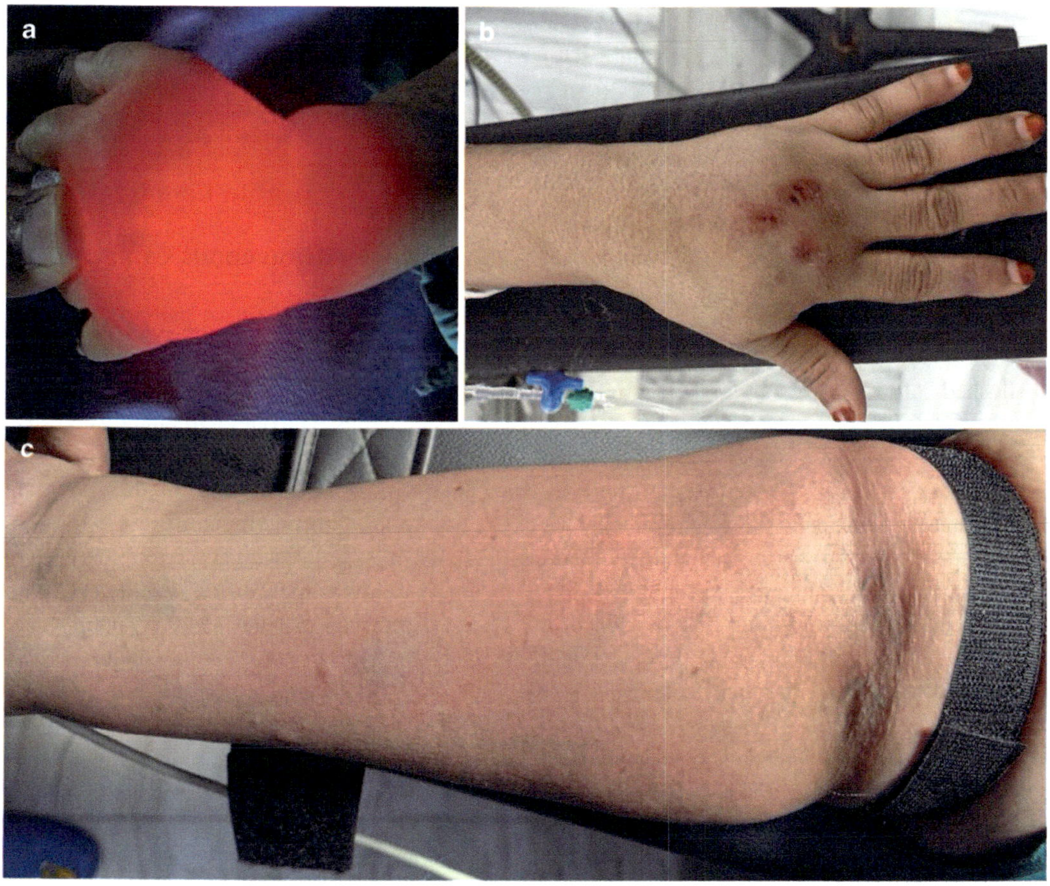

Fig. 1.2 Showing difficult venous cannulation. (**a**) No veins visible in a child even after doing transillumination with a vein finder. (**b**) Edematous hand due to trauma. (**c**) Small tortuous veins and limb pricked multiple times

veins in locations which are not usually noticed by the nurses or other medical practitioners.

(b) Lower limb veins, especially saphenous vein is often available. It's easier after induction of anesthesia and painful in awake patients. *Lower limb veins are useful for the second or additional cannula in major surgeries, especially if the procedure is in the upper part of the body.*

(c) Use of smaller size cannula, like 20 G, before induction and placement of additional cannula after induction when the veins become more prominent.

1.3.4 Use of Extension Lines, 3-Way Stopcocks and Maintenance of Lines and Cannula

- Extension lines are required when the access to the venous cannula is difficult due to its location, surgical position or procedure. Use of an extension provides access to the circulation through a 3-way connection. Different lengths of extension are available and include 10 cm, 15 cm, and 100 cm. The longer the extension, the slower the speed of infusion. Also, when infusions or bolus drugs are injected through long extensions, the effect can become unpredictable (Fig. 1.3).
- If a 3-way stopcock is used, it should be flushed before the use so that there is no dead space left. Sometimes, an additional infusion is attached to the 3-way, but this slows down the rate of primary fluid being administered.
- The intravenous lines which are attached to the cannula need to be flushed and the chamber filled before connecting to cannula. When more than one intravenous line is used in a patient, each should be labelled properly and documented. This becomes all the more important when patient is receiving multiple infusions and is in an unstable condition. Also, the intravenous connection should not be confused with the arterial line flush which should also be clearly labelled.

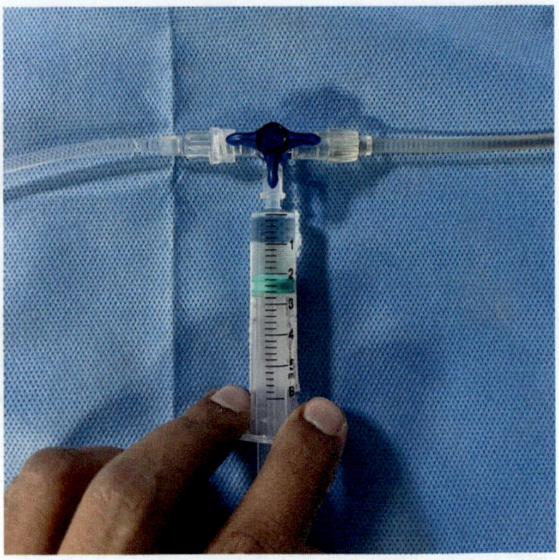

Fig. 1.3 Extension line with 3-way stopcock

- If a cannula is kept without any fluid in the postoperative period, it should be flushed with saline or very small dose of heparin (*hemlock),* to maintain the potency. *According to NABH standards, all cannulas should be flushed with saline before and after antibiotics injection.*

1.3.5 Newer Intravenous Cannula Designs

- The traditional intravenous cannula come with or without (*Jelco cannula)* injection ports and the side wings. The ones without ports are also used for arterial pressure monitoring.
- Needle stick injury is one of the important professional hazards for the anesthesiologist. Hence, it is recommended to avoid re insertion of cannula into the catheter and also to properly dispose the needle.
- Newer cannula come with unique needle design wherein the needle automatically gets distorted loosing it's sharpness, the movement it is withdrawn from the cannula. It cannot be re inserted, e.g., Venflon Pro Safety shielded catheters (B–D).
- Latex free material.

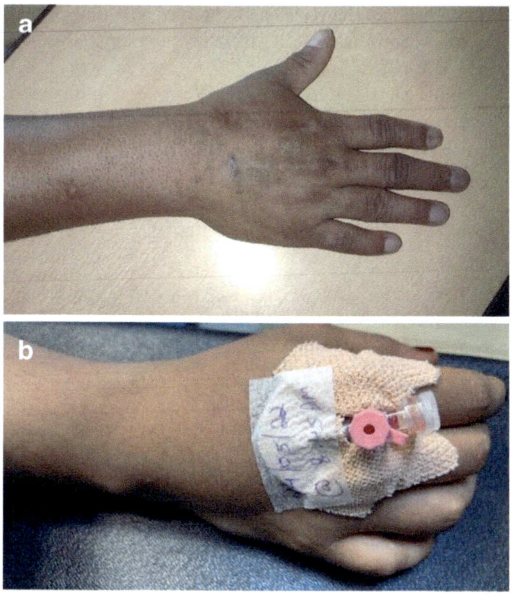

Fig. 1.4 Complications of peripheral venous cannulation. (**a**) Thrombosed veins. (**b**) Swelling due to extravasation of fluid into subcutaneous tissue

1.3.6 Complications with Intravenous Cannulas (Fig. 1.4)

- Counter puncture causing extravasation and hematoma.
- Accidental arterial placement. Easy to detect due to the high pressure with which the flow comes out in case of artery. One has to be very careful when a cannula is inserted in a location which is known to have an artery, like radial artery near the wrist.
- Thrombophlebitis is related to the size of the cannula, duration for which it is left in place, maintenance of the potency, and also the injection if certain drugs.
- Cannula blockade.
- Air embolism and paradoxical air embolism in children with congenital left to right heart communication.
- Needle stick injuries.

1.4 Peripheral Venous Access in Children

Principles are similar to the adult venous access as described above.

Main differences in children are:

(a) Technically may be more difficult requiring specific expertise.
(b) Small veins requiring small size cannula.
(c) Visibility or identification of the vein can be difficult.
(d) Transillumination can be helpful and commonly used.
(e) Maintenance of the cannula is more difficult.
(f) Since the child can't understand, it can't cooperate. Hence awake cannulation is more difficult.

How to achieve cannulation in a child:

- Try to establish rapport with the child and parents.
- Identify the site clearly.
- Apply EMLA (eutectic mixture of local anesthetics) cream, 45 min prior to cannulation to make the procedure painless. Vasoconstriction resulting from the medication could make the technique more difficult.
- Stabilize the hand.
- Use Transillumination with a "cold light" source. *Though it is called cold light, one has to be extremely careful to prevent burns which can readily occur.* It is safer to cover it with a layer of gauze and use for as minimum time as possible.
- Once inserted, fixing the cannula and preventing the child from removing it is often a challenge and might need covering of entire hand beyond wrist, especially in small infants.

1.5 Use of Ultrasound and Vein Detectors

Ultrasound scanning and guidance helps in locating the veins even when no vein is otherwise visible. Similarly, vein detector can be helpful in locating the veins. By applying color doppler, it is possible to distinguish vein and artery which otherwise become difficult in situations such as shock or patients with cyanotic heart diseases.

Suggested Reading

1. Bledsoe BE. Atlas of paramedic skills. Englewood Cliffs, NJ: Prentice-Hall; 1987. p. 124–42.
2. Mahler SA, Wang H, Lester C, et al. Ultrasound-guided peripheral intravenous access in the emergency department using a modified Seldinger technique. J Emerg Med. 2010;39(3):325–9.
3. Mbamalu D, Banerjee A. Methods of obtaining peripheral venous access in difficult situations. Postgrad Med J. 1999;75:459–62.
4. Hambrick EL, Georges GC. Peripheral intravenous access. In: Roberts JP, Hedges JP, editors. Clinical procedures in emergency medicine. 3rd ed. Philadelphia, PA: Saunders; 1998. p. 322–33.
5. Millam DA. Tips for improving your venipuncture techniques. Nursing. 1987;17:46–9.

Oxygen Therapy

2

Santosh Kumar Sharma

"Oxygen therapy is the administration of oxygen at concentrations greater than those found in ambient air." A continuous transfer of oxygen is needed to replace this consumption at the cellular level.

2.1 Goals of Oxygen Therapy

1. To treat or prevent hypoxemia
2. To decrease work of breathing
3. To decrease myocardial work

Oxygen therapy improves patient comfort, increases the body's oxygen reserve, and raises the partial pressure of oxygen in the tissues and blood. It has symptomatic, supportive, and specific roles.

2.2 Indications of Oxygen Therapy [1]

Oxygen therapy is indicated when PaO_2 is less than 60 mmHg or SpO_2 is less than 90% in a previously normal patient. The oxygen therapy increases lung reserve (preoxygenation), helps to correct hypoxemia, helps meet an increased demand (high altitude, shivering, hyperthermia), increases dissolved oxygen in the blood (like anemia, cyanide and CO poisoning), and may help to tide over increased cardiac work (myocardial infarction, angina).

S. K. Sharma (✉)
Department of Anesthesia, BRD Medical College, Gorakhpur, Uttar Pradesh, India

2.3 Physiology of Oxygen Therapy

2.3.1 Oxygen Content

It is the amount of oxygen carried by 100 mL of blood, combined with hemoglobin and in dissolved form. Normal O_2 content is 20 mL/100 mL. Most of the oxygen carried in the blood is transported bound to hemoglobin. A very small amount of oxygen is transported dissolved in the plasma (Table 2.1).

2.3.2 Oxygen Flux

It is the amount of oxygen delivered to the tissues per unit time, equal to the amount of oxygen leaving the left ventricle per minute. Any decrease in cardiac output, saturation, or hemoglobin level will affect oxygen flux (OF) adversely.

OF = C.O. × (SaO_2/100) × 1.31 × (Hb conc ./100) = 5500 × (95/100) × 1.31 × (14.5/100) = 1000 mL (taking SaO_2 95% and Hb 14.5 g/dL)

N. Gupta et al. (eds.), *Techniques in Anesthesia, Intensive Care and Emergency Medicine*,
https://doi.org/10.1007/978-981-96-1202-4_2

Table 2.1 Variables for deriving at an oxygen content

Hb bound O_2	$= SaO_2 \times Hb\% \times 1.39$ mL/dL
Plasma dissolved O_2	$= 0.003$ mL/dL/mmHg $\times PO_2$
Arterial oxygen content (CaO_2)	$= SaO_2 \times Hb\% \times 1.39$ mL/dL + 0.003 mL/dL/mmHg $\times PaO_2$ **~20 mL**
Venous oxygen content (CvO_2)	$= SaO_2 \times Hb\% \times 1.31$ mL/dL + 0.003 mL/dL/mmHg $\times PvO_2$ **~15 mL**
O_2 delivery (DO_2)	$= CaO_2 \times$ cardiac output = 850 to 1200 mL/min (500–700 mL/min/m^2)
O_2 consumption (VO_2)	$= (CaO_2 - CvO_2) \times$ cardiac output = 240–270 mL/min (120–160 mL/min/m^2)
Extraction fraction $(VO_2/DO_2) \times 100$	$= (CaO_2 - CvO_2)/CaO_2$ ~25%

2.3.3 Oxygen Cascade

It refers to steps by which partial pressure of O_2 decreases progressively from highest level in inspired gas to a lower level in mitochondria.

The partial pressure of any component gas in a mixture is calculated as:

$$\text{Partial pressure} = \text{total absolute pressure} \times \text{volume fraction of gas component.}$$

For the oxygen component, $PO_2 = P \times FO_2$, where PO_2 = partial pressure of oxygen (160 mmHg), P = total pressure at sea level (760 mmHg), FO_2 = volume fraction of oxygen content (21%). Air reaching the trachea gets humidified hence the water vapor pressure (47 mmHg) must be subtracted from the total atmospheric pressure (760–47 = 713 mmHg). The partial pressure of oxygen in trachea is thus (0.21 × 713) = 150 mmHg.

Dry atmosphere air (influenced by barometric pressure)
(160 mmHg)
↓
Humidified air in trachea
(150 mmHg)
↓
Alveoli (influenced by alveolar ventilation)
(104 mmHg)
↓
Arterial blood (influenced by V/Q mismatch)
(95–100 mmHg)
↓
Tissue extraction
↓
Venous blood (40 mmHg)
↓
Mitochondria (1–3 mmHg)

The successive step-down in PO_2 can be altered in hypoventilation, ventilation/ perfusion inequality, or diffusion abnormality, resulting in tissue hypoxia (Table 2.2).

2.3.3.1 Pasteur Point

It is the critical mitochondrial PO_2 below which metabolism becomes anaerobic. This represents the last point of oxygen cascade. The range is 0.15 to 0.3 kpa (1.4 to 2.3 mmHg).

2.3.4 Hypoxia

Hypoxia is defined as a condition in which a part of the body or the whole body is deprived of adequate oxygen supply. Different types of hypoxia are described in Table 2.2.

There are several methods, techniques, and devices for oxygen therapy. Oxygen therapy is not necessarily a primary treatment for most of the patients, but an essential supportive treatment. Oxygen administration alone, in the absence of management of the primary pathology/disease may be ineffective.

Primary goal of oxygen therapy is to increase FiO_2, by using appropriate device and flow. FiO_2, is the first step, or starting point in oxygen cascade and the benefits of high FiO_2 may be countered by the factors affecting subsequent steps of oxygen cascade. FiO_2 depends on patient and device factors. Patient factors include respiratory rate and depth, adequacy of ventilation, inspiratory flow, presence or absence of respiratory depression and the presence and severity of airway obstruction. Device factors are type of the device (fixed or variable performance), oxygen flow rate, tightness of mask, special effects, presence of a reservoir bag, and volume of mask.

Table 2.2 Types of hypoxia

Type of hypoxia	Pathophysiology	Examples
Hypoxic Hypoxia ($\downarrow PaO_2$)	Reduced supply	• $\downarrow FiO_2$—high altitude, oxygen poor air, hypoxic gas mixture • Hypoventilation (Ventilatory Failure)—$\uparrow PaCO_2$ • Pulmonary shunt (anatomical and physiological)—septal, vascular malformations; $\uparrow (PAO_2—PaO_2)$ • V/Q mismatch—pneumonia, lobar collapse; $\uparrow (PAO_2—PaO_2)$, $\uparrow PaCO_2$ • ↑ Oxygen demands—fever, shivering, convulsions • Diffusion defects
Anemic hypoxia (↓ oxygen content, PaO_2 normal))	Hb is reduced or functionally impaired, oxygen carrying capacity of blood is decreased	• Massive hemorrhage • Severe anemia • CO poisoning • Methemoglobinemia
Stagnant hypoxia	Transport failure, due to inadequate circulation and tissue perfusion	• LVF • Constrictive pericarditis • Myocardial ischemia • Arterial obstruction or thrombus, Pulmonary embolism • Hypothermia • Hypovolemia • Mitral stenosis
Histotoxic Hypoxia ($\uparrow PvO_2$)	Cells cannot utilise oxygen despite adequate delivery, due to paralysis of electron transfer system of cytochrome oxidase	• Cyanide • Arsenic poisoning

2.4 Source of Oxygen

There are several sources of oxygen supply which are used to deliver oxygen to the patient (Tables 2.3 and 2.4).

Table 2.3 Source of oxygen supply and their characteristics

Type	Characteristics and advantages	Limitations
1. Liquid medical oxygen—in plants or in smaller portable cryogenic containers (also known as reservoirs)	• Central piped system • Based on self-vaporization • Can be used for all oxygen needs • Does not need electricity	• Requires refill by liquid oxygen supplier • Requires back cylinder supply • Significant maintenance system • Need highly trained technicians and engineers
2. Pressure swing adsorption (PSA) plant—large central store based on adsorption technology	• Can be used for all oxygen needs • Central piped system	• Requires un-interrupted power supply • High capital investment • Requires back cylinder supply • Significant maintenance system • Need highly trained technicians and engineers
3. Oxygen concentrators—self-contained portable devices	• An electrically powered, electronically concentrator-controlled device • Produces oxygen from ambient air by absorption of nitrogen onto some type of alumina silicates (Zeolyte)	• Does not store oxygen when not in operation
4. Compressed gas cylinders used either directly at patient care area or through sub-central manifold systems with cylinders linked in parallel	• Black with white shoulders in India • Pin index = 2, 5, or bull nose • Filled by cryogenic distillation or pressure swing adsorption plants • Can be used as back-up for LMO and PSA plants • No power source needed	• Exhaustible supply • Highly dependent on supplier • Requires supply chain • Risk of leakage

Table 2.4 Various sizes of oxygen cylinders

Size	Capacity (L)	Pressure (psi)
B type	200	1900
D type	400	1900
E type	660	1900
F type	1300	1900
G type	3400	1900
M type	3450	2200
H type	6900	2200

2.5 Oxygen Therapy Devices [2]

These are classified into two categories: Low flow/variable performance (patient dependent) devices and high flow/ fixed performance (patient independent) devices (Table 2.5).

The low-flow (variable performance) devices have a flow rate less than the peak inspiratory flow rate (PIFR). The delivered FiO_2 (24–50%) depends on the respiratory rate (RR) and tidal volume (TV). So, rebreathing may occur, and all ventilatory requirements of the patient may not be met. Common examples are nasal cannulas and Hudson masks.

The high-flow/fixed-performance devices have a flow rate higher than PIFR, so they provide fixed and predictable FiO_2 (up to 100%) independent of RR/TV, without rebreathing and meets all the patient's ventilatory requirements. A Venturi mask is a commonly used fixed-performance device.

The low-performance devices are further classified based on their capacity:

(a) No capacity: have no reservoir volume like nasal cannula
(b) Low capacity: the reservoir volume is less than 100 mL, like a simple mask
(c) Medium capacity: the reservoir volume is 100–250 mL, like Hudson mask
(d) High capacity: the reservoir volume is 250–1500 mL; Facemask with reservoir bag
(e) Very high capacity: the reservoir volume is more than 1500 mL, like the oxygen hood

Table 2.5 Characteristics of oxygen delivery devices [3]

Oxygen delivery device	Salient features	Flow rates in L/min	Percentage of FiO_2 delivered	Indications	How to titrate	Advantages	Disadvantages
Nasal cannula (Fig. 2.1)	Two prongs placed in nose and tubings placed above ears	1–6	24–44 (each liter adds 4% FiO_2	Low flow low percentage oxygen supplementation	Titrate flow rate only	• Comfortable/well tolerated • No rebreathing • Can communicate, eat, drink, wear glass and read • Cheap • Useful for long term therapy	• Nasal irritation if flow >4 L/min without humidification • FiO_2 reduced by blocked nose • >4 L/min does not increase oxygenation further • Crusting • Wastage of oxygen during expiration
Simple face mask (Fig. 2.2)	Covers nose and mouth	5–8	35–60	High flow high percentage oxygen supplementation in post-op. recovery room, and transport of patients	Titrate flow rate only	• Increases the size of the oxygen reservoir beyond the limits of the anatomic reservoir • Lateral perforations allow escape of CO_2 • Permits humidification	• Flow rate <3–4 L/min may cause rebreathing of expired gas • Need to remove when speak, eat, or drink • Drying/irritation of eyes • Painful with facial burns/trauma • Application problem with Ryle's tube
Non rebreathing mask (Fig. 2.3)	Transparent plastic mask with reservoir bag under the chin having two unidirectional valves, one to prevent expired gas flow into reservoir bag and another to prevent air entrainment	10–15	60–100	Provide high FiO_2 to patients suspected with significant hypoxemia but normal respiration (short term use)	Non-titratable	• Disposable, light weight • Exhaled oxygen from anatomic dead space is conserved in the reservoir	• Short term use only • Insufficient flow rate may lead to rebreathing of CO_2 • Claustrophobia • Drying/irritation of eyes

Venturi-mask also called air entrainment venti masks or high air flow with oxygen-entrainment (HAFOE) (Figs. 2.4 and 2.5)	• O_2 is directed by a small bore tubing to a mixing jet Adapter entrains ambient air to provide fixed FiO_2	Fixed flow based on adapter chosen or graduated dial	Adapters available in 24 (blue), 28 (white), 31 (pink), 35 (yellow), 40 (orange), 60 (green)	Provides precise controlled percentage of oxygen supplementation (e.g., COPD patients where higher FiO_2 is dangerous)	Titrate FiO_2 only	• Weaning of oxygen support is easier • Due to high flow, excess gas flushes out the expired CO_2 through the holes on the sides of mask	
Oxygen hood	Transparent box which covers only head allowing access to the lower body	7–15	80–90	Short term use for neonates and infants	Titrate flow rate only		• Lot of wastage • Nebulisation not possible • Accurate concentration unpredictable
Oxygen tents	Transparent enclosures in larger sizes for adult pts	10–12	60–70	Short term use in adults	Non titrable	• Temperature and CO_2 levels regulated • Air changes regulated	• Clumsy and claustrophobic • FiO_2 can be very variable • Risk of infection
High flow nasal oxygen devices (HFNO)	• Delivery of supplemental oxygen to the nasopharynx during apnoea • Based on mass flow ventilation	15	Upto 100	Used for Apneic Oxygenation	Titrate FiO_2 only	• Simple and fast • Excellent pre-oxygenation	• Uncomfortable without heating/ humidification
Trans-nasal Humidified Rapid insufflation Ventilatory Exchange (THRIVE)	• Gaseous exchange through flow dependent dead space flushing • Provides apneic ventilation	Very high flow @ 70	21–100	• Perform tubeless surgeries • Non-hypercapnia acute hypoxemic respiratory failure	Titrate flow rate only	• Combines the benefit of apneic oxygenation and CPAP • Reduced rate of rise of CO_2 by approximately 1/3 of that expected	• Uncomfortable without heating/ humidification

(continued)

Table 2.5 (continued)

Oxygen delivery device	Salient features	Flow rates in L/min	Percentage of FiO_2 delivered	Indications	How to titrate	Advantages	Disadvantages
Bag Valve Mask systems • Self-inflating (AMBU bags) • Non-self-inflating (anesthesia bag)	• Have an oxygen inlet reservoir • Have a gas inlet and valve	Flow kept high enough so bags do not deflate	Constant FiO_2 of >90%	• Resuscitation • Surgical procedures	Titrate flow rate only	• Their masks provide comfortable leak free seal for manual ventilation	• In spontaneous Breathing person flow has to be adjusted with the valve • Chances of aspiration • Constant adequate flow of gases has to be maintained
Air Entrainment Nebulizers	• Large volume, High Output device	Flow kept high enough so that the mist is visible during inspiration (8 to 15)	21–100%	• Placed on patients following extubation • Can be applied with many devices: aerosol, tracheostomy dome/collar, face tents, T piece adapter	Titrate flow rate only		• Excess water may collect in tubing and may obstruct and develop resistance to flow • Sometimes Bronchospasm may occur due to irritant nature

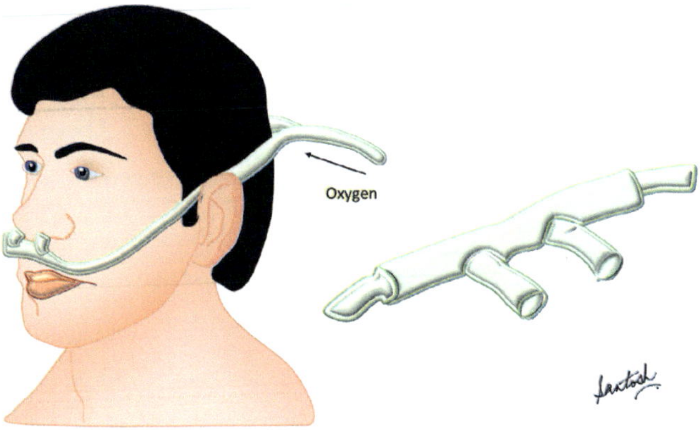

Fig. 2.1 A nasal cannula with two prongs

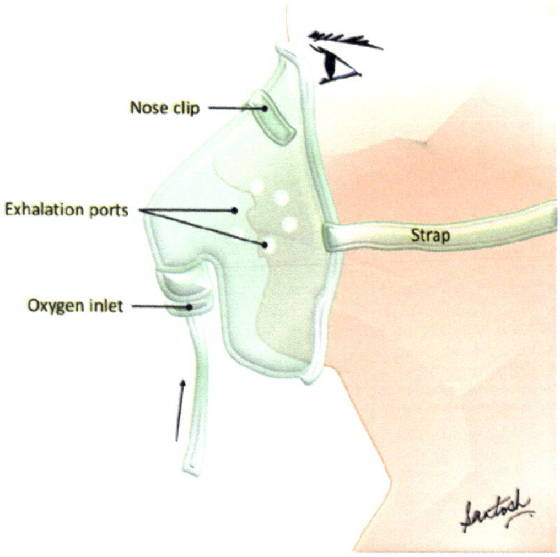

Fig. 2.2 A simple face mask

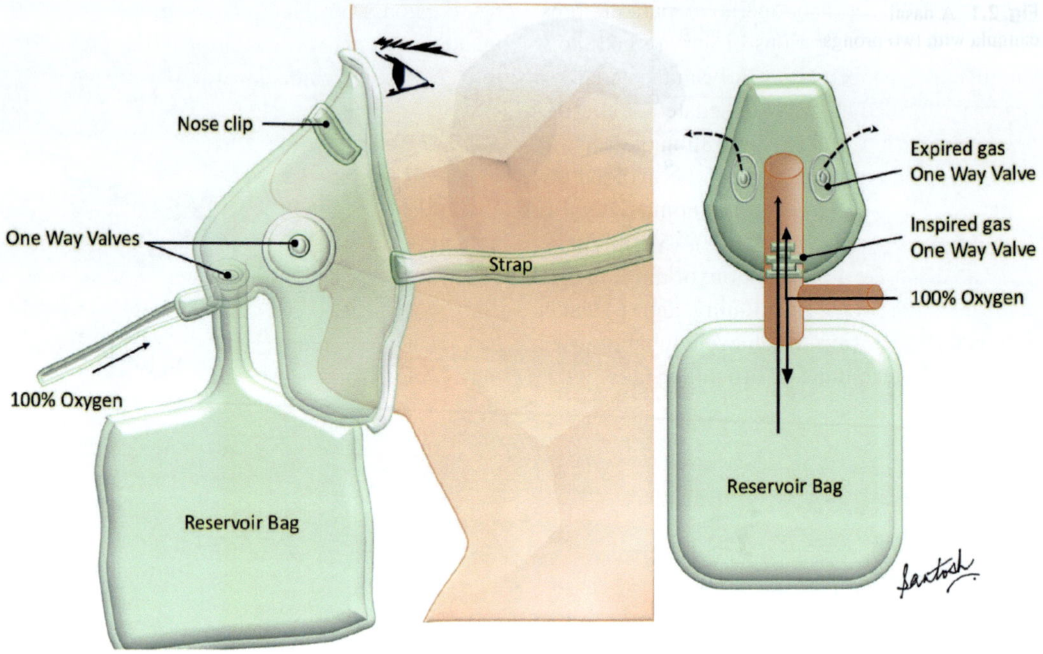

Fig. 2.3 A non-rebreathing face mask

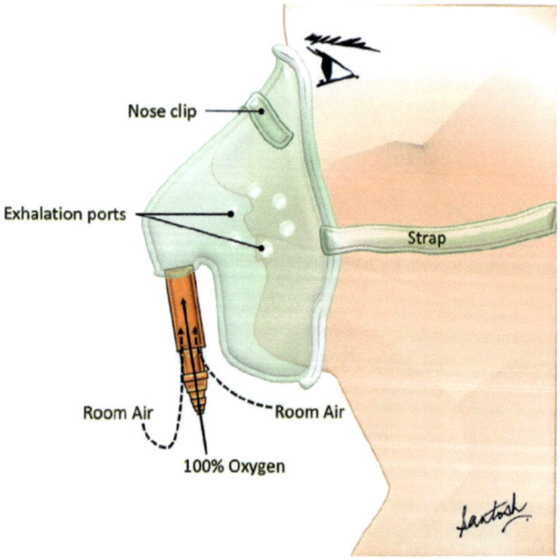

Fig. 2.4 A Venturi mask

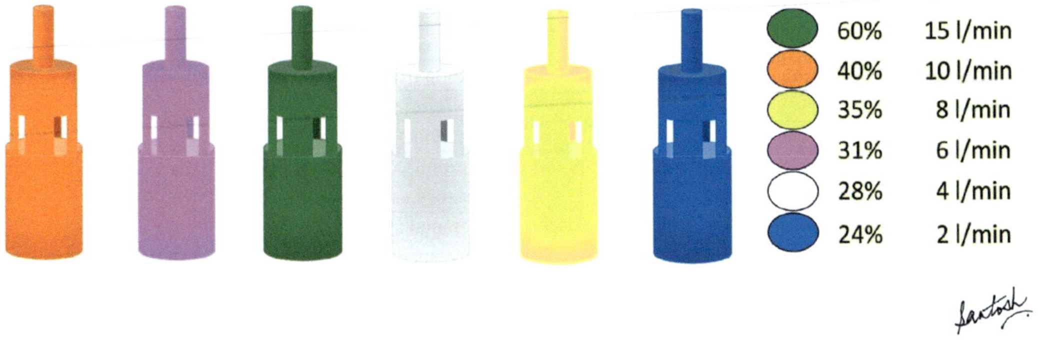
60% 15 l/min
40% 10 l/min
35% 8 l/min
31% 6 l/min
28% 4 l/min
24% 2 l/min
Santosh

Fig. 2.5 Various adapters of a Venturi mask

2.6 Hyperbaric Oxygen Therapy (HBOT)

2.6.1 Principle

It acts by increasing the O_2 dissolved in plasma. At rest, 5 mL O_2 is utilized/100 mL blood. Blood has 0.3 mL of dissolved O_2/dL/mmHg PO_2. The dissolved O_2 can increase if 100% O_2 is used above atmospheric pressure. At 3 atmospheric pressures (ATA), 5.6 mL O_2/dL blood. The metabolic demands of an average person can be met by dissolved oxygen alone when breathing 100% O_2 at 3 ATA (Table 2.6).

It follows Henry's Law, which states that at a constant temperature, the amount of a given gas dissolved in a liquid is proportional to the partial pressure of that gas in equilibrium with that liquid. So, increasing pressure increases the dissolved gas.

Similarly, based on Boyle's Law—at a constant temperature, the volume of that gas is inversely proportional to the pressure exerted on it. If pressure doubles, volume is halved. This principle is behind its use in decompression sickness and air/gas embolism in reducing the size of gas bubbles within tissues and circulation. It is also responsible for pain in the sinuses and ears.

2.6.2 Role in Carbon Monoxide (CO) Poisoning

The affinity of CO for Hb is 210 times that of O_2. The half-life of Carboxy-Hb is 320 min at room air, 90 min with 100% O_2, and 23 min with 100% O_2 at 3ATA. The mechanism is by competitive dissociation and increased amount of dissolved O_2.

2.7 Oxygen Toxicity

The primary targets of toxicity are the lungs and central nervous system and is dependent on two factors- PaO_2 and exposure time (Table 2.7).

1. Pulmonary toxicity (Smith Effect)
   (a) It is a chronic toxicity
   (b) 100% O_2 > 24–48 h produce a definite tissue injury
   (c) First sign appears about 10 h of O_2 at 1 ATA
   (d) Clinical features: carinal irritation after deep inspiration, uncontrolled cough, chest pain and dyspnea.
2. CNS toxicity (Paul Bert Effect)

Table 2.6 Indications of hyperbaric oxygen therapy

Primary therapy	Adjunctive therapy
Carbon monoxide poisoning	Radiation tissue damage
Air/gas embolism	Crush Injuries
Decompression sickness	Acute blood loss
Osteoradionecrosis	Compromised skin flaps/grafts
Clostridial myositis and myonecrosis	Refractory osteomyelitis
High altitude pulmonary oedema	Intracranial abscess
Extensive burns	Enhancement of healing of problem wounds

Table 2.7 Contraindications and adverse effects of oxygen therapy

Absolute contraindications
• Patient does not consent to receiving the oxygen
• The use of some O_2 delivery devices (e.g., nasal cannulas and nasopharyngeal catheters) in neonates and pediatric patients having nasal obstructions
Possible adverse effects [4]
• Oxygen toxicity
• Depression of ventilation in a select population with chronic hypercarbia
• Retinopathy of prematurity
• Absorption atelectasis
• Fire hazard

(a) These are acute effects
(b) Occurs at $O_2 > 3$ATA
(c) Clinical features: early signs and symptoms are quite variable
   - The most constant features are the twitching of perioral and small muscles of the hand
   - Facial pallor (intense peripheral vasoconstriction)
   - Cog-wheel breathing (diaphragmatic twitching)
   - Vertigo
   - Nausea
   - Altered behavior
   - Clumsiness
   - Finally, generalised convulsions

2.7.1 Management

These symptoms subside after 4 h of cessation of O_2. 100%—oxygen should not be used for more than 12 h, 80%—not more than 24 h, and 60%—not more than 36 h. The goal should be to use lowest possible FiO_2 compatible with adequate tissue oxygenation.

2.8 Adjuncts to Oxygen Therapy

1. Optimize cardiac output—infusions, transfusion, inotropes, diuretics, digoxin
2. Improve lung condition—humidification, antibiotics, bronchodilators, intubation, tracheostomy
3. Raise hemoglobin level
4. Reduce oxygen demand—prevent hyperthermia, paralysis, and IPPV

Suggested Reading

1. Shankar PS. Oxygen therapy. Q Med Res. 1980;30:1–20.
2. Jindal SK, Gupta D. Oxygen therapy. JIMSA. 1999;12:41–5.
3. Gibson RI, Comer PB, Backham RW, et al. Actual tracheal oxygen concentration with commonly used oxygen equipment. Anaesthesiology. 1976;44:71–3.
4. Petty TL. Clinical applications of oxygen in intensive and rehabilitative respiratory care, vol. 3. Philadelphia, PA: Lea & Febiger; 1982. p. 74–87.

3 Mask Ventilation

Anju Gupta and Parul Raina

Key Points
- Mask ventilation is a basic technique for airway management that all the anesthesiologists and health care workers should master.
- Masks of appropriate types and sizes should be used to achieve ventilation.
- It is important to master the technique of patient positioning and mask holding.

A LIFE SAVIOR ~ A SKILL OLD ENOUGH BUT YET RELEVANT TO SAVE LIFE !

Despite advances in airway management, ventilation by the mask remains an "Essential skill" every anesthesiologist must have. It's a noninvasive technique for airway management.

It's mainly used as a bridge to establish a more definitive airway. Despite wide advancement in anesthesia gadgets, mask ventilation remains to be an important skill. It is normally used during induction of anesthesia and when an anesthetic of short duration is administered; however, laryngeal mask airways have replaced it these days.

Table 3.1 Indications of mask ventilation

1. Preoxygenation
2. Induction of anesthesia via inhalation agent
3. To provide oxygen and anesthetic gases to a spontaneously ventilating patient and an anesthetized, apneic patient via PPV
4. As a rescue technique when tracheal intubation proves difficult
5. Cardiac arrest
6. Respiratory failure

Still, mask ventilation is a valuable rescue technique when definitive airway management proves difficult and an important part of all difficult airway algorithms. The advantages of mask ventilation are that it helps to maintain oxygenation, increases safe apnea time, easy to learn, and prevents hypoxia till more advanced techniques are available.

Various indications of mask ventilation are summarized in Table 3.1.

3.1 Contraindications

There are no absolute contraindications of mask ventilation. The relative contraindications are:

1. When there is an increased risk of regurgitation.
2. Caution in case of patients with severe facial trauma.

A. Gupta (✉) · P. Raina
Anesthesiology, Pain Medicine, Critical Care, All India Institute of Medical Sciences, New Delhi, Delhi, India

N. Gupta et al. (eds.), *Techniques in Anesthesia, Intensive Care and Emergency Medicine*, https://doi.org/10.1007/978-981-96-1202-4_3

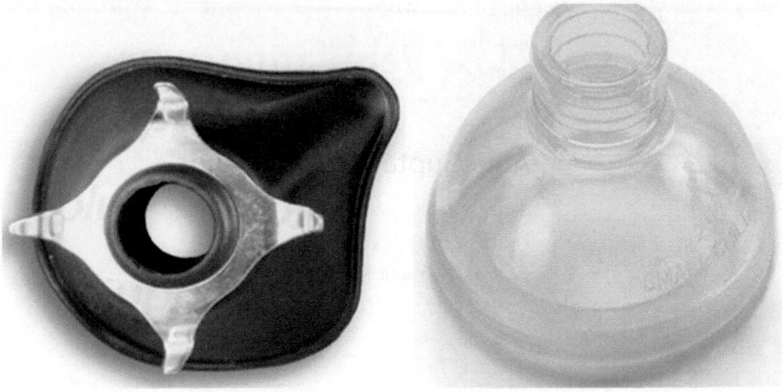

Fig. 3.1 Various types of masks

3. Those with an unstable cervical spine fracture where the head and neck manipulation must be avoided.
4. Face deformity leads to ineffective mask ventilation because of anatomical obstructions.

3.2 Types

The facemasks are available in various shapes and sizes. In addition, they may be made of different materials like silicon, black rubber, or transparent PVC. The transparent designs have an additional advantage that one can visualize blood, secretions, or vomitus along with exhaled moisture (Fig. 3.1).

3.3 Techniques for Face Mask Ventilation

Prerequisites:

1. For good mask ventilation, an appropriate size of face mask is important for a tight seal on the patient's face.
2. The back/ spine of an anesthetist at the head end should be straight and the body as close to the table such that the head of the patient lies at the level of the xiphisternum.

If the technique is not followed, it can result in

(a) Cramps in the hands of the user either because of an ill-fitting mask or wrong position.

Table 3.2 Various methods of holding a mask

One-hand technique	Single operator with the left-hand grip method
Two-hand technique	Operator using two hands in case of inadequate mask ventilation with one hand and assistance/ventilator providing ventilation
Two-handed jaw thrust	Operator with assistance. In case of inadequate mask ventilation with two hands
Claw hand technique	Useful for children undergoing short-duration ophthalmic procedures

(b) An inadequate seal will cause air dilution and inadequate gas exchange during spontaneous and controlled ventilation, respectively.
(c) Leak of anesthetic gases due to improper seal can lead to OT pollution.

There are various methods for holding a mask to ensure an open airway and tight seal (Table 3.2).

3.3.1 One-Hand Technique

The operator stands on the patient's head end. A properly held mask enables no or minimal leakage. On either side of the connector, the thumb and index finger of the hand are positioned on the facemask's body. The little finger is placed on the angle of the mandible, the ring finger is placed on the mandibular ridge, and the middle finger is positioned on the chin. The thumb and index finger make the C in what is known as the standard **C and E grip**, while the other three fingers form the E. While the E grip assists in tilting the head, the C grip assists in keeping a tight pressure over the nose and chin to prevent any leakage.

The chin-lift grip technique is another one-hand non-E-C technique that has been mentioned. The web space between the thumb and index finger is put just around the connector while using the "chin lift grip," and the remaining fingers are placed below the chin. This produces a strong grip that controls the whole mask and creates a reliable seal. This grip applied force along the sagittal plane, whereas the "E-C chnique" applied torque off the sagittal plane, maintaining head extension. In this strategy, the "airway maneuver first, seal second" order is used. For inexperienced airway managers, this approach is reported to produce an effective seal that is simpler to apply because it allows for the long-term maintenance of ventilatory parameters.

Alternatively, the right hand can also be used for holding a mask where the anesthesia machine is on the left side so that bag holding and ventilation are easy.

3.3.2 Two-Hand Technique

The body of the mask is held in place by two thumbs. Bilateral mandibular rami are under the index and other fingers. A forward thrust on the angle of the mandible lifts the jaw anteriorly while the head is dorsiflexed at the atlantooccipital joint. This grip is also referred to as a double C and E grip or a two-handed claw grip, and the move is termed the **Esmarch-Heiberg** maneuver.

A different two-handed mask hold is known as the V-E grip (or a two-handed vice grip), in which the thumbs and thenar eminences are put over each side of the mask while the second through fifth digits pull the jaw upward.

3.3.3 Two-Handed Jaw Thrust

One person stands at the head of the patient and performs a jaw thrust at the angle of the left mandible while the right-hand compresses the reservoir bag. The second person stands at the patient's shoulder, facing the first person. This second person's right-hand covers the left hand of the first person, and the left hand achieves a right-sided jaw thrust and mask seal.

3.3.4 Claw Hand Technique

Facing the child, the face mask is applied to the face by using the right hand with the palmar surface facing upward. The ring finger goes under the jaw angle, and the middle finger is placed under the angle of the jaw on the left. The index finger and the thumb circle the body of the mask. The anesthesia provider then tightens the grip on the mask to achieve a good fit. The little finger is kept free.

3.3.5 Special Situations

Beard Patient Technique: Place the round end of the mask between the lower lip and the alveolar ridge. Beard can be covered with clear adhesive tape, plastic wrap, gauze, or gel.

Another option is to use a supraglottic airway device. If feasible, shave the beard.

Mask Ventilation of the Tracheostomy Stoma: A Rendell-Baker-Soucek mask is placed around the stoma with the nasal portion pointing in a caudal direction so that the mandibular curve rests on the tracheal region and the apex on the suprasternal notch.

Advantages of Face Mask

- Minimal occurrence of sore throat.
- Less anesthetic depth than using a supraglottic device or an endotracheal tube.
- Muscle Relaxants can be avoided.
- Economical method to manage the airway for short cases.

Disadvantages of Face Mask

- One person is always occupied during mask holding.
- Higher fresh gas flows are often needed.
- In remote locations, anesthesia like Computer Tomography (CT scan), Magnetic Resonance Imaging (MRI), mask ventilation is difficult due to poor airway access.
- Mask ventilation cannot be used longer and requires more intraoperative airway manipulations to maintain a patent airway.
- In facial abnormality, Laryngeal Mask Airway (LMA) is a better option than mask ventilation.

3.4 Complications

1. *Eye injury*: Corneal abrasion can occur if a facemask is inadvertently placed on an open eye. Pressure on the medial angles of the eyes and supraorbital margins can cause eyelid edema, chemosis of the conjunctiva, and rarely blindness if placed for a long time.
2. *Skin allergy*: Skin allergy to mask materials can lead to dermatitis around the area of contact between mask and skin. Also, chemicals used for sterilization of reusable masks can cause allergic reactions. If the mask is made of rubber, serious reactions can occur in patients with latex allergies.
3. *Skin necrosis*: Undue pressure on the face to keep a tight seal for a long period can cause skin laceration and necrosis, especially in elderly patients.
4. *Nerve injury*: Pressure for a long duration by face mask on the underlying nerve can lead to nerve damage. So, the mask should be removed from the face periodically to avoid continuous pressure on one particular area.
5. *Cervical spine movement*: Mask ventilation can lead to more cervical spine movement than LMA or tracheal intubation. This is significant in patients with an unstable cervical spine injury.
6. *Gastric inflation*: Gastric insufflation is more with mask ventilation when used for positive pressure ventilation. Thus, it's advisable to use inspiratory pressure below 20 cmH_2O.
7. *Jaw pain*: Postoperative jaw pain is more common after mask ventilation.
8. *User Fatigue*: Holding a mask for a long time may result in operator fatigue.

3.5 Difficult Mask Ventilation

Defining difficult mask ventilation has always been debated since its subjective phenomena. Mask ventilation which is difficult for a trainee, must not be for an anesthesiologist who has been practicing for over 20 years. Thus, a definite definition for difficult mask ventilation hasn't still come. Various studies have been done, and various grading systems have been developed to identify and predict difficult mask ventilation and its severity.

Due to this, a range of incidence has been reported due to a lack of consensus in definition, a wide range of 0.08% to 15%. The most extensive studies have shown the incidence of difficult mask ventilation at approximately 1.4% and impossible MV approximately 0.15%.

American Society Of Anesthesiologists Task force defines difficult mask ventilation as when "it is not possible for the unassisted anesthesiologist to maintain oxygen saturation more than 90% using 100% oxygen and positive pressure mask ventilation in a patient whose oxygen was more than 90% before anesthetic intervention, and/or it is not possible for the unassisted anesthesiologist to prevent or reverse signs of inadequate ventilation during positive pressure and mask ventilation."

3.5.1 Factors Affecting Mask Ventilation

To understand the cause and reason for difficult mask ventilation, knowledge of airway anatomy and how the airway is kept patent under anesthesia is of utmost importance.

Thus, factors affecting mask ventilation can further be divided into operator factors (errors in technique, equipment, anesthesia, positioning) and patient factors.

3.5.2 Operator Factors

The clinician's experience and equipment use play an important role in mask ventilation. MV is a skill that is achieved through training and maintained through regular practice. This, in turn, helps address various issues like patient positioning, airway maneuvers, and equipment sizing. *An incorrectly sized oropharyngeal or nasopharyngeal airways* will lead to difficult MV and can cause trauma and bleeding. Similarly, an *improper size mask* can also lead to a difficult MV. Many times *faults with the anesthesia machine or breathing circuit,* if left unchecked, can cause a difficult/impossible MV. Thus, a prior checklist and appropriate size of masks and airways need to be kept ready before starting any case.

General anesthesia itself plays a role in appropriate mask ventilation. Inadequate depth of anesthesia and inadequate muscle relaxation may lead to increase muscle rigidity, reduced chest wall compliance, and difficult MV. Chest wall rigidity is also seen with high doses of opioids. Muscle relaxants can make mask ventilation easy, by eliminating rigidity and laryngospasm. But in a suspected difficult MV, it's better to check if one can ventilate or not before administering muscle relaxants as sometimes loss of tone and upper airway collapse by giving muscle relaxants can make mask ventilation difficult.

The 4th National Audit project by the royal college of Anesthetists and Difficult Airway Society (DAS) found in some cases that a lighter plane of anesthesia and a reluctance to administer muscle relaxants may have caused patient harm.

3.5.3 Patient Factors

Identifying the risk factors for difficult MV on pre-operative assessment can minimize the episode of the "can't ventilate" situation while administering anesthesia and thus reduce the morbidity and mortality of the patient by taking necessary steps. So, it's imperative to identify the risk factors related to the patient (Table 3.3).

Table 3.3 Risk factors for difficult mask ventilation

Facial deformity	Upper or lower airway tumors
Edentulous	Extrinsic compression of airway
Foreign bodies	Obesity
Beard	Airway edema
Large tongue/epiglottis	Pneumothorax
Tonsillar hyperplasia	Bronchopleural fistula
Laryngospasm/ bronchospasm	Chest wall deformity
Male gender	Previous neck irradiation

Langeron et al. identified five criteria were considered as an independent risk factor for difficult MV:

Obese (BMI > 26 kg/m^2)
Bearded
Edentulous
Snoring
Elderly (>55 years)

Kheterpal et al. reviewed over 50,000 anesthetics. It showed that neck radiation, male sex, sleep apnea, Mallampati 3–4, and the presence of beard were independent predictors of difficult mask ventilation.

> *Mallampati 3–4, obesity, and neck radiation are risk factors for difficult mask ventilation and intubation.* Also, careful consideration of airway plans needs to be done for patients with previous neck radiation as surgical access may also be difficult.
> *The mandibular protrusion test* indicates the ability to perform an adequate jaw thrust, thus reliable in identifying patients with risk of airway collapse and difficult MV and predicting difficult intubation.

3.5.4 Management

If difficult mask ventilation is predicted:

(a) Consider rapid sequence induction ensuring optimal preoxygenation. Back-up plan to keep supraglottic airway devices ready.
(b) Proper patient positioning will help improve the apneic time by decreasing dependent atelectasis. In obese individuals, the ear should be at the same level as the sternal notch (RAMP Position), So that the oral, pharyngeal, and laryngeal axes are aligned.
(c) Simple measures like shaving the beard, keeping dentures in situ to improve the seal, and removing them immediate before intubation helps. In cases where the beard couldn't be shaved, slicking down the beard with jelly helps improve the seal.
(d) Use of airway adjuncts such as oropharyngeal and nasopharyngeal airways, continuous positive airway pressure, maintaining the depth of anesthesia and muscle relaxation.
(e) Keeping difficult airway trolley ready in all situations.

Preoxygenation is one of the utmost and mandatory steps before inducing a patient suspecting of a difficult airway. It gives additional time to change the approach to ventilation by decreasing the desaturation episodes.

If difficult mask ventilation is unexpected:

Management in an unexpected difficult mask ventilation becomes a dynamic process. From rechecking the position, using an airway, and above said management methods, if the difficulty remains, a call for help to allow a 2-person technique and/or operator change should be made. If this also doesn't improve saturation and it has fallen to less than 90%, consider putting a supraglottic airway device for ventilation and use this as a conduit for intubation. If relaxant is given, an attempt to intubation should be taken and a difficult airway cart needs to be ready simultaneously. Consider waking up the patient if an attempt to put supraglottic airway is failed. Rescue techniques like a cannula or surgical cricothyroidotomy need to be kept ready.

Suggested Reading

1. Gropper MA, Miller RD, Eriksson LI, Fleisher LA, Wiener-Kronish JP, Cohen NH, et al. Miller's anesthesia, 2-volume set E-book. Amsterdam: Elsevier Health Sciences; 2019.
2. Baheti DK, Laheri VV. Understanding anesthetic equipment & procedures: a practical approach. London: JP Medical; 2018.
3. Dorsch JA. Understanding anesthesia equipment. Lippincott Williams & Wilkins; 2012. Martindale, Berkow. Manual of emergency airway management, 3rd edition. Anesthesiology. 2009;111(3):683.
4. Ririe DG. Airway management. Anesthesiology. 1996;85(2):448.
5. Podder S, Dutta A, Yaddanapudi S, Chari P. Challenges in paediatric mask holding; the "claw hand" technique. Anaesthesia. 2001;56(7):697.
6. Moore EW, Cowan CM. A close shave. Anaesthesia. 1999;54(3):305.
7. Kheterpal M, Shanks T. Prediction and outcomes of impossible mask ventilation: a review of 50,000 anesthetics. Anesthesiology. 2009;110(4):891–7.
8. Difficult mask ventilation [Internet]. WFSA Resour Libr 2020. https://resources.wfsahq.org/atotw/difficult-mask-ventilation/. Accessed 18 Sep 2022.
9. El-Orbany M, Woehlck HJ. Difficult mask ventilation. Anesth Analg. 2009;109(6):1870.
10. Langeron O, Masso E, Huraux C, Guggiari M, Bianchi A, Coriat P, et al. Prediction of difficult mask ventilation. Anesthesiology. 2000;92(5). Kheterpal, Martin, Shanks, Tremper. Prediction and outcomes of impossible mask ventilation: a review of 50,000 anesthetics. Anesthesiology. 2009;110(4):891–7.

4 Laryngeal Mask Airways: Insertion Techniques

Anju Gupta and Karthik V. Iyer

Key Points

- The mask of SGA should generally be completely deflated and well lubricated, without folds in its surface for its smooth placement.
- In general, for a patient whose weight falls in between two categories, the bigger size should be chosen.
- If initial SGA placement is not successful and results in leakage, the next larger size should be attempted.
- Generally, "pen-holding" technique has a high success and results in satisfactory placement for most devices, but alternative insertion techniques are desirable to know as they help in trouble shooting inadequate placement in many cases.
- Second generation devices should be preferred whenever available for all but most superficial and very brief procedures.
- If insertion is unsuccessful with cricoid pressure, release pressure and reattempt insertion.
- SGA are useful and life-saving rescue devices for ventilation in case of failure of Bag-mask ventilation and intubation.

Appropriate patient, SGA type and size selection, maintaining adequate depth of anesthesia during and after insertion, and regular monitoring of cuff pressure ($\leq$ 60 cmH_2O) are needed for successful use of SGAs.

4.1 Introduction

Supraglottic airways (SGAs) are commonly used as primary airway devices during anesthesia and are an important rescue device in case of failed bag-mask ventilation. Learning the indications and practicing the techniques of SGA insertion are an integral part of training in anesthesiology.

SGAs were pioneered by *Archibald Brain*, a British anesthetist who first developed the prototype of the Laryngeal Mask Airway in 1981, which became commercially available in 1987 and subsequently was introduced into clinical practice in 1988 as the LMA® Classic™ (cLMA). Over the years, supraglottic airways have become commonplace in anesthesia and as a part of difficult airway guidelines and during cardiopulmonary resuscitation.

Nomenclature

- Supraglottic airways also referred to as extra glottic airways are devices with their ventilation port being over the glottis in the hypopharyngeal space. Based on the various types, they seal the pharyngeal space superiorly and

A. Gupta (✉) · K. V. Iyer
Anesthesiology, Pain Medicine, Critical Care, All India Institute of Medical Sciences, New Delhi, Delhi, India

N. Gupta et al. (eds.), *Techniques in Anesthesia, Intensive Care and Emergency Medicine*, https://doi.org/10.1007/978-981-96-1202-4_4

the esophagus inferiorly to enable effective ventilation through the glottis.
- Laryngeal masks refer to SGAs having a cuff which occupy the hypopharyngeal space and form a seal around the periglottic tissues.
- The acronym LMA® (and not the term laryngeal mask airway) is trademarked and used for devices manufactured by the LMA® Group of companies.

This chapter seeks to explain the insertion techniques of laryngeal mask airways.

4.2 Classification of Supra Glottic Airways

The commonly used classification of SGAs was given by *Cook*. They are classified as follows with examples in Table 4.1:

- First generation: These SGAs are "simple airway tubes." They are not specifically designed to prevent regurgitation and aspiration of gastric contents.
- Second generation: They are specifically designed to reduce risk of aspiration of gastric contents, usually through a gastric draining port.

Cook has further suggested adding suffix "i" if the SGA enables intubation with >50% success, and further adding "d" for direct intubation and "g" for guided intubation.

A previous system of classification given by *Miller* is based on sealing mechanism of the SGAs:

- Cuffed peri-pharyngeal sealers.
- Cuffed peri-laryngeal sealers.
- Cuffless anatomic pre-shaped sealers.

All laryngeal mask airways, as per the above classification, are cuffed peri-laryngeal sealers.

Miller modified this classification in 2014, wherein the term "generation" gave a chronological context along with the sealing mechanism. Each generation is further classified into base-of-tongue sealers and peri-laryngeal sealers based on the site of sealing:

- First generation: These devices have an inflatable sealing mechanism. (Table 4.2).
- Second generation: These devices have a wedge mechanism of sealing and can be either base-of-tongue and peri-laryngeal sealers. They do not have an inflatable cuff.
- Third generation: These devices have a self-energizing or self-pressurizing cuff which ensures that cuff pressure increases dynamically with an increase in airway pressure, contributing to reduced aspiration risk and a better seal. The term "3rd generation" is also used when the SGA has added features like presence of integral bite block, novel drain tube, and improves ease of intubation.

The presence or absence of gastric decompression mechanism are denoted by (+) and (−) respectively. (I) is used to denote use of SGA as a conduit for intubation.

Table 4.1 Classification of SGAs based on classification given by Cook[a] [7]

Classification	Examples
First generation	LMA® Classic™, LMA® Flexible™, LMA® Unique™, LMA® Fastrach™ (ILMA-*intubating LMA*) Ambu® Aura40™, Air-Q® Intubating Laryngeal Airway, Laryngeal Tube (LT™), Cobra Perilaryngeal Airway (CobraPLA™), Combitube®
Second generation	LMA® ProSeal™, LMA® Supreme™, i-gel®, Ambu® AuraGain™, LTS™, SLIPA™

[a]Please note that the table includes commonly used SGAs and is not an exhaustive list

Table 4.2 This table includes examples of SGAs based on the modified classification by Miller[a]

Classification	Base-of-tongue sealers	Peri-laryngeal sealers (examples)
First generation (inflatable mechanism of seal)	Combitube®(+), LT™(−), LTS™(+), CobraPLA™(−)	LMA® Classic™ (−), LMA® Flexible™ (−), LMA® Unique™ (−), LMA® Fastrach™ (ILMA) (−)(I), LMA® CTrach™ (−)(I), LMA® ProSeal™ (+), LMA® Supreme™ (+),Ambu® Aura40™ (−), Air-Q® Intubating Laryngeal Airway (−)(I)
Second generation (wedge mechanism of seal)	SLIPA™(+)	i-gel®(+)(I)
Third generation (self-energizing mechanism of seal)	–	Baska Mask®(+)(I)

[a]Please note that the table does not include an exhaustive list

Table 4.3 Important characteristics of commonly used laryngeal mask airways

Type of LMA®	Important design characteristics
LMA® Classic™ (cLMA)	• Curved shaft that connects to the spoon shaped mask • Aperture bars to prevent epiglottis from blocking the tube
LMA® Unique™ (uLMA)	• Single use; same as cLMA
LMA® Flexible™ (fLMA)	• Flexible, wire-reinforced shaft
LMA® ProSeal™ (PLMA)	• Drain tube for insertion of suction tube • Dorsal cuff which improves peri-laryngeal seal • Introducer pocket (locating strap) over the anterior distal end of the tube • Flexible, wire-reinforced shaft with inbuilt bite block • Curved metal introducer to aid in insertion
LMA® Fastrach™ (ILMA)	• Short curved stainless steels shaft with metal handle at the connector end • Mask contains a V-shaped ramp to guide tube endo-tracheal tube into the glottis and a single mobile epiglottic elevator • Flexible, wire-reinforced tracheal tube for intubation via ILMA, along with stabilizer rod
LMA® Supreme™ (SLMA)	• Preformed curve • Integrated bite block • Special fixation tab posterior to the drain tube insertion port • Specially designed cuff with FirstSeal™ (perilaryngeal seal) and SecondSeal™ (esophageal seal) technology • Lesser cuff inflation volumes

Tips:
- *Knowledge of device characteristics is important for proper device selection in an individual case to optimize outcomes with SGA*
- *SGAs with gastric port should be used for majority of cases when available*

4.3 Important Characteristics of Commonly Used Laryngeal Mask Airways

The following table (Table 4.3) gives important design characteristics of commonly used laryngeal mask airways. These are included as brief points, as details regarding individual devices is beyond the scope of the chapter.

4.4 Indications

Indications for LMA use have been evolving ever since its introduction. The following are the appropriate routine indications for its use:

1. Any elective short procedure in supine position in an ASA I or II case that does not involve the gastrointestinal or respiratory tract

(e.g., minor orthopedic, gynecologic, urologic or breast, inguinal and other superficial procedures.
2. Non-operating room anesthesia (e.g., MRI/radiation therapy).
3. Some ophthalmic and ENT procedure.
4. Difficult airway management (primary or rescue device).
5. Alternative device to intubation for airway management in the cardiac arrest.
6. Conduit for intubation.
7. Prehospital airway management.

4.5 Contraindications

Absolute:
1. No mouth opening.
2. Total airway obstruction.

Relative:
1. Increased risk of aspiration (e.g., Full stomach, pregnancy, morbid obesity, upper gastrointestinal bleed etc.)
2. Suspected or known abnormalities in supraglottic anatomy.
3. Poor pulmonary compliance.

Tips
- Patient selection is important to ensure successful outcomes with SGA.
- SGAs have emerged as an important rescue device in managing difficult airway (DA) patients and must be included as a component of DA cart.
- American heart association recognizes SGA as an acceptable alternative to intubation.
- Though the list of indications is ever expanding, its non-conventional uses, e.g., prone position surgeries should be limited to only experienced operators.

4.6 Device Preparation

1. Examine the LMA® to look for any obvious damage to the integrity of the device. Look for holes in the cuff especially in the area of welding and the pilot balloon. Cuff damage can happen following expansion of the residual air or fluid in the cuff during sterilization. The interior of the shaft should not have any particulate matter. This step is crucial for fLMA where part of the wire used in reinforcement of the shaft can break and project into the tube. The aperture bars should be intact.
2. Deflation of the cuff—Air from the cuff should be withdrawn fully and the cuff should not spontaneously re-inflate. If the latter happens, it may suggest a faulty valve in the pilot balloon or a hole in the cuff. In PLMA, ensure that the red plug on the pilot balloon is closed. If open, this can lead to partial re-inflation causing difficulty in insertion.
3. Inflation of the cuff—The cuff should then be inflated up to the recommended volume for the size. There should be no herniation or abnormal shape of the cuff. Inflating the cuff to more than 50% of the recommended volume can detect small leaks that occur at the welding of the cuff following inadvertent expansion during sterilization. The cuff should sustain the pressure for at least 2 min.
4. Just prior insertion, the cuff should be fully deflated such that the rim of the LMA® faces toward the dorsal part of the cuff. Pressing the ventral part of the cuff against a sterile surface can help produce the needed shape of the cuff (Fig. 4.1a). Manufacturer provided deflation tool can be used at this time (Fig. 4.1b).
5. Water-soluble lubricant should be applied on the posterior surface of the cuff. Lubrication of the anterior surface should be avoided as it causes aspiration of the lubricant and drying of the lubricant can obstruct the air entry.

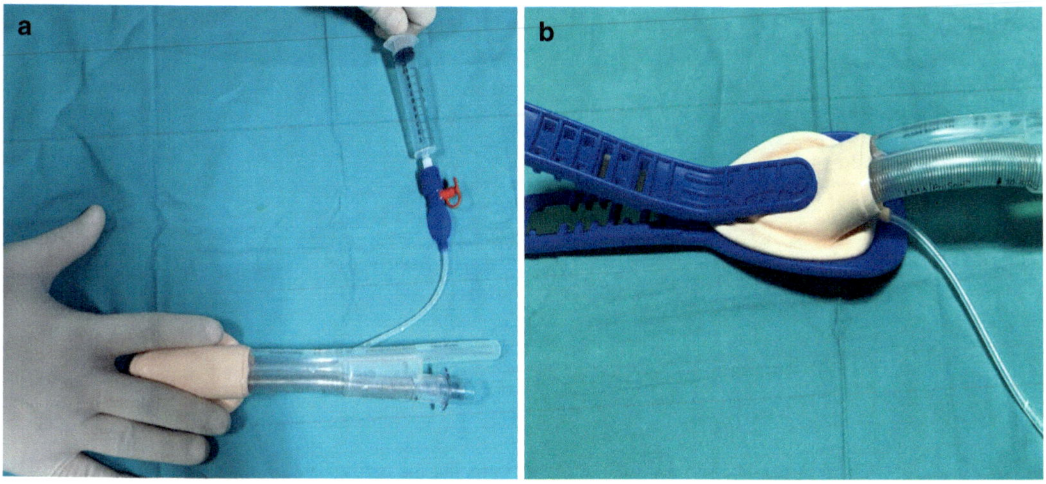

Fig. 4.1 (**a**) Note how the SGA is held with one hand, while deflating with the other; (**b**) Manufacturer supplied deflation tool for PLMA. Different types of deflation tools may be available

4.7 Patient Preparation

Adequate depth of anesthesia is required prior insertion of the LMA®. This can be ensured by checking for absence of jaw tone or absent withdrawal during trapezius squeeze. A functional intravenous line should be secured prior to airway insertion. Muscle relaxation is not necessary, prior to insertion.

Patient's head is placed in a sniffing position like that during laryngoscopy. The jaw can be held open or jaw thrust can be applied by an assistant to increase pharyngeal space which is especially required for PLMA, SLMA and ILMA as they have larger cuffs.

> **Tip**
> - Appropriate level of anesthetic depth is a must during insertion and while the surgery is undergoing with SGA in situ.

4.8 Techniques of Insertion

The following techniques are described for cLMA but can be used other laryngeal mask airways as well.

4.8.1 Standard Technique

1. The laryngeal mask airway is held in a "pen-holding" fashion with the index finger of the dominant hand placed at the junction between the anterior part of the shaft and the deflated cuff and the thumb posteriorly (Fig. 4.2a).
2. The non-dominant hand, meanwhile, maintains head extension, with the anesthesiologist standing at the head end of the patient.
3. The LMA® is then inserted along the midline of the oral cavity or slightly lateral from the midline along the hard palate with a cranio-posterior direction of force applied via the index finger, such that the ventral surface of the LMA® faces the chin and then the dorsal surface of the tongue (Fig. 4.2b).
4. The dorsal surface of the LMA® then slides along the hard palate, soft palate and moves caudally along the posterior pharyngeal wall. As the tip of the device engages in the upper esophageal sphincter (UES), a resistance is felt to its passage and the anesthesiologist should stop pushing it any further.
5. Then, the shaft is held by the non-dominant hand after which the index finger is removed. Removing the index finger without stabilizing the shaft can lead to displacement or

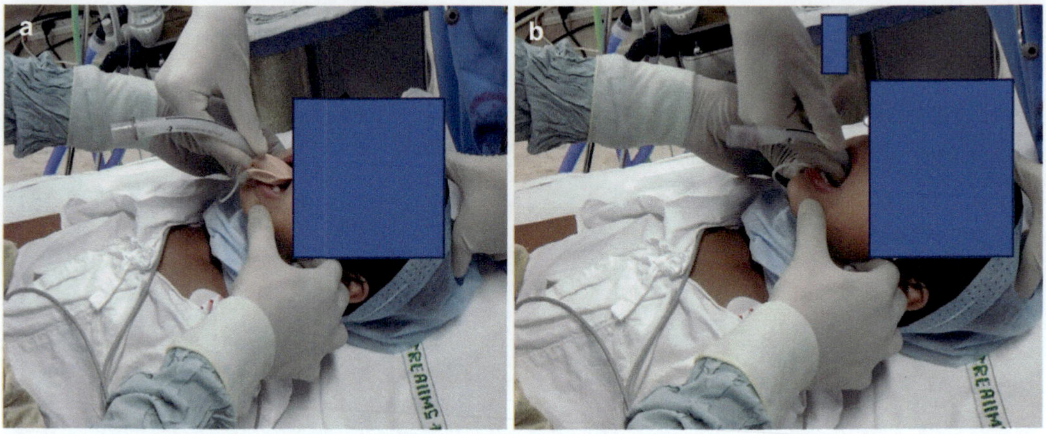

Fig. 4.2 (**a**) cLMA held in pen-holding fashion with cuff tip facing the hard palate; (**b**) The index finger guides the cLMA into the hypopharynx with force being applied in the cranio-posterior direction

axial rotation of the airway. The cuff is then inflated with air as per the defined volume for the specific LMA®. This is noted on the shaft of the LMA®. During inflation, the airway should be left free. The LMA® might rise slightly.

6. Once the LMA® position is confirmed by ventilating through it, the shaft is then fixed using a tape to both the maxillary prominences.
7. The standard technique ensures that the deflated cuff leads to minimal airway stimulation and can pass through the oropharyngeal space without much resistance.
8. Leaving the shaft free during inflation of the cuff ensures that the tip of the LMA® rises slightly above the UES. If this is not done, the cuff can expand within the UES can reduce its tone thereby increasing risk of aspiration.
9. The soft tip of the LMA® may fold posteriorly during insertion. The anesthesiologist can confirm this by moving the index finger along the dorsal surface of the airway before removing the index finger. If the tip has folded, then the LMA® should be removed and reinserted.
10. Alternately, once the LMA® has crossed the palate, the shaft can be held by the non-dominant hand and the index finger of the dominant hand can be moved along the dorsal surface and then back to its initial position. This can be done dynamically during insertion, and the index finger along the dorsal surface can prevent the posterior folding of the tip. This has been described in pediatrics, where the tip is more likely to hit the base of tongue, hypertrophied tonsils or epiglottis leading to folding of tip due to limited pharyngeal space.

Tips

- Standard technique is suitable in majority of cases and rest of the techniques are usually indicated for trouble shooting.

4.8.2 Partial Cuff Inflation Technique

Another technique is to partially inflate the cuff and then follow the same steps as the standard technique (Fig. 4.3). Partially inflating the cuff provides strength to the cuff and may prevent posterior folding of the tip. It can also reduce trauma to the peripharyngeal tissues, but studies have shown that the standard technique has a higher success rate than partial inflation of successful placement of LMA®. In pediatrics, partial cuff inflation has shown to increase success of

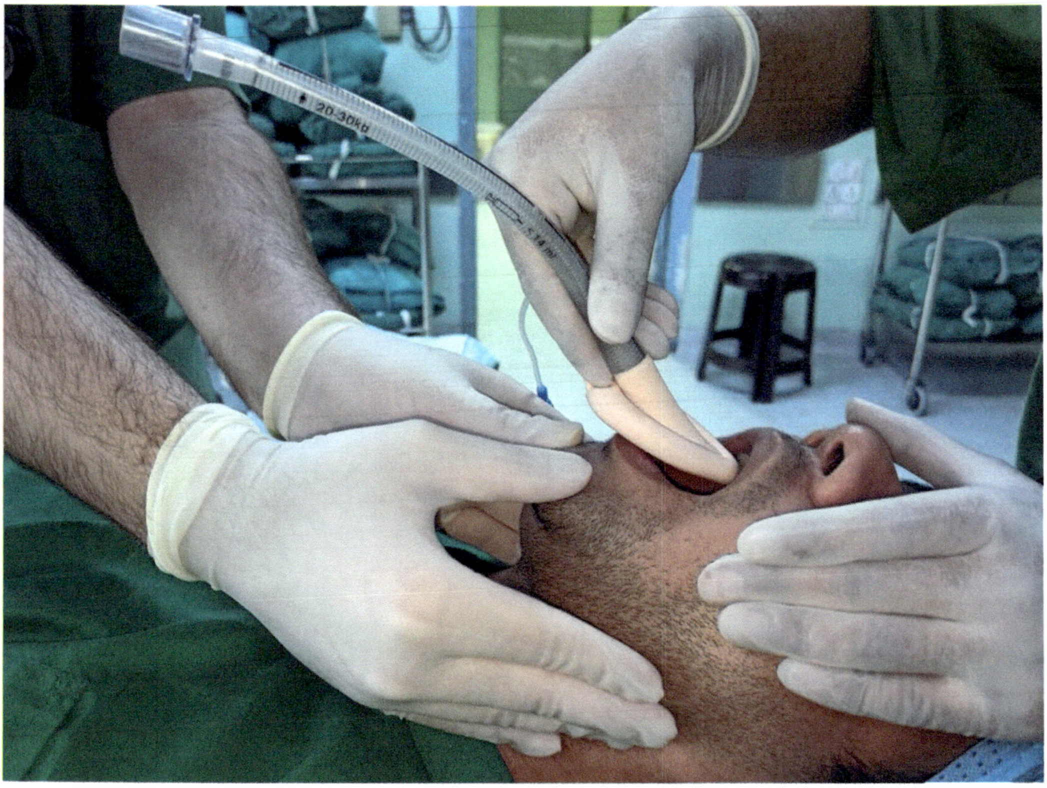

Fig. 4.3 Note the partially inflated cuff. fLMA used here for simulation

LMA® placement. Partial cuff inflation can also be done by attaching a syringe without piston and engaging the valve in the pilot balloon such that the cuff pressure equalizes with the atmospheric pressure. Following placement, one can check for leak to determine additional inflation, thereby preventing hyperinflation.

> **Tips**
> - Partial inflation of cuff means inflating cuff up to the point that there are no wrinkles in the cuff.

4.8.3 Rotational (Reverse) Technique

The reverse technique of LMA® insertion was described by rotating the LMA® by 180°, with the cuff partially inflated, then inserted up to the hypopharynx in this reverse way (Fig. 4.4) and then turned again by 180° such that the aperture faces the glottis. This was called the "Charlottetown twist." The reverse or 180° rotational technique has shown to increase success rate of insertion in pediatrics when compared to the standard technique.

4.8.4 Thumb Insertion Technique

This is done with the anesthesiologist facing the patient, rather than being in the head end. Here the LMA® is held with the thumb of the dominant hand in the junction between the shaft and cuff and it guides insertion of the airway (Fig. 4.5a). The shaft can be supported by the non-dominant hand (Fig. 4.5b), and the assistant can provide jaw thrust and maintain head extension to increase the oropharyngeal space. This is particularly useful when access to the head end is restricted.

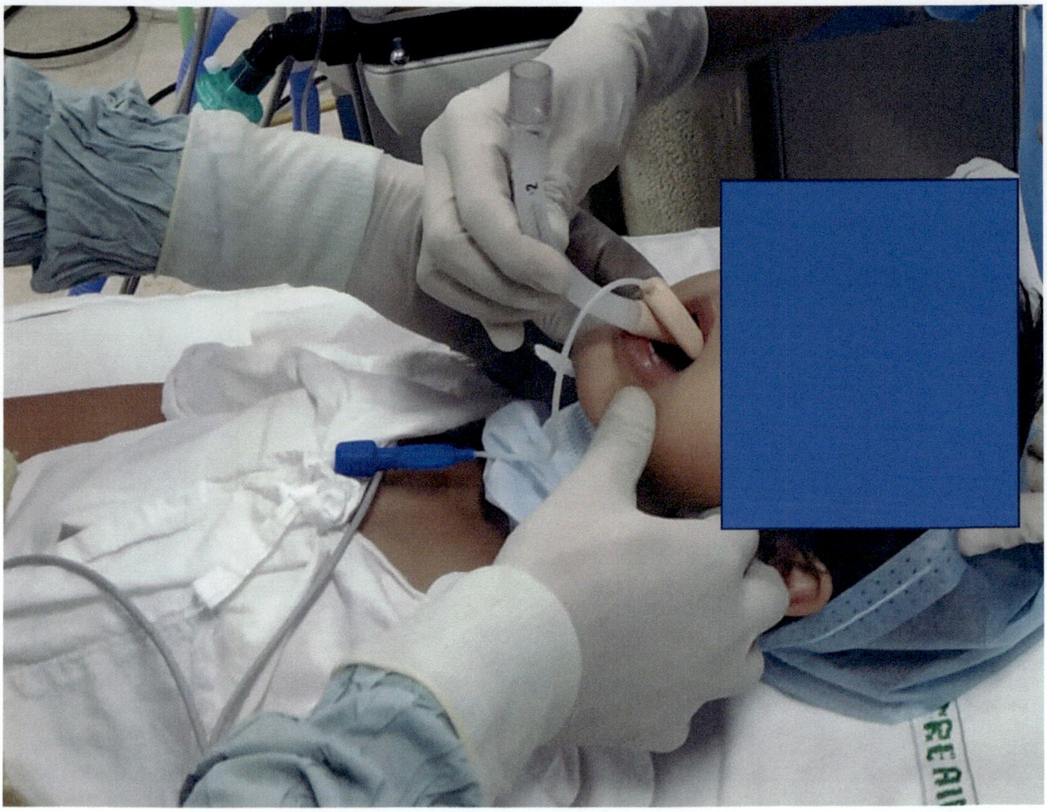

Fig. 4.4 Rotational technique. The bowl of the cuff faces the palate

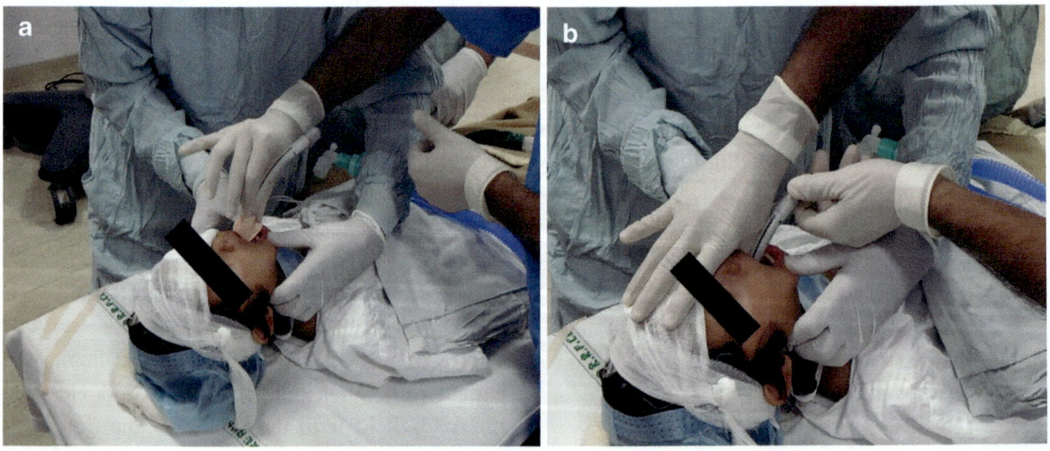

Fig. 4.5 (**a**) The anesthetist stands facing the patient. Note that the thumb is between the shaft and the deflated cuff; (**b**) The thumb guides the cLMA into the pharynx, while the other fingers are spread out over the patient's face. The non-dominant hand can support the shaft during insertion

4.9 Other Modifications

Kundra et al. studied a lateral approach, wherein the LMA® with a partially inflated cuff was rotated by 45° after inserting in the mouth such that the LMA® skips the epiglottis and the base of tongue. Once in the hypopharynx, it was rotated back to neutral midline position. They showed a reduction in the time and attempts at insertion. The LMA® can be inserted without guidance of the airway with index finger, as the shaft is firm, although success is more with the standard technique.

Similarly, it can also be inserted with the anesthesiologist facing the patient without thumb guidance.

4.9.1 Techniques for LMA® Flexible™

The technique for fLMA insertion remains the same as the standard "pen-holding" technique. Alternately, the flexible wire-reinforced shaft can be stabilized by using a rigid stylet or a tracheal tube inserted within the shaft to act as a stylet. Such modifications are generally not indicated as the standard technique has good success rate in itself.

4.9.2 Techniques for LMA® ProSeal™

Preparation of the patient and the device is similar as described above. The PLMA has a soft, malleable cuff and posterior folding is common during insertion. This should be confirmed before inflation of the cuff as described above in the standard technique. The various insertion techniques are as described:

1. *Digital technique*: Like the standard technique described above, the digital technique involves stabilizing the PLMA in a "pen-holding" fashion between the index finger and thumb of the dominant hand. The index finger is positioned in the introducer pocket present at the junction of the distal part of the anterior shaft and the mask (Fig. 4.6). The digital technique can be guided by a gentle laryngoscopy aimed at identifying the posterior glottis and hypopharynx.

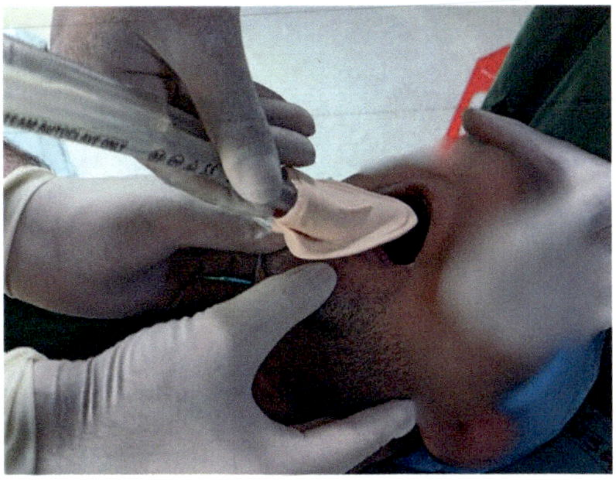

Fig. 4.6 Digital technique for PLMA. Note that the index finger is placed within the introducer pocket

2. *Introducer technique*: The metal introducer tip is inserted into the introducer strap and the shaft of the PLMA is opposed against the convex posterior surface of the introducer and is fixed to the introducer proximally at the superior portion of the bite block. The handle of the introducer is then held with the dominant hand such that the handle is parallel to the patient's chest, and PLMA inserted with the PLMA tip facing the hard palate and with a smooth rotational movement at the wrist, the PLMA is pushed along the palate into the hypopharynx till a resistance is felt (Fig. 4.7). Following stabilization of the shaft with the non-dominant hand, the introducer is then carefully removed.
3. *Guided techniques*:
   - This was first described using gum-elastic bougie, wherein, the straight end of the bougie is inserted into the esophagus under laryngoscopy guidance, and the PLMA was then railroaded over the bougie with the digital technique. This was modified by inserting the bougie through the drain tube of the PLMA first and then inserting it into the esophagus rather than rail-roading the PLMA after the bougie was inserted (Fig. 4.8).

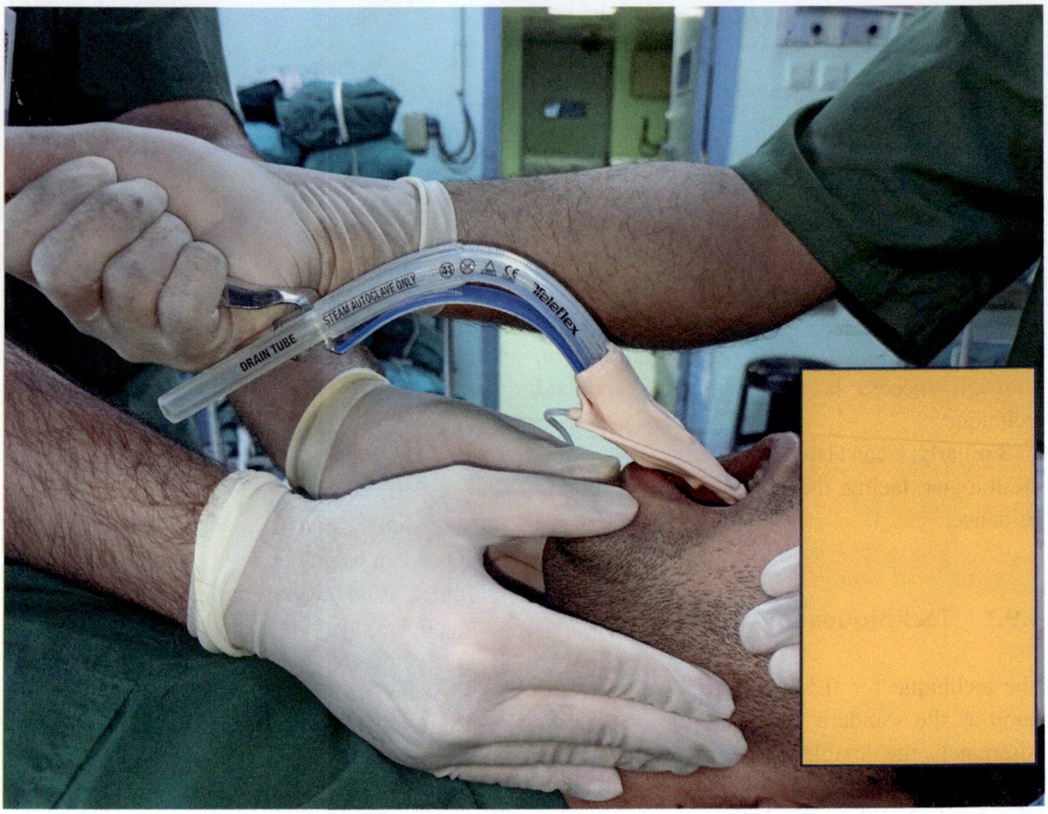

Fig. 4.7 Introducer technique for PLMA. The tip faces the hard palate and the handle is parallel to the patient's chest

- *Martinez-Pons* described the use of a gastric tube inserted within the drain tube and followed by PLMA insertion with the digital technique, without initial laryngoscopy. This avoided the risk of posterior folding of the PLMA tip during insertion.
- A suction catheter can be inserted through the drain tube of the PLMA overshooting the distal end of the drain tube by 15 cm which is inserted blindly into the hypopharynx followed by guiding the PLMA with the digital technique (Fig. 4.9). This can reduce number of attempts as the suction catheter avoids posterior folding of the tip, and laryngoscopy is also avoided.

4. *90° rotational technique:* Here, the PLMA cuff is fully inserted into the mouth like the digital technique and then rotated 90° anticlockwise (Fig. 4.10), is further pushed into the hypopharynx and then rotated back such that the ventral surface of the mask faces the glottis.. This has been shown to improve insertion success and reduce mucosal trauma. A reverse (180°) rotational technique like the one described for cLMA above is difficult for the PLMA due to its large and soft cuff.
5. *Other techniques:* A novel technique using a rigid stylet inserted in the drain tube up to its tip followed by shaping the PLMA similar to that with the introducer in-situ has been shown to improve insertion success when compared to the introducer technique (Fig. 4.11).

4.9.3 Technique for LMA® Fastrach™ (ILMA)

The ILMA can be inserted with the head in neutral or sniffing position. Insertion technique is

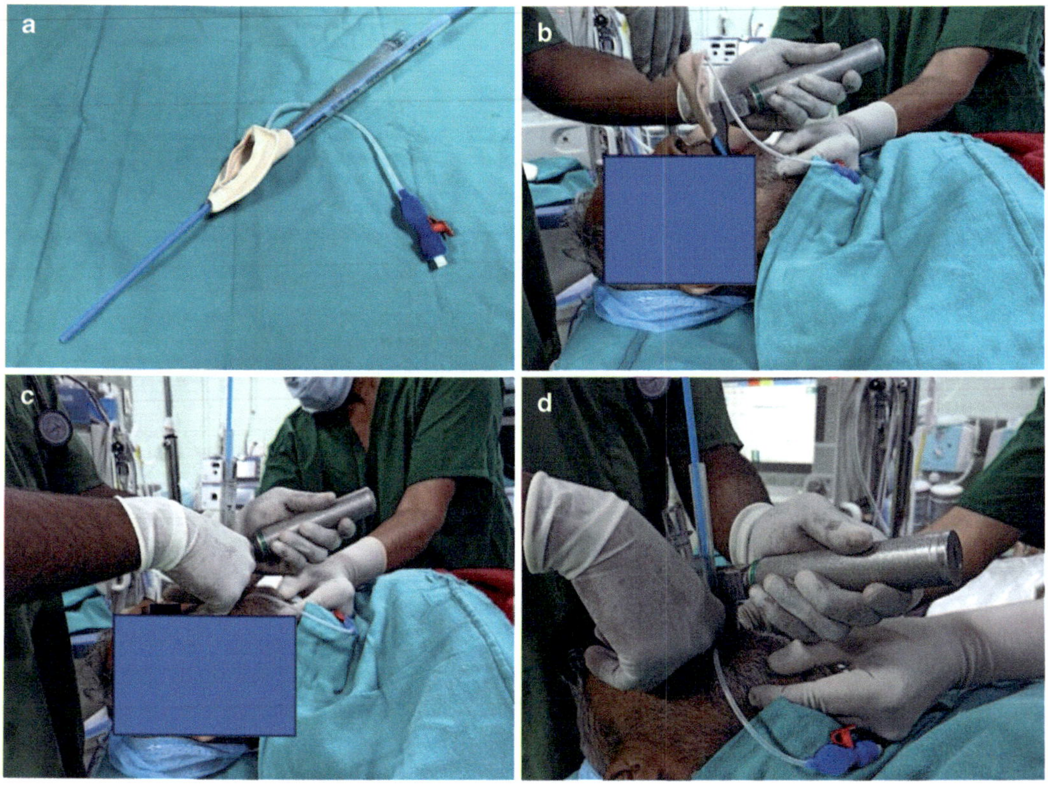

Fig. 4.8 (**a**) Straight end of bougie inserted through the drain tube of PLMA; (**b**) PLMA being inserted under laryngoscopy guidance. The laryngoscope identifies the hypopharynx and not the glottis. Bougie inserted first into hypopharynx followed by PLMA; (**c** and **d**) Further steps during insertion

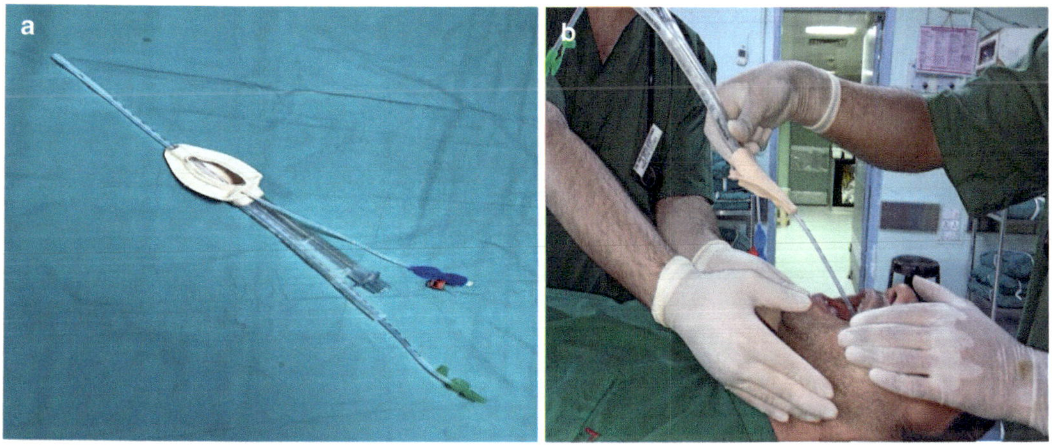

Fig. 4.9 (**a**) Suction catheter introduced through the drain tube. (**b**) Advance the suction catheter through the mouth followed by the PLMA. The suction catheter enters the upper esophagus and guides the PLMA into the hypopharynx while preventing posterior folding

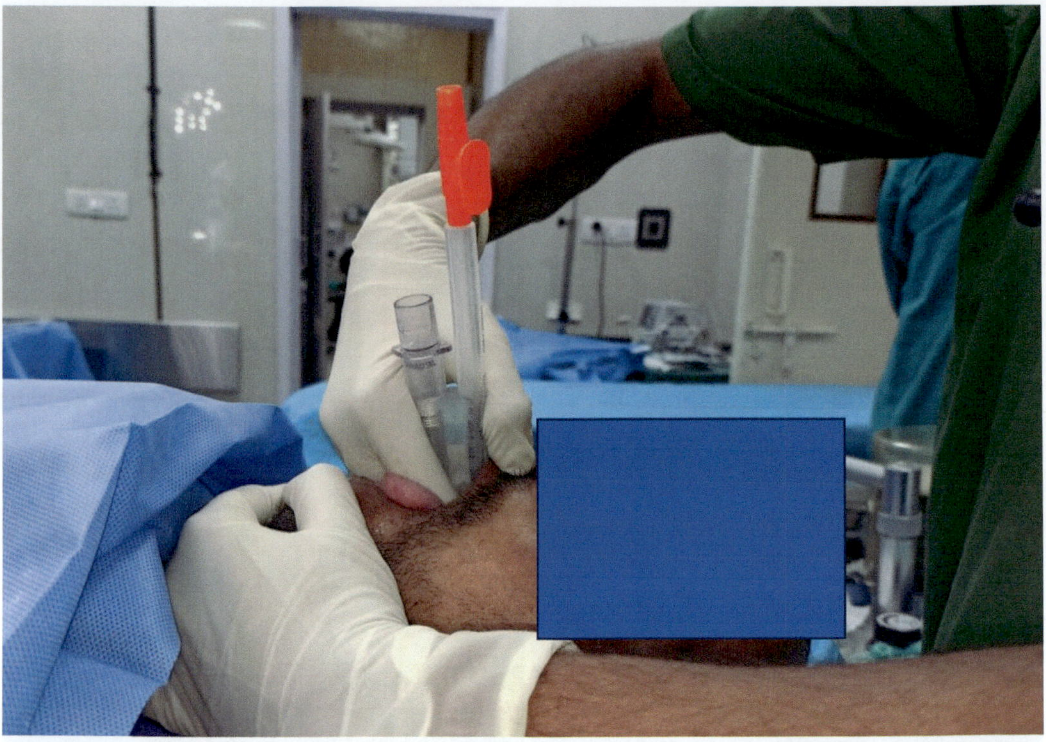

Fig. 4.10 PLMA being inserted after intra-oral 90° anti-clockwise rotation. This image also shows presence of suction catheter through drain tube

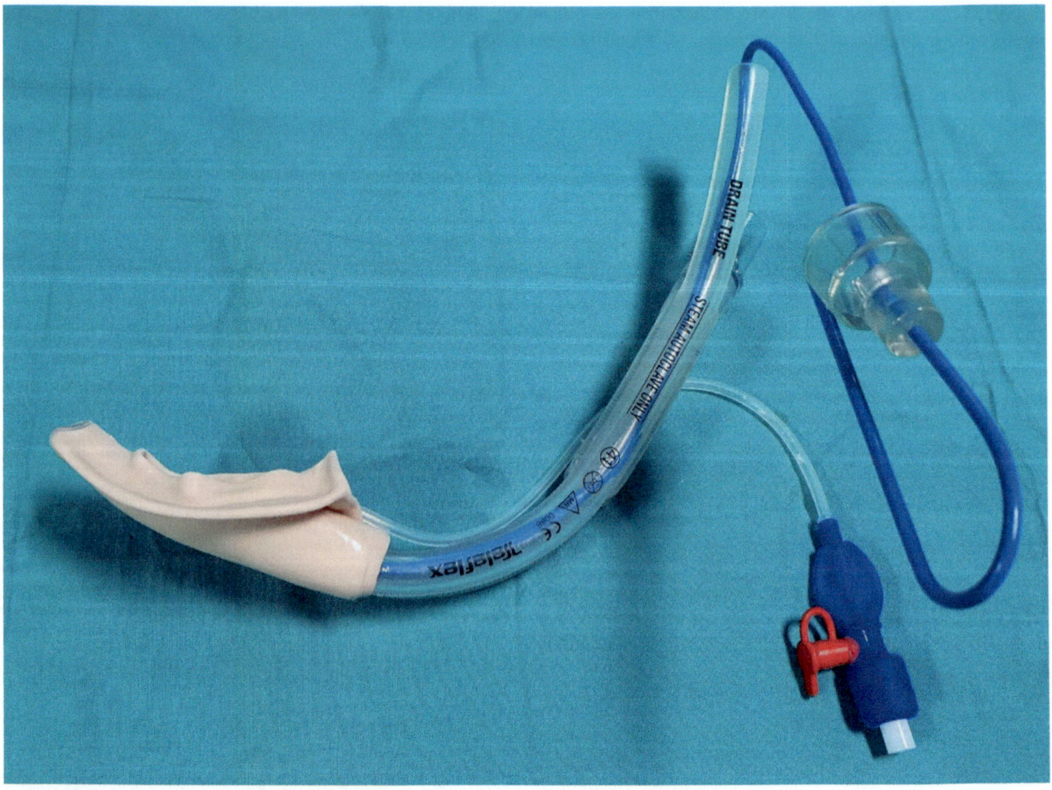

Fig. 4.11 Rigid stylet inserted into the drain tube and PLMA shaped appropriately

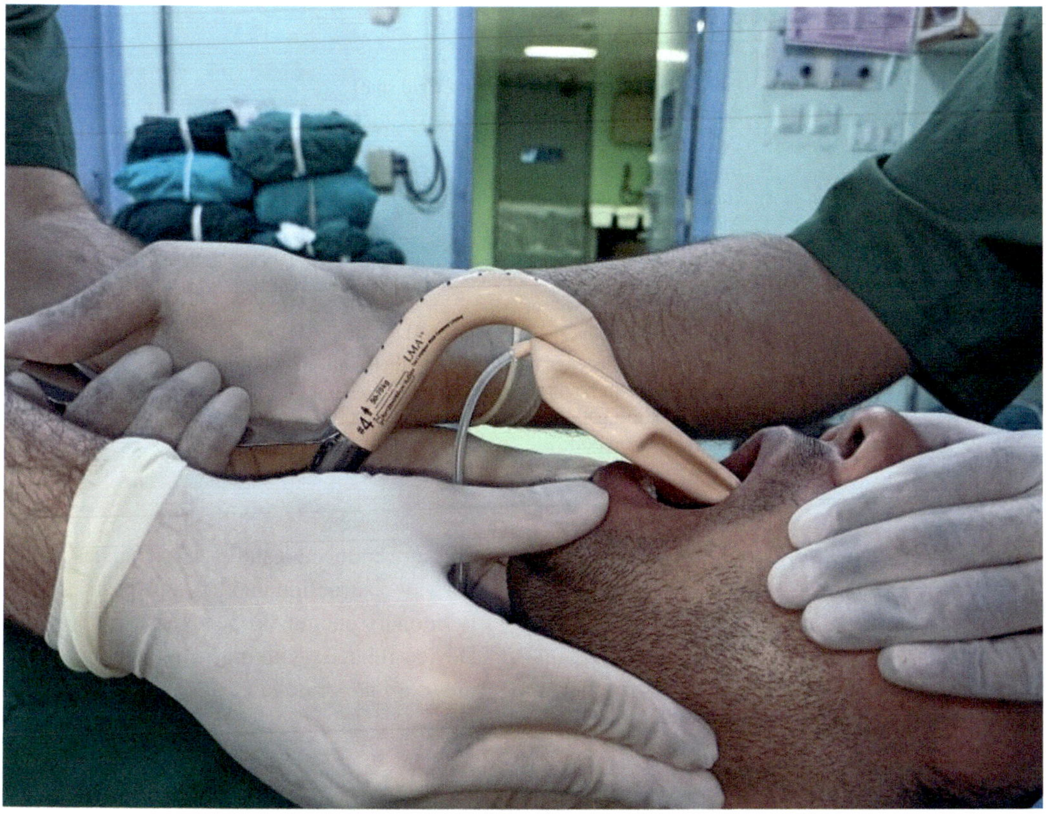

Fig. 4.12 Insertion of ILMA. Similar to introducer technique of PLMA

like the introducer technique for PLMA described above (Fig. 4.12). The technique of intubation through the ILMA is beyond the scope of this chapter.

4.9.4 Technique for LMA® Supreme™

The SLMA has a preformed rigid curve. Thus, introducer or digital technique ("pen-holding") is not needed. The SLMA is held at its shaft around the bite block and the tip is directed toward the hard palate and then inserted in a single smooth rotational movement with the cuff being directed in the cranio-posterior direction. To prevent the tip from folding, a suction catheter may be inserted in the gastric deflation port similar to that of PLMA.

4.10 Important Characteristics and Techniques of Insertion of Other Commonly Used SGAs

The following table (Table 4.4) gives important design characteristics of these SGAs.

4.10.1 Techniques of Insertion for Ambu® Laryngeal Masks

Insertion technique is similar to the standard and partial cuff inflation techniques described earlier for cLMA. As the shaft is rigid and preformed, the shaft can be held similar to the SLMA and the SGA can be inserted, without using the "pen-holding" technique to guide the SGA.

Table 4.4 Important characteristics of commonly used SGAs

Type of SGA	Important design characteristics
Ambu® Aura40™	• Preformed anatomical curve with rigid shaft • Reinforced tip
Ambu® AuraGain™	• Preformed anatomical curve • Integrated bite block • Gastric access channel • Aids intubation
Air-Q® Intubating Laryngeal airway (ILA)	• Dark blue mask bowl • Rigid shaft with color coded connectors for various sizes • The glottic surface of the Air-Q® has ridges to make a better seal • The airway tube has a keyhole-shaped outlet
i-gel®	• Preshaped perilaryngeal cuff made of thermoplastic elastomer • Wide shaft with integrated bite block • Allows for intubation • Gastric suction port

4.10.2 Techniques of Insertion for Air-Q® ILA

Both standard technique and 180° rotational technique similar to the cLMA have been described for Air-Q®.

4.10.3 Techniques of Insertion for i-gel®

i-gel® has a relatively rigid shaft and the preshaped, non-inflatable cuff cannot fold easily. During insertion, the head is laced in neutral or sniffing position, the i-gel® is held at its bite-block and is inserted with its tip facing the hard palate pushing it in a cranio-posterior direction. A 180° reverse insertion technique similar to the one described for cLMA previously has been used for i-gel.

4.11 Complications

Complications due to SGA use are rare (0.15%) in elective setting and include the following:

- Gastric aspiration.
- Sympathetic response to insertion (milder than endotracheal intubation).
- Local trauma and sore throat.
- Pressure-induced lesions, nerve palsies.
- Airway obstruction and laryngospasm.
- Pulmonary edema, bronchospasm.
- Device related: Kinking, fragmentation, failure to inflate or deflate etc.

Suggested Reading

1. Cook TM, Woodall N, Frerk C. Major complications of airway management in the UK: results of the fourth National Audit Project of the Royal College of Anaesthetists and the difficult airway society. Part 1: Anaesthesia. Br J Anaesth. 2011;106(5):617–31.
2. van Zundert TCRV, Brimacombe JR, Ferson DZ, et al. Archie brain: celebrating 30 years of development in laryngeal mask airways. Anaesthesia. 2012;67(12):1375–85.
3. Frerk C, Mitchell VS, McNarry AF, Mendonca C, Bhagrath R, Patel A, et al. Difficult airway society 2015 guidelines for management of unanticipated difficult intubation in adults. Br J Anaesth. 2015;115(6):827–48.
4. Link MS, Berkow LC, Kudenchuk PJ, et al. Amercan heart association cardiopulmonary resuscitation and emergency cardiovascular care. Part 7: adult advanced cardiovascular life support. Circulation. 2015;132(suppl 2):S444–64.
5. Lindsay HA, Cook TM, Russo SG, et al. Supraglottic airway techniques: layngeal mask airways. In: Hagberg CA, Artime CA, Aziz MF, editors. Hagberg and Benumof's airway management. 4th ed. Philadelphia, PA: Elsevier; 2018. p. 339–40.
6. Cook T, Howes B. Supraglottic airway devices: recent advances. Contin Educ Anaesth Crit Care Pain. 2011;11(2):56–61.

7. Cook TM. A further plea for a unified classification of supraglottic (extraglottic) airway devices. Br J Anaesth. 2016;117(1):136–7.
8. Miller DM. A proposed classification and scoring system for supraglottic sealing airways: a brief review. Anesth Analg. 2004;99:1553–9.
9. Michálek P, Miller DM. Airway management evolution—in a search for an ideal extraglottic airway device. Prague Med Rep. 2014;115(3–4):87–103.
10. Asai T. Airway obstruction due to a damage to the laryngeal mask. Anesth Analg. 2005;100(5):1549.
11. Sinha R, Ray B. Difficulty in proseal laryngeal mask airway insertion: an unusual cause. J Anaesthesiol Clin Pharmacol. 2013;29(3):401.
12. Keller C, Brimacombe J. Failed gastric tube insertion with the ProSeal laryngeal mask airway (PLMA). Anaesthesia. 2003;58(7):713–4.
13. Asai T, Koga K, Morris S. Damage to the laryngeal mask by residual fluid in the cuff. Anaesthesia. 1997;52(10):977–81.
14. Krishnappa S, Kundra P. Optimal anaesthetic depth for LMA insertion. Indian J Anaesth. 2011;55(5):504–7.
15. Dinesh Kumar K, Bhardwaj N, Yaddanapudi S. Comparison of trapezius squeeze test and jaw thrust as clinical indicators for laryngeal mask airway insertion in spontaneously breathing children. J Anaesthesiol Clin Pharmacol. 2017;33(1):71–5.
16. Asai T, Morris S. The laryngeal mask airway: its features, effects and role. Can J Anaesth. 1994;41(10):930–60.
17. Dorsch JA, Dorsch SE. Supraglottic airway devices. In: Understanding anesthesia equipment. 5th ed. New Delhi: Wolters Kluwer; 2008. p. 463–5.
18. Renu S, Rajeshwari S. Failed laryngeal mask insertion—another technique. Pediatr Anesth. 2008;18(6):571–2.
19. Southern DA, Lake APJ, Wadon AJ. The laryngeal mask: a modification in its use and design. Anaesthesia. 1992;47(6):530.
20. Brimacombe J, Berry A. Insertion of the laryngeal mask airway—a prospective study of four techniques. Anaesth Intensive Care. 1993;21(1):89–92.
21. An J, Shin SK, Kim KJ. Laryngeal mask airway insertion in adults: comparison between fully deflated and partially inflated technique. Yonsei Med J. 2013;54(3):747–51.
22. O'Neill B, Templeton JJ, Caramico L, Schreiner MS. The laryngeal mask airway in pediatric patients: factors affecting ease of use during insertion and emergence. Anesth Analg. 1994;78:659–62.
23. Moon B-E, Kim M-S, Lee JR. A simple method of partial inflation of the LMA cuff before insertion in children to allow cuff pressure without adjustment after insertion. Korean J Anesthesiol. 2012;62(6):524–8.
24. Dubois J, Farmer S, Fitzpatick T. The Charlottetown LMA twist. Can J Anaesth. 1998;45(8):823.
25. Soh CR, Ng ASB. Laryngeal mask airway insertion in paediatric anaesthesia: comparison between the reverse and standard techniques. Anaesth Intensive Care. 2001;29(5):515–9.
26. Nakayama S, Osaka Y, Yamashita M. The rotational technique with a partially inflated laryngeal mask airway improves the ease of insertion in children. Pediatr Anesth. 2002;12(5):416–9.
27. Ghai B, Makkar JK, Bhardwaj N, Wig J. Laryngeal mask airway insertion in children: comparison between rotational, lateral and standard technique. Pediatr Anesth. 2008;18(4):308–12.
28. Goyal M, Dutt A, Khan Joad AS. Laryngeal mask airway insertion by classic and thumb insertion technique: a comparison. F1000Research. 2013;2:123.
29. Dorsch JA, Dorsch SE. Supraglottic airway devices. In: Understanding anesthesia equipment. 5th ed. New Delhi: Wolters Kluwer; 2008. p. 465.
30. Kundra P, Deepak R, Ravishankar M. Laryngeal mask insertion in children: a rational approach. Pediatr Anesth. 2003;13(8):685–90.
31. Krishna HM, Kamath S, Shenoy L. Insertion of LMA classic™ with and without digital intraoral manipulation in anesthetized unparalyzed patients. J Anaesthesiol Clin Pharmacol. 2012;28(4):481–5.
32. Philpott B, Renwick M. An introducer for the flexible laryngeal mask airway. Anaesthesia. 1993;48(2):174.
33. Chawla AV, Newton NI. Machine and monitoring failure from electrical overloading. Anaesthesia. 2002;57(11):1134–5.
34. Nalini K, Shivakumar S, Archana S, Sandhya Rani D, Mohan CR. Comparison of three insertion techniques of ProSeal laryngeal mask airway: a randomized clinical trial. J Anaesthesiol Clin Pharmacol. 2016;32(4):510–4.
35. Lindsay HA, Cook TM, Russo SG, et al. Supraglottic airway techniques: Layngeal mask airways. In: Hagberg CA, Artime CA, Aziz MF, editors. Hagberg and Benumof's airway management. 4th ed. Philadelphia, PA: Elsevier; 2018. p. 340.
36. Howath A, Brimacombe J, Keller C. Gum-elastic Bougie-guided insertion of the ProSeal™ laryngeal mask airway: a new technique. Anaesth Intensive Care. 2002;30(5):624–7.
37. Matioc AA, Arndt GA. Unassisted gum elastic Bougie—guided insertion of the Proseal laryngeal mask airway. Anesthesiology. 2004;101(5):1240–1.
38. Brimacombe J, Irving S. Ease placement of LMA ProSeal with gastric tube inserted. Anesth Analg. 2004;98:1816–7.
39. García-Aguado R, Viñoles J, Brimacombe J, et al. Suction catheter guided insertion of the ProSeal™ laryngeal mask airway is superior to the digital technique. Can J Anesth. 2006;53(4):398–403.
40. Hwang J, Do S-H. Comparison of two insertion techniques of ProSeal™ laryngeal mask airway. Anesthesiology. 2009;110:905–7.
41. Myatra S, Khandale V, Pühringer F, Gupta S, Solanki S, Divatia J. A novel technique for insertion of ProSeal™ laryngeal mask airway: comparison of the stylet tool with the introducer tool in a prospective, randomised study. Indian J Anaesth. 2017;61(6):475–81.

42. Gaddam M, Sethi S, Jain A, Saini V. Comparison of air-Q® insertion techniques in pediatric patients with fiber-optic bronchoscopic assessment: a prospective randomized control trial. Korean J Anesthesiol. 2019;72(6):570–5.
43. Sharda M, Kapoor MC, Atray R, Garg S. Insertion of i-gel™ by the reversed technique improves the success rate and reduces the time taken for its placement: a prospective, randomized, controlled, interventional trial. J Anaesthesiol Clin Pharmacol. 2017;33(2):226–30.

Endotracheal Intubation: Gold Standard of Airway Care

5

Raveendra Shankaranarayana Ubaradka
and Muralishankar Bhat

Key Points

- Endotracheal intubation is a core skill in airway management and requires technical proficiency.
- Successful and rapid intubation can be lifesaving in emergencies.
- In elective situations, the procedure should be planned with due consideration to various factors involved such as drugs, equipment, patient preparation, and intubation aids.
- Anticipation of difficulty and failure and having backup plan to manage such situations is critical.
- Procedure is not without complications which can range from mild and insignificant to life threatening.

5.1 Introduction

Endotracheal intubation (ETI) is the placement of an endotracheal tube in the trachea for safe and effective management of airway, ventilation and to protect the lungs from soiling. ETI could be elective, urgent, or lifesaving. It could be technically easy, difficult or can fail. Consequences of difficulty or failure can vary from being insignificant to fatal depending on the way the whole process is managed. **Technique is only a part of overall airway management, which in turn is a part of patient management.** Different aspects of ETI are covered here.

Correct placement of a cuffed endotracheal tube in the trachea is considered as the gold standard of airway protection and management. It provides an unobstructed pathway for gas exchange and ventilation. Broad categories of indication are *management of airway obstruction, facilitation of ventilation, protection of airway and or lungs and isolation of lungs.* ETI is performed primarily in operation theatre, intensive care and emergency department. In life saving situations, it can be performed in the ward, or site of accident, or in any other location.

It must be remembered that while ETI is a critical procedure and often life-saving, it could endanger the patient's life or brain if not performed properly or when the technique fails. Success depends on technical skill, availability of equipment and personnel, location, appropriate use of airway aids and management of oxygenation during the procedure. Management of failure to intubate situations is equally important. For every intubation, irrespective of the experience and skill, there must be a proper plan, prepa-

R. S. Ubaradka (✉)
Jerudong Park Medical Centre,
Brunei Muara, Brunei Darussalam

M. Bhat
Department of Anaesthesiology, KS Hegde Medical College, Mangalore, India

N. Gupta et al. (eds.), *Techniques in Anesthesia, Intensive Care and Emergency Medicine*,
https://doi.org/10.1007/978-981-96-1202-4_5

ration, a back-up plan (also referred to as Plan B), and execution.

5.2 Equipment, Indications, and Drugs (Fig. 5.1)

Equipment

Visualization: Direct laryngoscope (DL) or video laryngoscope*.

Endotracheal tubes: proper size and type.

Airway aids: Oral and nasal airway, stylet, boogie, Magill's forceps.

Ventilation: Oxygen source, mask, AMBU bag or anaesthesia machine.

Back up ventilation device: Supraglottic airway device like I gel or laryngeal mask airway (LMA).

Apneic/supplemental oxygenation: nasal prongs or high flow O_2 devices.

Monitors: Pulse oximeter for monitoring oxygen saturation (SpO_2), noninvasive blood pressure (NIBP), electrocardiogram (ECG), end tidal carbon dioxide ($EtCO_2$) and ultrasound (USG).

Suction: a wide bore catheter or with Yankeur tip, especially in patients who are at risk of aspiration.

*Video laryngoscope (VL) is an alternate to DL which has a different technique of using it. VL provides an image of the airway on a screen and the technique can be observed by others. "Seeing is not intubating" is a common caution regarding VL usage. It implies that ability to visualize the glottis need not translate into successful intubation. There are different models,

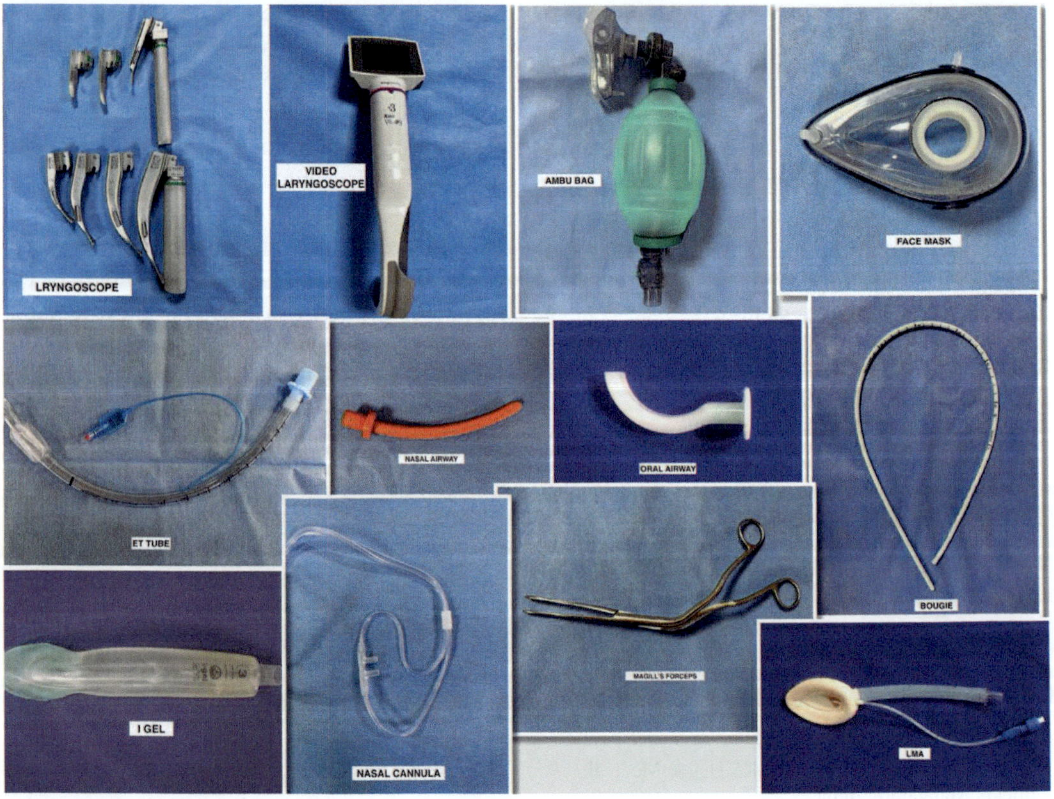

Fig. 5.1 Different airway equipment: The equipment shown here are representative of each category and different sizes and types are available in each group

sizes, and types of blades available and clinicians should be familiar with the equipment available in their workplace.

Standardized airway trolleys should be kept ready in critical locations and regularly must be checked for functional status. Should be assembled properly before procedure.

5.2.1 Endotracheal Tubes (Fig. 5.2) and Description of a Typical Endotracheal Tube

Conventional endotracheal tubes used in adults are made up of polyvinyl chloride, with a low-pressure high-volume cuff. They can be used for oral or nasal route. Specialized micro cuff ETT are used in children above 3 months and uncuffed tubes are used in infants less than 3 months of age. There are several types of specialized endotracheal tubes varying in their shape, thickness, length, cuff and material from which they are made up of. Specialized tubes are indicated in specific situations.

Drugs (Fig. 5.3)**: Dose of drugs varies depending on situation and are not covered here**.

Drug/group	Deciding factors	Remarks
Induction agents: Propofol, thiopentone, ketamine, etomidate and ketofol (mixture of ketamine and propofol)	Effect on hemodynamics, presence of contraindications, comorbidity, familiarity	Not required in unconscious patient and cardiac arrest. On other patient's sedatives may be used instead of induction agents
Analgesics: Fentanyl or others	Hemodynamic stability and level of consciousness	May be given after intubation also
Muscle relaxants	Succinylcholine, rocuronium or atracurium	Depending on ability to ventilate after paralysis and preference of performing persons
Others: depending on the patient condition	Atropine, ephedrine, metoclopramide	Depends on clinical situation
Choice of drugs, combination, sequence and dose depends on the performer (emergency physician, anaesthesiologist, intensivist, other medical professionals or emergency/paramedical technicians) location (emergency department, ICU or ward) and patient factors (polytrauma, agitation, full stomach etc.)		

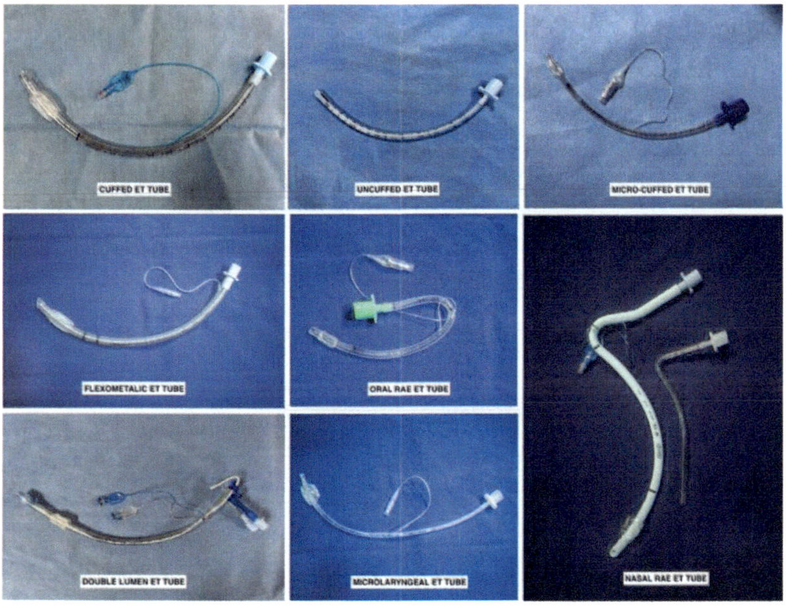

Fig. 5.2 Different endotracheal tubes

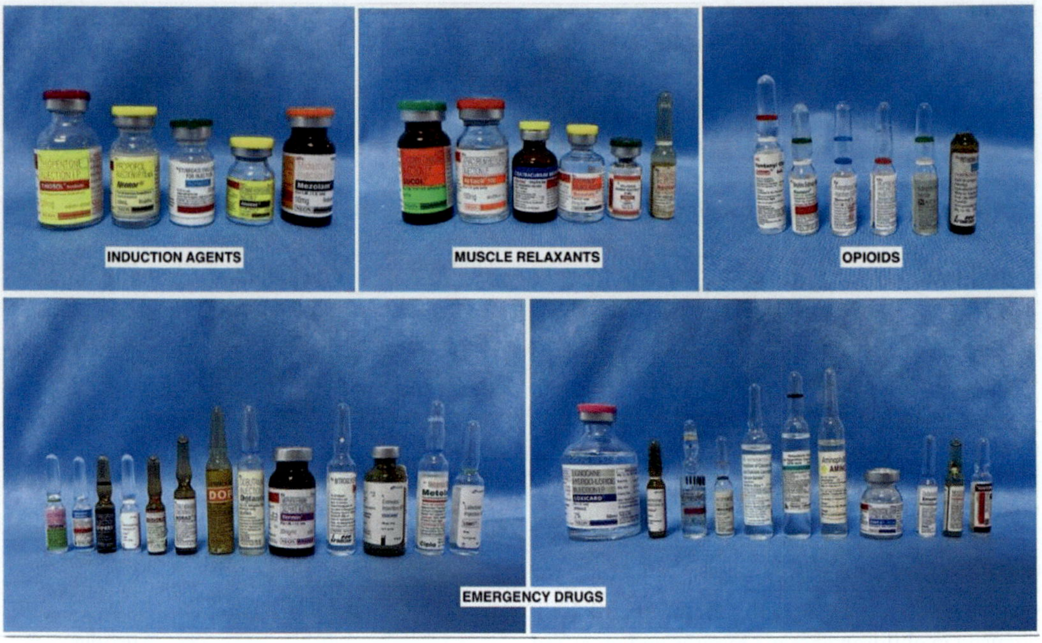

Fig. 5.3 Commonly used drugs during intubation

Indications for ETI

Airway obstruction	Unconscious or semiconscious patient Obstruction due to disease, infection, inflammation and trauma
Facilitate breathing/ ventilation	Cardiac or respiratory arrest, increased work of breathing, neuromuscular disorders, spinal cord injury
Airway protection or protection of one lung	Soiling of lung due to infection, hemorrhage, bronchopulmonary and broncho cutaneous fistulas
Anaesthesia	General anaesthesia and management of complications

5.2.2 Alternates to Endotracheal Intubation

Airway can be managed by mask ventilation (MV), supraglottic airway device (SGAD) or surgical airway either as alternate to intubation or when intubation is difficult or fails. MV is the technique used before intubation and subsequently in between attempts if more than one attempt is required. Ability to ventilate with a face mask (bag mask ventilation) reassures about the ability to provide oxygenation, even if intubation becomes difficult.

5.2.3 Techniques

A common sequence of events for an elective ETI is (a) recognition of indication for airway management, assessment of the airway and patient. This should lead to identification of normal vs. difficult airway and high-risk patients due to comorbidities. (b) preparation: equipment, drugs and monitors and help (c) plan for oxygenation (d) proper positioning of patient with C-spine protection if needed (e) anticipating complications and (f) performing the procedure and (g) post intubation management. Good intravenous access, monitors, facility for ventilation and emergency drugs are mandatory for every intubation.

When choosing the drugs for intubation, consider the adverse effects of the drugs in every patient, presence of contraindications and experience of the performer with those drugs. A person performing the ETI must be equipped with reasonable knowledge related to airway assessment, airway insertion and bag mask ventilation, monitoring, techniques and importance of oxygenation, importance of trained assistant/ experience colleague and basic airway algorithm.

Details of Critical Points Related to Endotracheal Intubation: Positioning, Preparation of Endotracheal Intubation and Oxygenation Vs. Intubation

Positioning: It is one of the key determinants of successful ETI irrespective of the techniques. For conventional techniques using DL and VL, extension of the neck with flexion of atlantooccipital joint is preferred for adult non-obese patients. This can be achieved by a small pillow or with a head ring. For obese patients, "stacked pillows" or a ramp position is useful. This "Head Elevated Laryngoscopy Position (HELP)" improves patient comfort and functional residual capacity. In this position and sternal notch and external auditory meatus are in the same line. Lastly, for infants less than 2 years a rolled towel under the shoulder helps in more effective laryngoscopy. Sometimes in emergency department, intubation may have to be performed in lateral position or even in sitting position. In such cases, specialized techniques and physicians with airway experts may be required. "Face to face" or "Inverse" intubation is rarely used to intubate patients stuck under building or landslide, etc. who need to be approached from the front only.

Preparation of endotracheal tube: This can be performed by an experienced assistant. It includes (a) ensuring sterility (b) proper size selection (c) checking the integrity of the cuff (d) lubrication of the tube and (e) "pre-shaping the tip with a malleable stylet. For adult males, common size is 7 for nasal and 7.5/8 for oral intubation. For females, one size less from the corresponding sizes for males. For every selected size, tubes with one size smaller diameter should be available for using in case of inability to pass the appropriately sized tube.

Oxygenation vs. Ventilation: Twin goals of intubation are to provide oxygenation and ventilation, simultaneously protecting the airway. However, ETI is not equivalent to oxygenation. Oxygen reserves are built up prior to intubation by preoxygenation or mask ventilation in patients with respiratory arrest. This alone may not be sufficient to maintain oxygenation during the process of intubation which usually involves a varying period of apnea. Process of administering additional oxygen, mainly by passive flow, during this apnea is called apneic oxygenation and also referred to as peri oxygenation. In addition, individual such techniques are referred to by different names. They include use of simple nasal oxygen with nasal prongs (Fig. 5.6), with a flow of 3 to 15 L during the laryngoscopy (NO-DESATS: Nasal Oxygenation During Attempts at Securing Tracheal tube), and use of specific equipment for apneic oxygenation like Trans nasal Humidified Oxygenation with Rapid Insufflation Ventilatory exchange (THRIVE).

In this context, prolonged laryngoscopy, multiple intubation attempts, failed intubation, unrecognized intubation and aspiration are the "technique related" causes of hypoxia. Measures to prevent hypoxia due to/during intubation include (a) preoxygenation, apneic oxygenation, (b) mask ventilation before laryngoscopy and in between the attempts and (c) optimizing the other factors affecting oxygenation. Further, it is important for an assistant or colleague or a nurse to time the procedure during laryngoscopy and keep alert the performer when the time exceeds 30–45 s or when the saturation level drops to less than 94% (in patients with previously normal values). Thus, oxygenation (restoration of saturation in an already hypoxic patient or prevention of hypoxia in a patient whose airway is being managed) is an independent primary objective of airway management. Failure of oxygenation is a more serious cause of hypoxia than failure to intubate.

5.2.3.1 Technique 1: Elective Orotracheal Intubation: Conventional Technique (Fig. 5.4)

Description
ETT is passed under direct visualization of the glottis, position is confirmed and connected to appropriate ventilation device.

Steps
Position the patient and connect the monitors (SpO_2, NIBP and ECG), connect nasal oxygen at 3 L/min flow rate and Preoxygenate with 100% for 3 min. Inj. propofol, 2–3 mg/kg followed by inj. Succinylcholine (2 mg/kg) or rocuronium (1–1.5 mg/kg) Mask ventilate till fasciculations disappear for succinylcholine or for 1 min with rocuronium. Increase nasal oxygen flow to 10 to 15 L. Direct Laryngoscopy: with the laryngoscopy blade in open position and light on, insert the blade into the oral cavity from the left angle of mouth and bring it to the midline positioning the tongue under the blade. Tip of the blade should be at the valleculum. Next, open the mouth further with anterior force without using the upper teeth as fulcrum. Alternately, video laryngoscope (VL) can be used.

Visualize glottis or glottis opening. in addition to the above-described technique of Laryngoscopy, external laryngeal manipulation or boogie (Fig. 5.5) may be required for intubation. The tip of the tube should be positioned proximal to carina. Remove the Laryngoscopy, inflate the cuff (Fig. 5.14), connect the Ambu bag or ventilator and ventilate. Confirm proper position by bilateral chest expansion and breath sounds, normal capo gram ($EtCO_2$), normal inflation pressure and ultrasound. Fix the tube properly. Measure the cuff pressure and maintain it at less than 20 mmHg using a cuff pressure monitor (Fig. 5.14).

Remember
Esophageal intubation per se need not be harmful. Failure to recognize the same can be lethal. When in doubt, remove the tube. Hypoxia is a late sign. Absence of normal capnography waves and ultrasound are the real time most reliable diagnostic tools for detection of esophageal intubation (Figs. 5.7, 5.8, and 5.9). Duration of laryngoscopy should not exceed 30–45 s and certainly not more than 60 s. When a novice is intubating a patient, it is better to monitor the time and remind him/her when it exceeds 30 s and again at 45 s. First attempt failure should be followed by mask ventilation, assessment of oxygenation, analysis of cause of failure and need for changes in patient position, blade size, tube size or use of boogie before the second attempt. Failure of second attempt should lead to activation of failed intubation algorithm. Multiple attempts can cause significant trauma and Seema of airway leading to life threatening complications. Intubation may be important but oxygenation is more important. Intubation is performed or intubation attempts are repeated only if it is going to facilitate oxygenation rather than becomes an impediment.

Variations
Propofol may be avoided if patient is in profound hypotension or is deeply unconscious due to any reason. Muscle relaxant may not be always required and its use is dependent on clinical judgement. Video laryngoscope can be used in place of the direct laryngoscope.

5.2.3.2 Technique 2: Elective Nasotracheal Intubation (NTI)—Conventional Technique

Nose is prepared with vasoconstrictor drops (oxymetazoline or xylometazoline) to prevent bleeding. After patient becomes unconscious (and paralyzed, if applicable), ETT is passed through the nostril into oral cavity. DL is performed as described above. ETT is manipulated

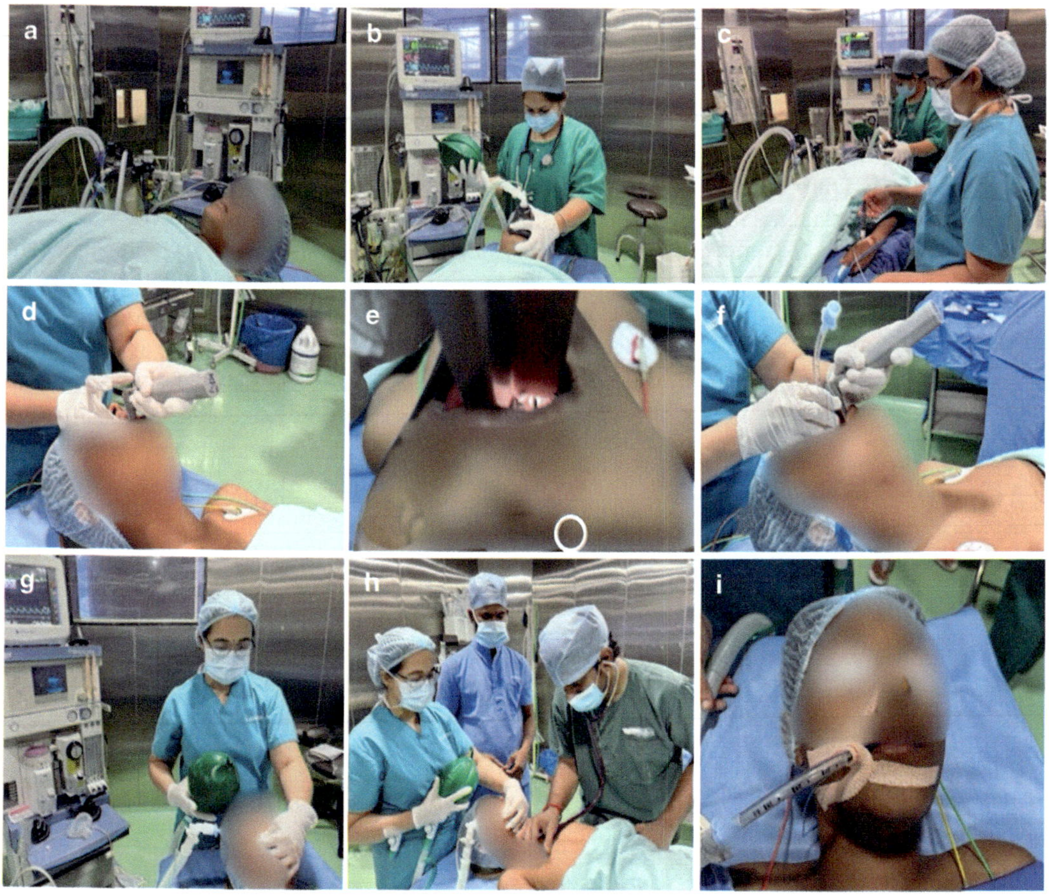

Fig. 5.4 Steps of intubation. (**a**) Pre-induction with monitors. (**b**) Pre-oxygenation. (**c**) Induction by giving inducing agent and muscle relaxant. (**d**) Direct laryngoscopy. (**e**) Visualization of the vocal cord. (**f**) Passing of ET tube. (**g**) Connecting breathing circuit to ET tube. (**h**) Confirming successful intubation and bilateral lung air entry with five-point auscultation method. (**i**) Fixing the ET tube. *Remember, in non anaesthesia related intubations, anaesthesia machines are replaced by ventilators or Ambu bags with oxygen insufflation*

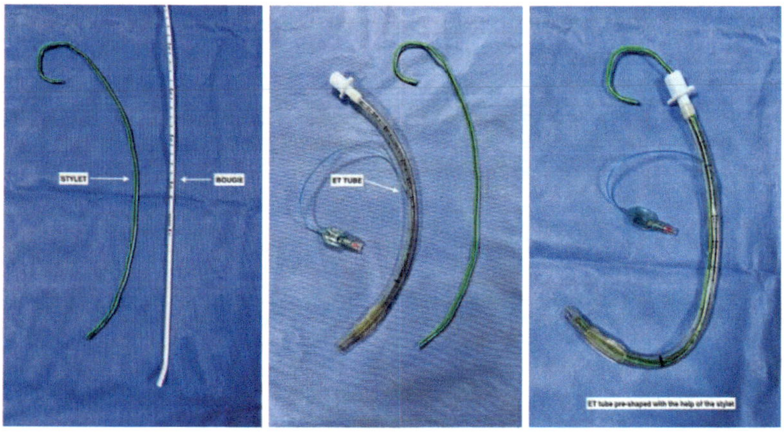

Fig. 5.5 Showing intubating bougie and stylet. A bougie can be used to rail road the ET tube in cases of difficult airway. A stylet is used to facilitate intubation by pre-shaping the ET tube tip at a desired angle

into the trachea, usually with the help of a Magill's forceps (Fig. 5.10).

Key Points

NTI is not routinely used in situations outside the operation theater, contraindicated in nasal bone fracture and base of skull fracture. Complications of NTI are risk of bleeding, injury to structures in nasopharynx and technical difficulty of negotiating the nasopharynx or manipulating the tube into the trachea.

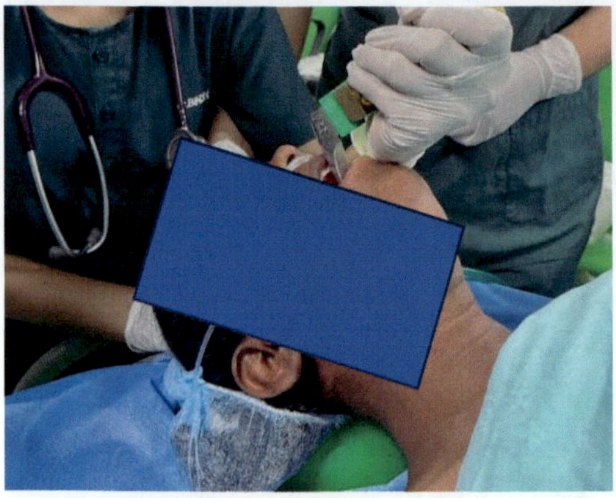

Fig. 5.6 During intubation, apnea time can be increased by providing oxygen with the help of a nasal canula

5.2.3.3 Technique 3: Emergency Orotracheal Intubation—Conventional Technique

Additional issues in emergency intubation are related to risk of pulmonary aspiration of gastric contents, increased risk of hypoxia, unstable patient or patient in cardiac arrest, urgency of the situation and increased risk of hypoxia and risk of technical failure. Measures to enhance the safety in such situations are use of cricoid pressure (CP), adequate preoxygenation, use of video laryngoscopy, administration of drugs to empty stomach such as metoclopramide or suction of gastric contents with a nasogastric or orogastric tube. Currently most used technique of intubation in emergency is called modified rapid sequence intubation (mRSI) or modified rapid sequence induction-intubation. In contrast, in agitated patients in emergency who cannot be oxygenated adequately before mRSI, an alternate

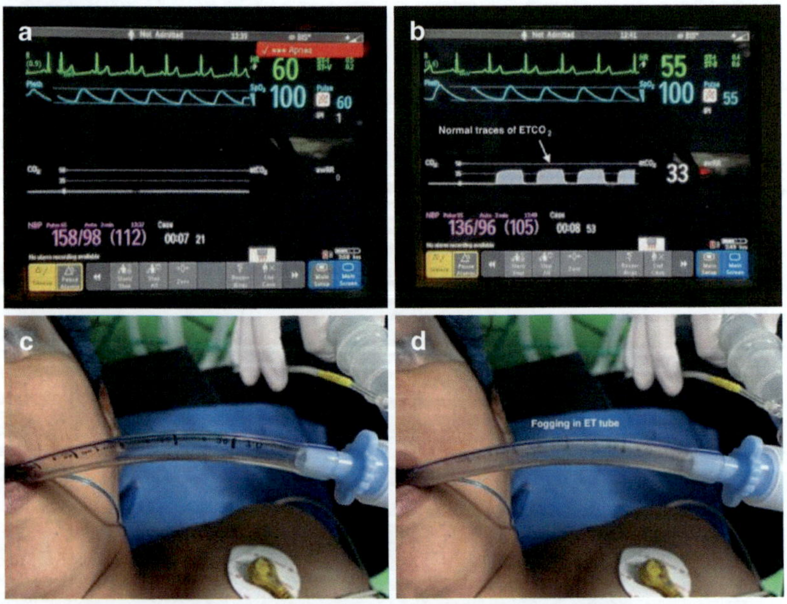

Fig. 5.7 Monitoring and confirmation of successful placement of ET tube with the help of $ETCO_2$ and detection of fogging in the ET tube. Although fogging in the ET tube is a crude method of confirmation of successful intubation, it can be taken as one of the signs which indicate ET tube is in the trachea. (**a**) Before intubation—no traces of $ETCO_2$. (**b**) Normal traces of $ETCO_2$ (Square wave capnogram) after successful intubation. (**c**) No fogging in ET tube raising doubts about successful intubation. (**d**) Fogging in the ET tube can be appreciated

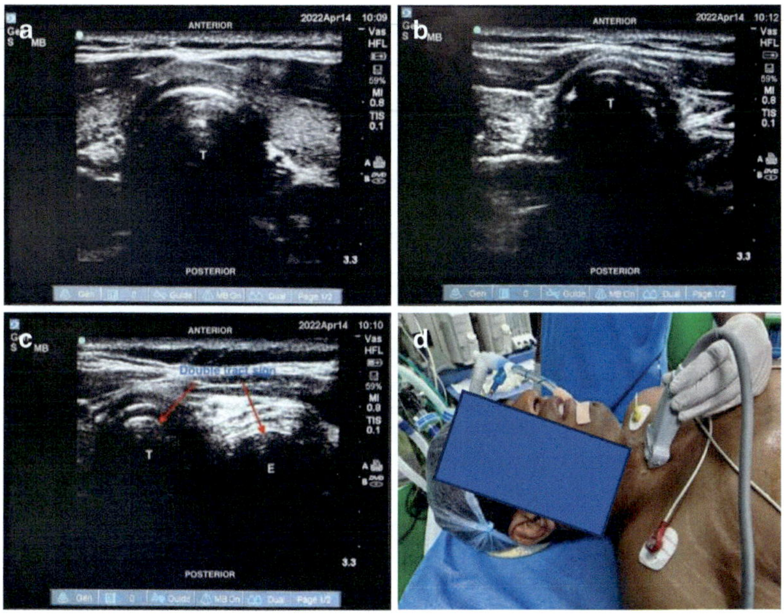

Fig. 5.8 Confirmation of intubation using tracheal ultrasound. (**a**) Normal ultrasound scan of trachea. (**b**) Post-intubation with ET tube in trachea—USG scan looks similar to normal tracheal scan. (**c**) ET tube in esophagus showing "double tract sign." (**d**) Placing a linear ultrasound probe transversely on the anterior aspect of the neck at the level to confirm endotracheal intubation

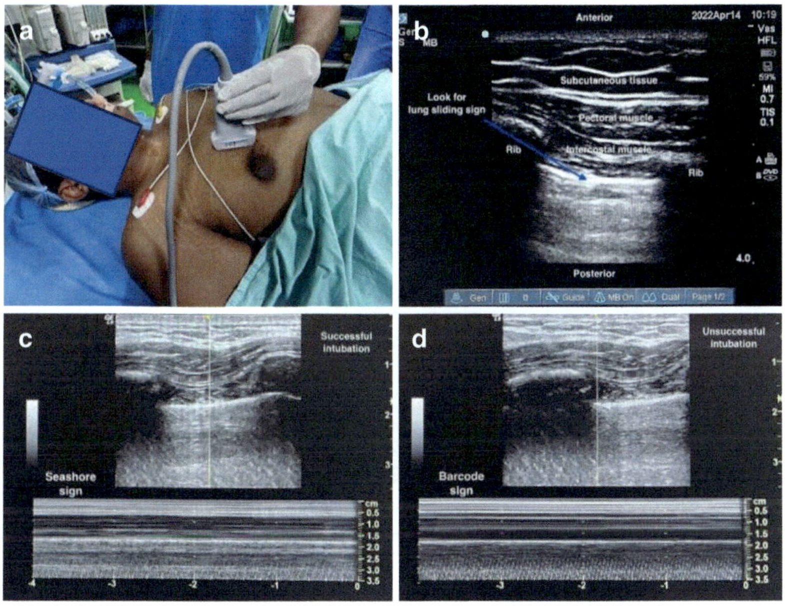

Fig. 5.9 Confirmation of intubation using lung ultrasound. (**a**) A linear transducer placed in the anterior chest wall along mid-clavicular line. (**b**) Presence of lung sliding sign confirms success intubation and ventilation. (**c**) M mode showing "seashore sign" indicating successful intubation. (**d**) M mode showing "barcode sign" indicating that lung is not being ventilated

approach called delayed sequence intubation (DSI) is also employed.

mRSI involves administration of specific drugs in fixed doses in sequence, use of cricoid pressure (Sellick's maneuver, Fig. 5.11), mask ventilation with a low inflation pressure and a quick laryngoscopy and intubation. Purpose of mRSI is to control and protect the airway within the shortest possible time in least traumatic manner without causing regurgitation and pulmonary aspiration of gastric contents. CP, also called Sellick's maneuver is effective only when the person applying the pressure is trained in doing it the right way.

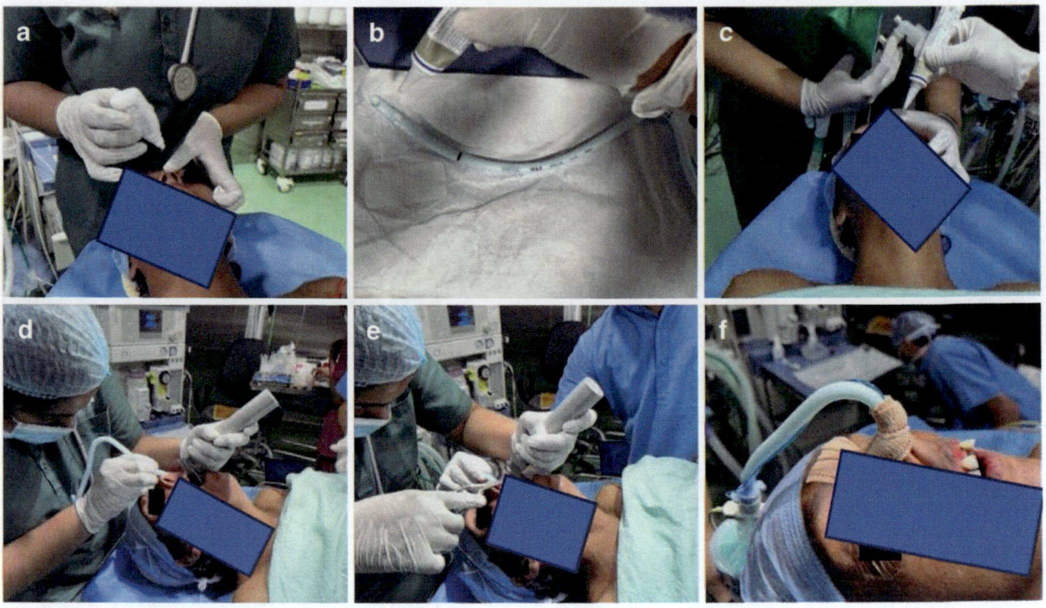

Fig. 5.10 Nasotracheal intubation. (**a**) Nose is prepared with vasoconstrictor drops. (**b**) Applying lubricant jelly to nasotracheal ET tube. (**c**) Applying lubricant jelly to nose. (**d**) Inserting the nasotracheal ET tube. (**e**) Manipulating the ET tube with the help of Magill's forceps. (**f**) Fixing of nasotracheal ET tube

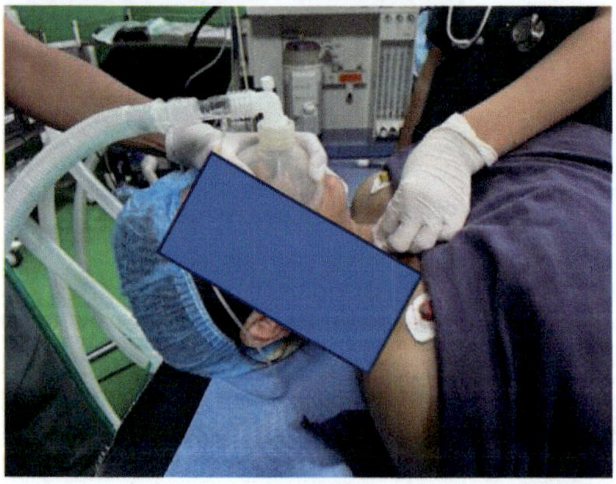

Fig. 5.11 Sellick's maneuver

Steps

1. If patient is conscious, explain the cricoid pressure in patient's language, in a non -threatening way.
2. Start with preoxygenation (ideally for 3 min, if not feasible, it can be for 8 vital capacity breaths).
3. Induce with pre-decided and fixed dose of drug (propofol 2 mg/kg or thiopentone 5 mg/kg). Increase cricoid pressure to compress the upper esophagus against the cervical vertebra.
4. Paralyze with IV succinylcholine (2 mg/kg) or rocuronium (1.2 mg/kg).
5. Mask ventilation with gentle inflation pressure for 60 s.
6. Intubate with a direct or video laryngoscope.
7. Inflate the cuff and confirm the placement of the tube and release the cricoid pressure.

Release the cricoid pressure if it is coming in the way of effective ventilation or laryngoscopy. Choice of drugs and dose can vary depending on hemodynamics and presence of contraindications.

5.2.3.4 Technique 4: Flexible Endoscopic Guided Intubation (Fig. 5.12)

Endoscopy guided intubation (fibreoptic intubation is a common term) is used when conventional techniques fail or are contraindicated or not ideal. Examples are patients with difficult airway or those who cannot be put to sleep safely before airway control. It requires skill which can

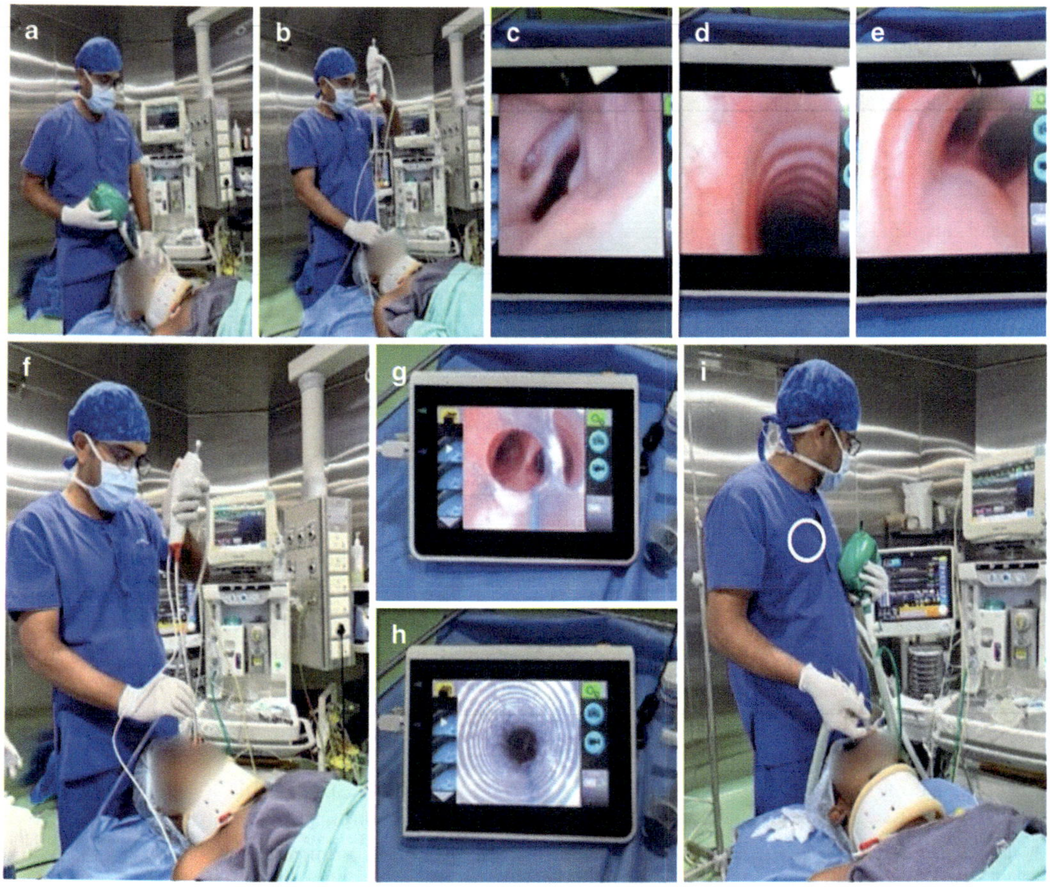

Fig. 5.12 Flexible endoscopy guided intubation. (**a**) Preoxygenation. (**b**) Inserting the flexible scope (with flexometalic ET tube mounted) through nose. (**c**) Visualizing the vocal cords. (**d**) Visualizing the trachea—tracheal rings can be appreciated. (**e**) Tracheal bifurcation at carina. (**f**) Passing the flexometalic ET tube. (**g**) ET tube inserted into trachea. (**h**) Withdrawing flexible endoscope by visualizing the ET tube. (**i**) Successful ventilation confirmed with $ETCO_2$ waveforms

be acquired only by proper training and equipment. Agitated or uncooperative patient, presence of blood or secretions or airway pathology can increase risk of failure. Advantages are (1) it can be performed in awake or sedated or anesthetized patients, (2) direct visualization of the entire airway, (3) neck movement can be avoided, (4) patient can be in any position (supine, lateral or even prone when it is inevitable), (5) simultaneous and accurate confirmation of intratracheal placement and proper positioning, and (6) can be used in different ways to achieve intubation when conventional technique is difficult or fails.

Technical details are not discussed here as it is reserved only for the clinicians trained in airway management and with additional training in flexible endoscopic guided airway management.

5.2.3.5 Technique 5: Video Laryngoscopy

Video laryngoscope is a laryngoscope which transmits the image of the laryngeal inlet indirectly via a prism, lenses, optical fibre, or video clips (Fig. 5.13). It provides an improved laryngeal view, reduces the risk of failure and may prolong intubation time. The accumulating

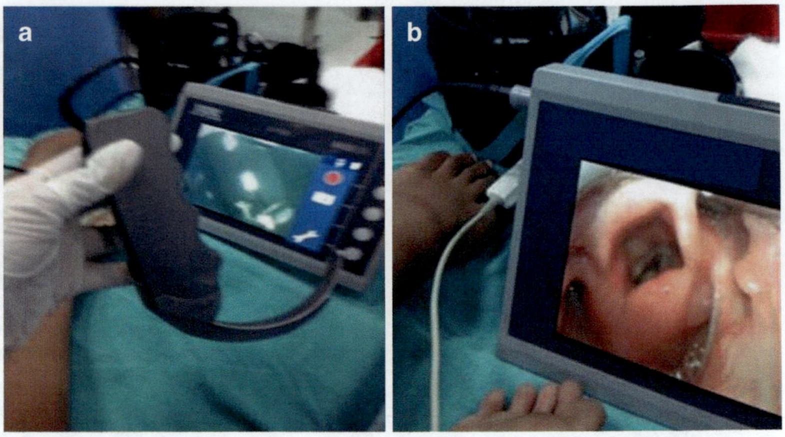

Fig. 5.13 (**a**) Video laryngoscope; (**b**) High-resolution image of glottis on the screen

evidence of improved success, better visualization (with its associated reduction in injury), reduced number of attempts, and even improved learning has recently led to recommendations for the universal adoption of video laryngoscopy.

It is a four-step procedure—mouth-screen-mouth-screen

1. Look at the **mouth** as you insert the video laryngoscope to avoid injury.
2. Visualise the epiglottis on the **screen.**
3. Look in the **mouth** as you introduce the ETT.
4. Visualise the ETT entering the glottis on the **screen.**

Levitan had described steps to intubate using a VAL.

Step 1: visualization of the epiglottis.

The blade of VAL is introduced through midline into the mouth till epiglottis is identified. For curved blade, tip is placed in the vallecula whereas for straight blade, blade is passed beyond the epiglottis lifting it directly.

Step 2: lifting force is applied to open the hypopharynx, maximize the laryngeal exposure.

Step 3: tilting the optics toward the ET tube will help the delivery of tube.

Step 4: advance the ETT slowly across the glottis, withdraw the stylet, and push the non-stylleted tube further into the trachea.

The only difference from the normal laryngoscope is that the laryngeal inlet is visualised indirectly on the screen and there is no need to align oropharyngeal curve and the pharynx-glotto-tracheal curve in one line.

Trouble shooting:

- In the unchanneled variety, an angulated stylet may be required to direct the tube into the glottic opening.
- Sometimes difficulty may be encountered while delivering the ETT. If the tube is impinging into the cricoid cartilage, withdraw the tube and rotate by 90 degrees.
- In some cases, manipulation of head and neck of patient with application of jaw thrust may be required to improve the view.

5.2.4 Confirmation of Endotracheal Intubation (Figs. 5.7, 5.8, and 5.9)

This is the final critical step and may not be always easy. Optimal position of the tip of endotracheal tube is approximately 1 to 2 cm proximal to carina. In this position, both lungs are equally ventilated and the risk of tube coming out with changes in position or patient movement is remote. Too proximal placement can cause damage to subglottic region or can predispose to partial or complete inadvertent extubation. When the tip of ETT is close to carina, it can lead to sympathetic stimulation whenever the tip touches the carina leading to tachycardia, hypertension and arrythmia. In addition, ETT can easily migrate to one of the mainstem bronchi (more frequently to right). Endobronchial intubation renders ventilation difficult, can cause rapid hypoxia and stimulate bronchospasm. Patient does not die per se because of esophageal intubation, but can certainly die or suffer hypoxic brain damage due to failure to recognize the esophageal placement.

Confirmation of endotracheal intubation

1. Bilateral and equal chest expansion.
2. Five-point auscultation.
3. Humidified gas across the ETT during ventilation.
4. Continuous square wave capnogram—at least six continuous waves.
5. Ultrasound.
6. X-ray chest.
7. Flexible video endoscopy.

5.2.5 Managing the Patient During Intubation

It is important to ensure the physical and physiological safety of the patient during intubation. Every patient should have a free-flowing intravenous access. Minimum mandatory monitors should always be used in every patient. Patient with suspected C spine injury require additional maneuvers such as manual inline stabilization during laryngoscopy. Agitated patient may need physical restraint. Emergency drugs should be used according to the patient's condition to prevent or treat the appropriate clinical conditions.

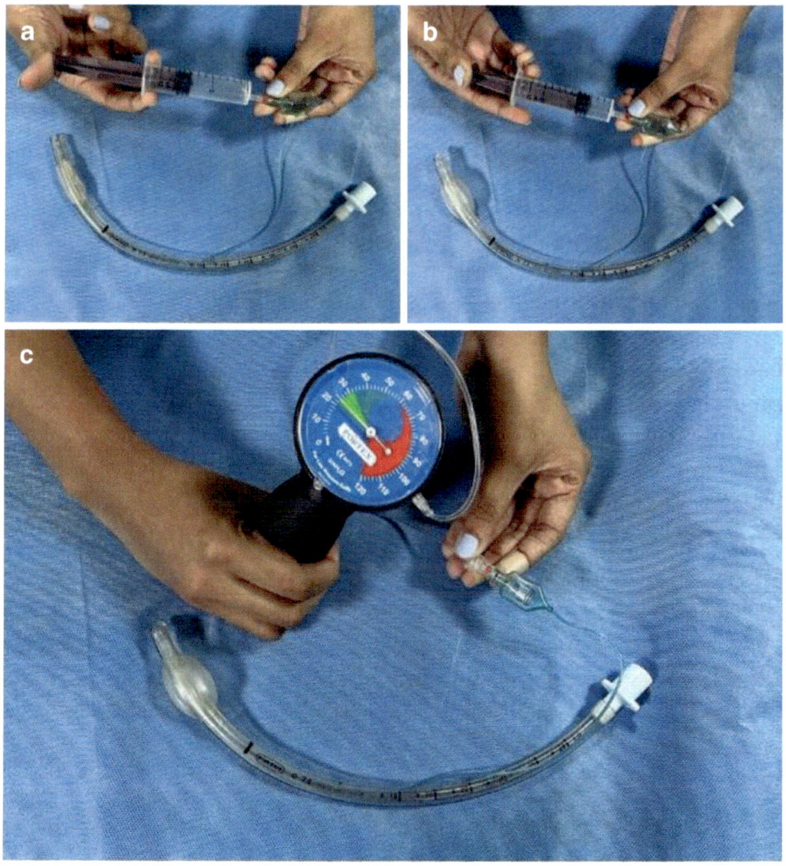

Fig. 5.14 (**a**) and (**b**) Showing the inflation of the cuff of the ET tube. (**c**) Measuring the cuff pressure with the help of a pressure gauge

5.3 Summary of Differences Between the Intubation in Different Locations

	Emergency	ICU	Ward/others
Patient	Incomplete history and assessment Potentially unstable Agitation and restlessness: could be due to hypoxia, hypovolemia, trauma, alcohol intoxication, drugs, pain Full stomach Violent behavior (patient or bystanders) Consent	Critically ill Potentially unstable May be on multiple drugs Positioning difficulty Hypoxemia	Cardiac or respiratory arrest Unconscious patient
Equipment	Usually well equipped	Usually well equipped	Crash trolley may have limited type of devices
Drugs	Available	Available	+/−
Expertise	Usually available	Usually available	May not be available
C-spine protection	Always provide till injury is ruled out	Depending on the patient	Usually not encountered
Help	Available	Available	Not available

5.4 Complications of Endotracheal Intubation

Complications can arise due to factors related to patient, equipment, skills, and drugs. They include soft tissue injury, damage to teeth, arytenoid laceration, bleeding, aspiration, esophageal intubation, failed intubation, bronchospasm, hypoxia, hypertension, tachycardia, and arrythmia. Most important for the physician is to recognize the esophageal intubation and rectify it and to manage a failed intubation. Sore throat, persistent cough, voice changes etc. are some of the post extubation complications and risk of tracheal stenosis in patients who had prolonged intubation should be kept in mind.

Adherence to proper technique and cautious use of medications appropriately would greatly reduce the complications. When they occur, early recognition and management are key to reducing the adverse outcomes. Detailed discussion of the complications is out of scope of this chapter.

Suggested Reading

1. Collins SR. Direct and indirect laryngoscopy: equipment and techniques. Respir Care. 2014;59(6):850–62; discussion 862–4.
2. Levitan RM, Mechem CC, Ochroch EA, Shofer FS, Hollander JE. Head -elevated laryngoscopy position: improving laryngeal exposure during laryngoscopy by increasing head elevation. Ann Emerg Med. 2003;41:322–40.
3. Endotracheal intubation following trauma. J Trauma. 2012;73(5):S333–40.
4. Patterson H. Emergency department intubation of trauma patients with undiagnosed cervical spine injury. Emerg Med J. 2004;21:302–5.
5. The Airway Manual. Practical approach to airway management. Berlin: Springer; 2023.
6. Teaching and training in fibreoptic bronchoscope guided endotracheal intubation. Indian J Anaesth. 2011;55(5):451–5.
7. Cook TM, Kelly FE, Boniface N, Seller C. Universal videolaryngoscopy: the importance of choosing the right device. Reply to: cognitive re-engineering after a 15-year experience with routine videolaryngoscopy. Br J Anaesth. 2019;122:e59–60.
8. Levitan RM, Heitz JW, Sweeney M, Cooper RM. The complexities of tracheal intubation with direct laryngoscopy and alternative intubation devices. Ann Emerg Med. 2011;57:240–7.
9. Henderson JJ, Suzuki A. Rigid indirect laryngoscope insertion techniques. Anaesthesia. 2008;63:323–4.

6 Percutaneous Tracheostomy

Nishant Sahay and Nishkarsh Gupta

6.1 Definition

Tracheotomy is an opening in the trachea.

A tracheostomy is a surgical opening into the trachea below the larynx, through which an indwelling tube is placed to overcome upper airway obstruction, facilitate mechanical ventilator support and/or removal of tracheo-bronchial secretions.

Tracheotomy resulting in a communication between the trachea and the outer air space by means of a stoma (tracheostomy) allows the person to breathe as described above.

6.2 History

Earliest tracheostomies were performed in Egypt in 3000 BC. Alexander the Great is fabled to have saved a soldier's life from suffocation by opening up his trachea using the tip of his sword.

Hippocrates, however, criticized the practice for fear of carotid lacerations.

For more than 200 hundred years, it was considered an unsafe procedure. No attempt was made to tracheostomise President George Washington even as he died of supraglottitis.

In the early twentieth century, Chevalier Jackson (scientist who invented a laryngoscope with light incorporated in it) standardized this surgical procedure showing that lower mortality rates could be achieved with a proper technique and meticulous post procedure care.

6.3 Types

Surgical Tracheostomy (ST): After an incision on the neck, dissection down to trachea is done and under vision an opening is created in the trachea which facilitates insertion of a tracheostomy tube.

Percutaneous Tracheostomy (PT): Often a bedside procedure involving a dilatation of the tracheal wall resulting in the placement of a tracheostomy tube without direct surgical visualization of the trachea.

N. Sahay
Department of Anesthesiology, AIIMS, Patna, India

N. Gupta (✉)
Department Onco-Anesthesiology and Palliative Medicine at DRBRAIRCH, All India Institute of Medical Sciences, New Delhi, Delhi, India

N. Gupta et al. (eds.), *Techniques in Anesthesia, Intensive Care and Emergency Medicine*,
https://doi.org/10.1007/978-981-96-1202-4_6

6.4 Indications

- In patients with prolonged translaryngeal intubation to prevent its complications
- To relieve upper airway obstruction
- To protect the airway in patients who are unable to do so independently
- In patients unable to maintain effective ventilation, e.g., due to motor neurone disease, Guillain Barre disease.
- Tracheo bronchial toileting and secretion management
- To facilitate certain surgical procedures
- To allow long-term ventilation or oxygenation support.

6.5 Contraindications

Absolute
- Informed consent not available
- Infection at the site of tracheostomy
- Neonates

Relative
- Coagulopathy
- Altered neck anatomy like thyroid mass/swelling
- Unstable cervical spine
- Morbid obesity
- Patients on ventilator support with high PEEP

Note: In patients with relative contraindications, only an experienced and skilled person should attempt percutaneous tracheostomy.

	Percutaneous tracheostomy	Surgical tracheostomy
1	Higher chances of minor bleeding during procedure	Incidence of minor bleeding less
2	Incidence of complications leading to major bleeding and hypotension is lesser	Incidence of major bleeding complications and hypotension more
3	Higher peri-procedural complications, e.g., false passage	Chances of peri-procedural complications lesser
4	Tracheostomy tube placement often more difficult	Tracheostomy tube placement is easier
5	Shorter procedure time	Procedure takes longer
6	Post procedure infections lesser	Higher post-operative infections rates/ stomatitis
7	Cosmetic sequelae better	Cosmetic sequelae worse
8	Lesser scarring of tissue noted	Scarring at incision site more
9	Less resource intensive in terms of cost per procedure, time and personnel involved	Higher cost per procedure, time and personnel involved
10	No Difference in mortality and serious, life-threatening adverse events directly related to the procedure	

6.6 Timing of Tracheostomy

Early vs. Late
- No consensus regarding a universal definition of early or late tracheostomy. Some consider early tracheostomy as within 7 days of intubation (range varies from 10 days to 21 days in literature). Late tracheostomy if done after 14 days of intubation (range 10 days to 21 days).
- No long-term or short-term advantage on survival or length of hospital stay.
- Early tracheostomy results in better nursing care, prevents laryngeal injury, reduction in use of sedative agents, more patient comfort and better communication with patients.
- Some authors reported a slight advantage of early versus compared to late tracheostomy as under
  - A higher likelihood of weaning from the ventilator (77 vs. 68%)
  - A higher likelihood of being discharged from the ICU within 28 days (48 vs. 39%)
  - A trend towards a lower rate of pneumonia

Tracheostomy is an aerosol generating procedure. In presence of contagious viral infection such as the COVID-19 pandemic, a delayed tracheostomy may be a justifiable consideration. In addition, when possible, tracheostomy should be performed in an airborne isolation environment.

6.7 Planning

- Technique as per available devices and expertise.
- STOP MAID:
  - S: Suction
  - T: Tools for intubation (laryngoscope blades, handle)
  - O: Oxygen
  - P: Positioning
  - M: Monitors (ECG, pulse oximetry, blood pressure, $ETCO_2$)
  - A: Assistant; Ambu-bag with face mask; airway devices (different sized endotracheal tubes 10 mL syringe, stylets); assessment of airway difficulty
  - I: Intravenous access
  - D: Drugs for pretreatment, induction, neuromuscular blockade (and any adjuncts)

6.8 Preparation

1. Place the patient in the tracheostomy position. Place a pillow under the shoulders which enables maximal extension of head and neck.
2. Elevate the head end of the patient's bed 20–40° as per operator preference.
3. Identification of site of puncture, between the cricoid and the first tracheal cartilage or between the first and second tracheal cartilages whenever feasible. USG helps in identification of site as well as aberrancies in the area.
4. Use ventilator changes and sedation to control patient's respiration. A PEEP level of 5 to 10 cmH_2O is recommended.
5. Endo tracheal tube fixation tapes to be loosened and cuff to be deflated.
6. Ventilator settings to be adjusted in view of the leak. May need to adjust inspiratory times, I:E ratio etc. to minimize air leaks.
7. Preoxygenation with 100% oxygen to be initiated.
8. Vigilant monitoring particularly in sick patients.
9. Prepare and drape the anterior neck area.

6.9 Procedure

PCT may be FIBREOPTIC BRONCHOSCOPE (FOB) guided or under ULTRASOUND guidance.

- FOB is the most commonly used method.
- Patient may be intubated or a supraglottic device may be used to manage airway during procedure.
- Endotracheal tube (along with the FOB) is pulled to below the vocal cord just before procedure. Red glow on the skin from the bronchoscope light may be used as a guide.
- Needle puncture is then visualized in real time to confirm entry of needle and then the guidewire entry is seen into the trachea.
- Posterior wall injuries may be prevented and if it occurs, may be seen real time.

Percutaneous tracheostomies use the Seldinger technique to gain access to the trachea. There are various methods of dilating the trachea to facilitate tube placement.

Based upon the dilatation techniques, percutaneous tracheostomies may be grouped as follows:

1	Serial Dilatation Technique 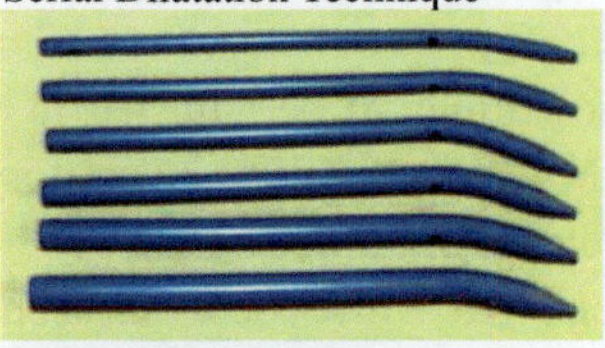	Ciaglia (pronounced chal-ya) Serial Dilator Technique 1985	Trachea entered using a needle, guidewire threaded. Tracheal stoma created by serial dilatations using progressively wider dilators
2	Single Dilatation Technique 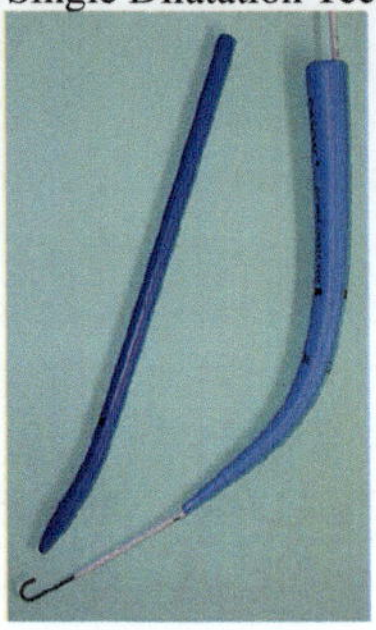	Ciaglia Single Dilator Technique (Blue Rhino) 1999	Trachea is entered using a needle, guidewire threaded. A single step, curved hydrophilic-coated Blue Rhino™ dilator is used for stoma creation
3		ULTRAperc Single Stage Dilator Technique Kit	Trachea entered using a needle, guidewire threaded. Portex Ultraperc™ (Smith Medical, Hythe, Kent, UK) comes with a single step, curved hydrophilic white dilator but in addition provides a tapered introducer for the tracheostomy tube
4	Rotational Dilatation Technique 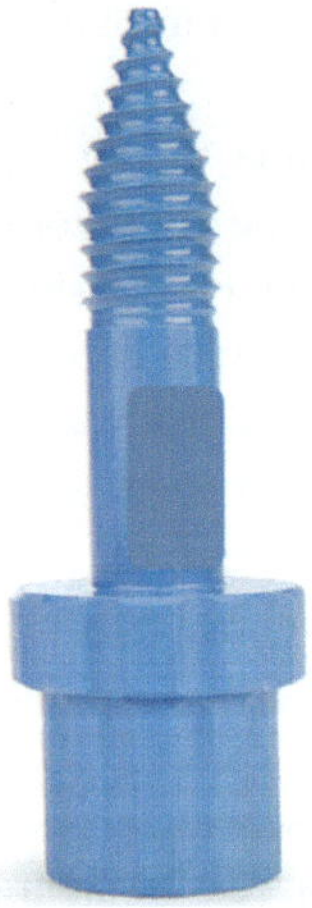	Frova's Technique (Percu Twist kit) 2002	Trachea entered using a needle, guidewire threaded. A screwlike dilating device that lifts the anterior tracheal wall during dilation thus keeping the tracheal lumen open and enabling an unrestricted bronchoscopic view of the dilation site at any given time
5	Balloon Dilatation Technique 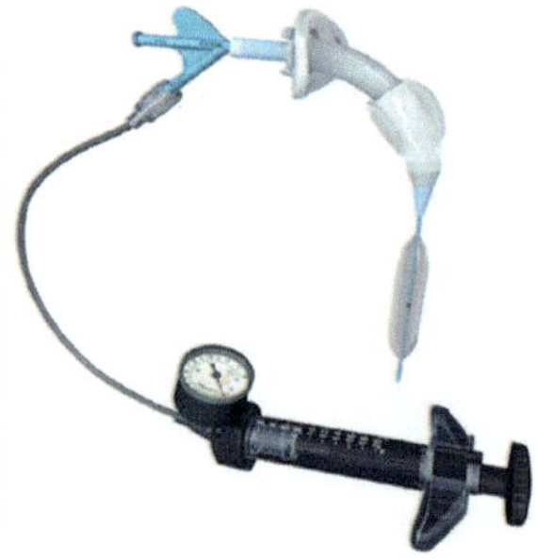	Ciaglia dilatational tracheostomy (Ciaglia Blue Dolphin, Cook) 2005	Trachea entered using a needle, guidewire threaded. Technique uses a combined dilator-tube introducer assembly, which uses a high-pressure balloon to dilate the stoma. The balloon-tipped catheter with tube-loading dilator assembly is a unique feature of this technique

6	Guidewire Dilator Forceps Technique 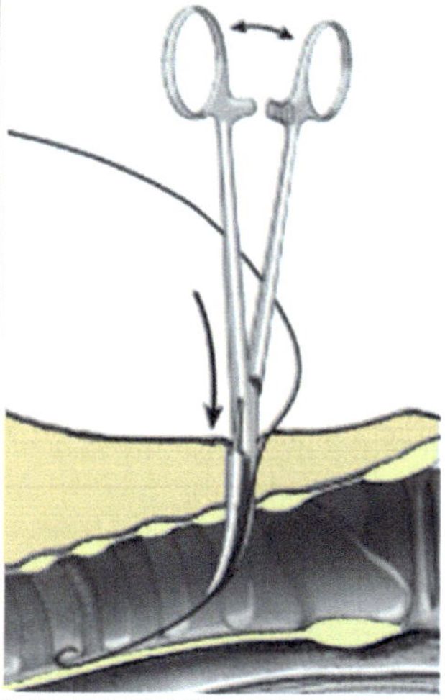	Grigg's Percutaneous Technique 1990	Trachea entered using a needle, guidewire threaded. Dilatation of the tracheal aperture is achieved by passing a special forceps (Howard Kelly forceps) over the guidewire, into the trachea. Opening these forceps, which resemble a nasal speculum, forcibly dilates the tracheal aperture and any intervening tissue
7	Fantoni's translaryngeal tracheostomy 1997	This is a complicated technique and involves passage of guidewire retrogradally through the vocal cords after needle puncture of trachea. This is followed by railroading the combined dilator and tracheostomy tube over the guidewire into the larynx and out through the anterior tracheal wall. Tracheostomy tube is then separated from the dilator and rotated by 180° such that it faces the carina	

6.9.1 UltraSound-Guided Percutaneous Tracheostomy

Some operators use USG just for pre procedure identification of site and scanning for site aberrancies. Others, in addition, use it for real time guidance during the procedure. This however, requires an additional trained operator.

Ultrasound may be useful, as it:

- Helps in identification of site of puncture

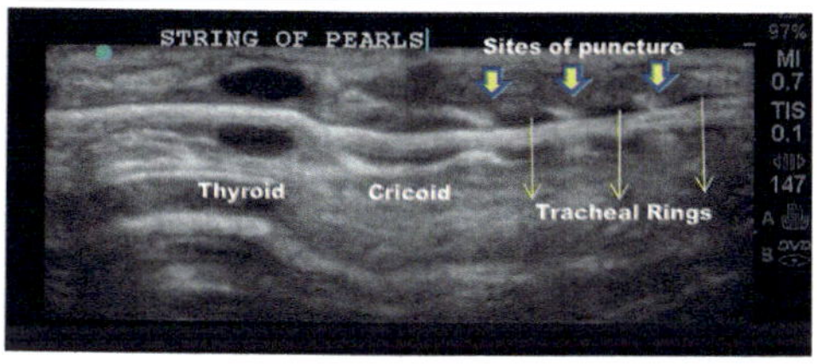

- Helps prevent complications due to aberrant blood vessels or the thyroid near the site
- Helps in delineating the airway
- Evaluates the thickness of skin over the neck, predicts depth of trachea from the skin
- Real time sonographic visualization of needle and guide wire passage

Use of USG has shown to reduce both the early complications like bleeding, pneumothorax, puemomediastinum, failure of procedure, and damage to the posterior wall.

Even some late complications like tracheal stenosis, tracheomalacia, and trachea-esophageal fistulae were reported to be lesser compared to conventional blind PCT.

6.9.2 Fiberscope Guided Percutaneous Tracheostomy

Good option when trachea is already intubated. Allows real time visualization of needle entry into the trachea. Endotracheal tube with fiberscope inside is withdrawn before needle puncture. Red glow on patient skin from the fiberscope light is used to guide distance of endotracheal tube to be withdrawn.

Needle entry at the delineated site is then seen on the fiberscope screen.

6.10 Complications

Early: those that take place within 1 week of placement (stoma takes a week to mature).

- Bleeding
- Infection of stoma
- Posterior membrane injury
- Subcutaneous emhysema
- Tracheostomy tube obstruction
- Early extubation

Late:

- Predisposing factors:
  - Prolonged placement in critically ill patients with multiple comorbidities.
  - Incidence may be approximately 65%.

- *Supra stomal complications*: Subglottic stenosis, tracheal stenosis, granulation tissue formation
- *Stomal complications*: Antero lateral stenosis, granulation tissue formation, anterior tracheal fracture, anterior tracheal wall depression, tracheomalacia
- *Infra stomal complications:* Localized in the cuff area or at distal end of tracheostomy tube: tracheoesophageal fistula, tracheo innominate fistula, tracheomalacia.

6.11 Special Consideration

Precautions to be taken in patients with highly infectious viruses such as novel Corona virus −19, which spread by the aerosol route.

Preparation
- Arrange full personal protective equipment.
- Ideally in a negative pressure operation theater. Consider turning off laminar flow.
- Use only cuffed non- fenestrated tracheostomy tubes and HME with viral filters.
- Elective is better, avoid delaying it till it becomes an emergency.
- Team briefing and explanation of all steps and clearly defined roles and responsibilities.

Planning
Some authors recommend to arrange three teams: all roles are well defined and rehearsed
- Performing the bronchoscopy
- Placement of the tracheostomy and
- Operation of the ventilator.

Performance
- Preoxygenate with PEEP
- Stop ventilation and stop all gas flows after painting and draping
- Confirm paralysis before entering the trachea
- Allow complete expiration with an open APL valve
- Double apnea technique when puncturing and dilating the trachea (patient paralyzed and operator holding breath, as much possible)
- Ensure adequate dilatation to allow easy insertion of tube
- Insert cuffed non fenestrated tube and immediately inflate the cuff
- Replace introducer with non fenestrated inner tube and HME
- Ventilation team promptly reattaches the circuit and initiates ventilation
- Confirm with $ETCO_2$ Only. Avoid contamination of stethoscope
- Fixation of tube
- Doffing of PPE

Post-Tracheostomy Care
- All personnel to wear appropriate PPEs
- Extreme care important during transfers and position changes
- Use HME with bacterial viral filters at all times
- Use in line closed suction system only
- Appropriate precautions and care whenever cuff is to be deflated

- No tube change for first week. Change always with a non fenestrated tracheostomy tube. Sequence: preoxygenate, stop ventilation and gas flows, reinsert tube and quickly reinflate cuff, connect to circuit with HME and viral filter
- Fenestrated tube only if negative for the virus

Suggested Reading

1. Brass P, Hellmich M, Ladra A, Ladra J, Wrzosek A. Percutaneous techniques versus surgical techniques for tracheostomy.Cochrane Database Syst Rev. 2016;(7):CD008045.
2. Rashid AO, Islam S. Percutaneous tracheostomy: a comprehensive review. J Thorac Dis. 2017;9(Suppl 10):S1128–38. https://doi.org/10.21037/jtd.2017.09.33.
3. Terragni PP, Antonelli M, Fumagalli R, Faggiano C, Berardino M, Pallavicini FB, et al. Early vs late tracheotomy for prevention of pneumonia in mechanically ventilated adult ICU patients: a randomized controlled trial. JAMA. 2010;303(15):1483.
4. Ciaglia P, Firsching R, Syniec C. Elective percutaneous dilatational tracheostomy. A new simple bedside procedure; preliminary report. Chest. 1985;87:715–9.
5. Byhahn C. Percutaneous tracheostomy: the Ciaglia techniques. In: Servillo G, Pelosi P, editors. Percutaneous tracheostomy in critically ill patients. Cham: Springer; 2016.
6. Patel PB, Ferguson C, Patel A. A comparison of two single dilator percutaneous tracheostomy sets: the blue RhinoTM and the UltrapercT. Anaesthesia. 2006;61:182–6.
7. Westphal K, Maeser D, Scheifler G, Lischke V, Byhahn C. PercuTwist: a new single-dilator technique for percutaneous tracheostomy. Anesth Analg. 2003;96(1):229.
8. Fantoni A, Ripamonti D. A non-derivative, non-surgical tracheostomy: the translaryngeal method. Intensive Care Med. 1997;23(4):386–92.
9. Sanabria A. Which percutaneous tracheostomy method is better? Respir Care. 2014;59(11):1660–70. A systematic review. [PubMed: 25185145].
10. Rajajee V, Fletcher JJ, Rochlen LR, Jacobs TL. Real-time ultrasound-guided percutaneous dilatational tracheostomy: a feasibility study. Crit Care. 2011;15:R67. https://doi.org/10.1186/cc10047.
11. Ravi PR, Vijai MN. Real time ultrasound-guided percutaneous tracheostomy: is it a better option than bronchoscopy guided percutaneous tracheostomy? MJAFI. 2015;71(158):164.
12. Wood DE, Mathisen DJ. Late complications of tracheotomy. Clin Chest Med. 1991;12:597–609.
13. Fernandez-Bussy S, Mahajan B, Folch E, Caviedes I, Guerrero J, Majid A. Tracheostomy tube placement: early and late complications. J Bronchol Interv Pulmonol. 2015;22(4):357–64.

7 Tracheostomy

Sriganesh Kamath

Key Points

- Mid tracheostomy is the most preferred site whereas high tracheostomy is done when total laryngectomy is planned.
- Reduces dead space by 30–50%.
- Loss of phonation, loss of air conditioning, inability to cough, and anosmia are the major disadvantages of a tracheostomy.
- Most common indication for tracheostomy is upper airway obstruction.
- During the surgery, it is mandatory to maintain midline dissection to reach the anterior wall of trachea quickly.
- End-tidal CO_2 detection from tracheostomy tube is advised to confirm the position of tube.
- Humidification of inspired air must be maintained to facilitate normal mucociliary mechanism.
- A fenestrated tube can facilitate speech by occluding the stoma.
- In the case of a permanent tracheostoma, patient and bystanders must be educated for tube care and emergencies.
- Pediatric tracheostomy is more challenging that adults as approach area is smaller and traches being more pliable.
- Vocal cord mobility is assured and recorded if decannulation is planned.

Tracheostomy is a standard procedure performed in critically ill patients requiring prolonged mechanical ventilation, weaning from assisted ventilation, airway suction, airway protection, or to relieve upper airway obstruction. It improves patient comfort compared with standard intubation.

7.1 History

Tracheotomy is one of the oldest known surgical procedures, dating back to ancient Egypt and India. The word tracheostomy is derived from two words meaning I cut trachea in Greek. The first written documentation of tracheotomy appears in the Rig Veda. Since then, the performance of this procedure has wavered between widespread acceptance and extensive rejection because of controversy over its safety, necessity, and technique selection. The historical development of tracheotomy can be divided into five periods.

S. Kamath (✉)
Department of ENT, KS Hegde Medical Academy, Mangalore, Karnataka, India
e-mail: shrinathkamath@nitte.edu.in

N. Gupta et al. (eds.), *Techniques in Anesthesia, Intensive Care and Emergency Medicine*,
https://doi.org/10.1007/978-981-96-1202-4_7

1. The Period of Legend (2000 BC to 1546 AD).
2. The Period of Fear (1546 to 1833), during which the operation was performed only by a brave few, often at the risk of their reputations.
3. The Period of Dramatization (1833 to 1932), during which tracheotomy was performed only in emergency situations on acutely obstructed airways.
4. The Period of Enthusiasm (1932 to 1965), during which the saying, "If you think of tracheotomy—do it!" became popular.
5. The Period of Rationalization (1965 to the present), during which the merits of tracheotomy versus intubation remain a topic of debate. The first scientific reliable description of successful tracheostomy by the surgeon who performed it was by Antonio Musa Brasavola in 1546. Chevalier Jackson is credited with the first clear open surgical (OS) description in 1909, and Ciaglia is credited with the first percutaneous dilatational tracheostomy (PDT) in 1985.

Today due to the advances in modern medicine and intensive care, tracheotomy is one of the most commonly performed surgical procedures.

Definition

A surgical opening made on the anterior wall of the trachea and converting it into a stoma on the skin surface to bypass the upper respiratory tract.

Classification

A. Depending on the timing.
   (a) Emergency
   (b) Elective
B. Depending on the cause
   (a) Temporary
   (b) Permanent
C. Depending on the site
   (a) High—above the isthmus of the thyroid gland, via first tracheal ring*
   (b) Mid—second and third tracheal rings**
   (c) Low—below the isthmus***

**: The only indication is malignancy larynx in stridor, planned for total laryngectomy.*

***: Preferred site.*

****: Laryngeal papillomatosis to prevent seeding.*

Functions of Tracheostomy

- Bypasses the upper airway obstruction.
- Reduces the dead space by 30–50%.
- Reduces the airway resistance.
- Protects against aspiration.
- Positive pressure ventilation.
- Eases the suctioning of lower airway.

Disadvantages of Tracheostomy

1. Unable to cough effectively.
2. Loss of phonatory function.
3. Loss of air-conditioning of inspired air.
4. Anosmia.
5. Inability to lift heavy weights.
6. The tracheostomy tube will act as a foreign body causing local inflammation.
7. Increased risk of infection.

Indications for Emergency Tracheostomy

Respiratory Obstruction

- Congenital-laryngeal web, subglottic stenosis, laryngomalacia, laryngeal cyst, laryngeal haemangioma, B/L cho-

anal atresia, craniofacial anomalies, cystic hygroma, B/L abductor palsy.
- Infections-Ludwig's angina, retropharyngeal abscess, parapharyngeal abscess, tongue abscess, acute epiglottitis, laryngeal diphtheria, acute laryngo-tracheobronchitis.
- Trauma—External laryngeal injury, stab injury of the neck, Fracture of maxilla and mandible.
- Neoplasms—Benign and malignant tumors of the larynx, oropharynx and hypopharynx.
- Foreign body larynx.

Indications for Elective Tracheostomy

(a) To provide mechanical ventilation.
(b) To prevent aspiration in the unprotected airway. Bulbar polio, polyneuritis, bilateral adductor paralysis, Congestive cardiac failure, pulmonary edema, chronic lung disease.
(c) To facilitate pulmonary toilet.
(d) Obstructive sleep apnoea.
(e) Ondine's curse.
(f) In anticipation of upper airway obstruction following major head and neck trauma.

Ondine's curse: A rare genetic condition, known as congenital central hypoventilation syndrome in which an individual completely stops breathing when falling asleep. Ondine's curse is named after a mythical tale in which a heartbroken water nymph curses her unfaithful husband to stop breathing should he ever fall asleep.

Relative Contraindications to Elective Tracheostomy

- Deranged coagulopathy.
- Inability to tolerate the procedure (from a medical perspective).
- Anatomic variations like the presence of aberrant vasculature, lower tracheal stenosis/obstruction, or tracheal fistula.
- Recent trauma/surgeries of the cervical spine.

7.2 Surgical Procedure

7.2.1 Anesthesia

Elective Tracheostomy—General Anesthesia/ Monitored Anesthesia/Local Anesthesia.

Emergency Tracheostomy—Local Anesthesia/ Monitored Anesthesia.

7.2.2 Position of the Patient

The patient is positioned supine with a sandbag placed transversely under the shoulders to extend the neck (unless the patient requires cervical spine precautions) (Fig. 7.1).

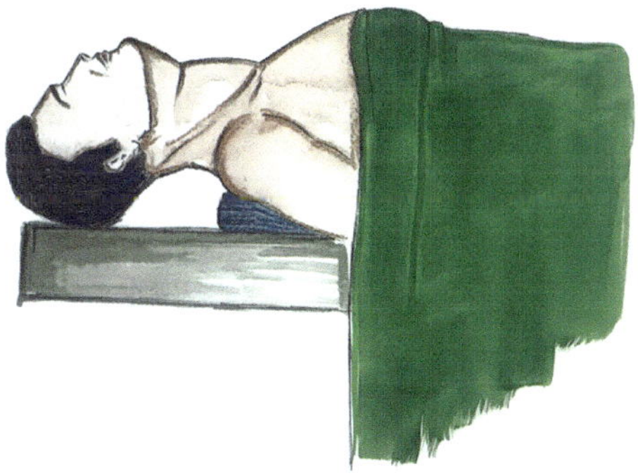

Fig. 7.1 Neck extension with the shoulder bag

While performing the tracheostomy for patients in stridor under local anesthesia, neck extension may further compromise the airway. In such cases, a compromised position, with which the patient feels comfortable can be used. The head of the bed is typically elevated 15°–20° to decrease venous engorgement. While using the cuffed tracheostomy tube, it should be tested prior to the procedure to ensure that the cuff is functional and has no air leak.

7.2.3 Infiltration

2% Lignocaine with adrenaline infiltrated into the extra tracheal tissues.

7.2.4 Incision

A 2–3 cm vertical or horizontal skin incision is made midway between the lower border of the cricoid cartilage and the suprasternal notch (Fig. 7.2).

A vertical incision in the midline can also be used to get a quick access to the airway in case of emergency tracheostomy.

7.2.5 Steps of the Procedure

Skin incision with no 15 scalpel. Division of subcutaneous tissue and fat (Fig. 7.3).

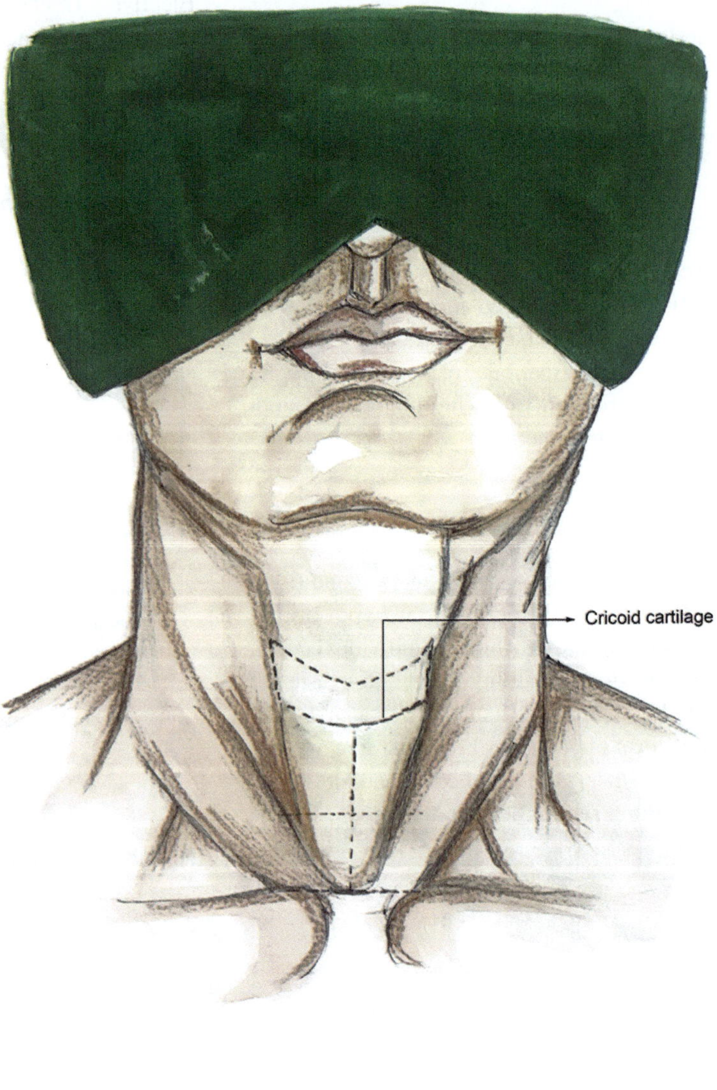

Fig. 7.2 Landmarks for infiltration and incision

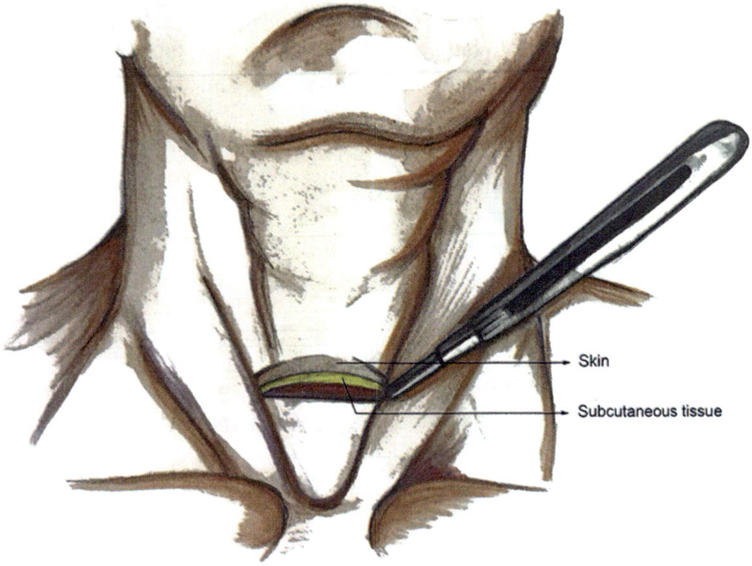

Fig. 7.3 Incision through the skin and subcutaneous tissue

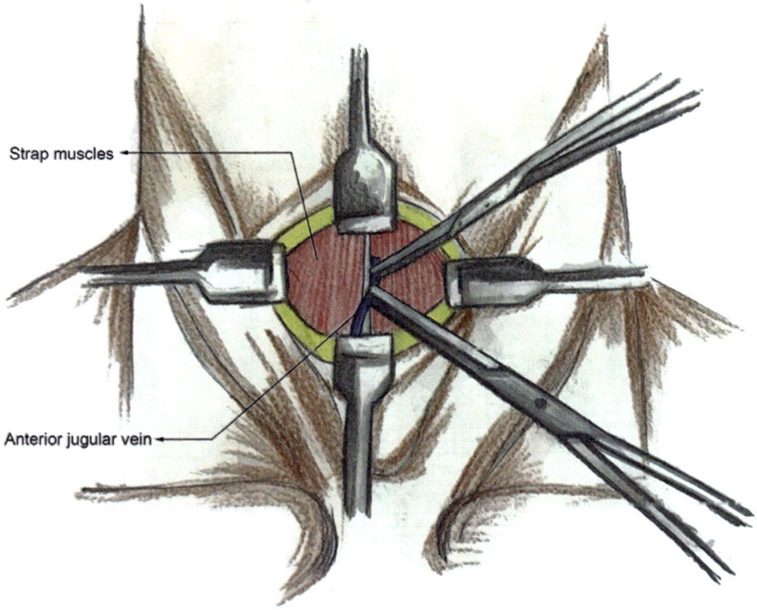

Fig. 7.4 Ligation of anterior jugular vein and exposure of the strap muscles

Retraction of the edges of the incision with retractors. (Keep changing the planes of retraction as one proceeds into the deeper planes) Ligation of the anterior jugular vein, if in the field (Fig. 7.4).

Cauterisation of the small vessels.

Throughout the procedure, we should keep palpating the trachea to ensure midline orientation is being maintained.

Division of Superficial facia with Platysma.

Division Superficial layer of deep cervical fascia.

Blunt dissection with artery forceps in the longitudinal plane on the median raphe to separate the strap muscles (stern hyoid and stern thyroid).

Retraction of thyroid isthmus with thyroid hook.

Retraction of cricoid using cricoid hook for fixation of the larynx, while performing tracheostomy under local anaesthesia.

Blunt dissection over the pretracheal fascia and fibro fatty tissue to expose the tracheal rings (2nd–5th) (Fig. 7.5).

Anaesthetist should remove the tapes used to secure the endotracheal tube and prepare to withdraw the tube slowly if the procedure is being done under GA.

2 mL of 4% lignocaine injected into the tracheal lumen to abolish cough reflex while performing tracheostomy under local anesthesia (Fig. 7.6).

The membranous part trachea is opened transversely in between second and third rings with no 11 scalpel.

Distally based inverted "U" shaped tracheal-wall flap (Bjork flap) may be created or a section of the anterior tracheal wall removed. (Other methods being cruciate incision, H incision, T incision or removal of circular/square shaped anterior wall of the trachea) (Fig. 7.7).

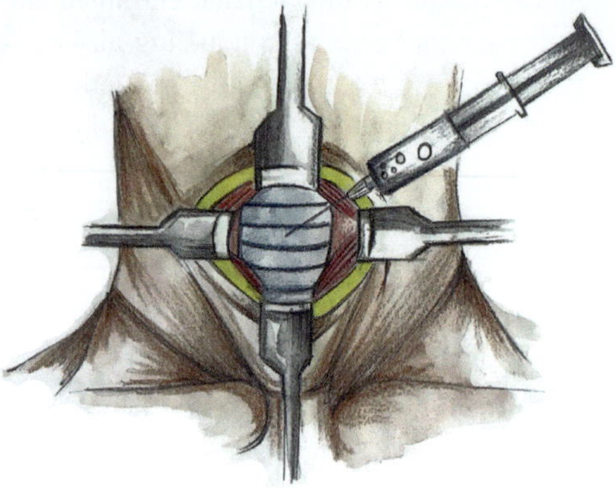

Fig. 7.6 Infiltration of 4% lignocaine into the trachea

Fig. 7.5 Retraction of strap muscles, pretracheal facia and thyroid gland

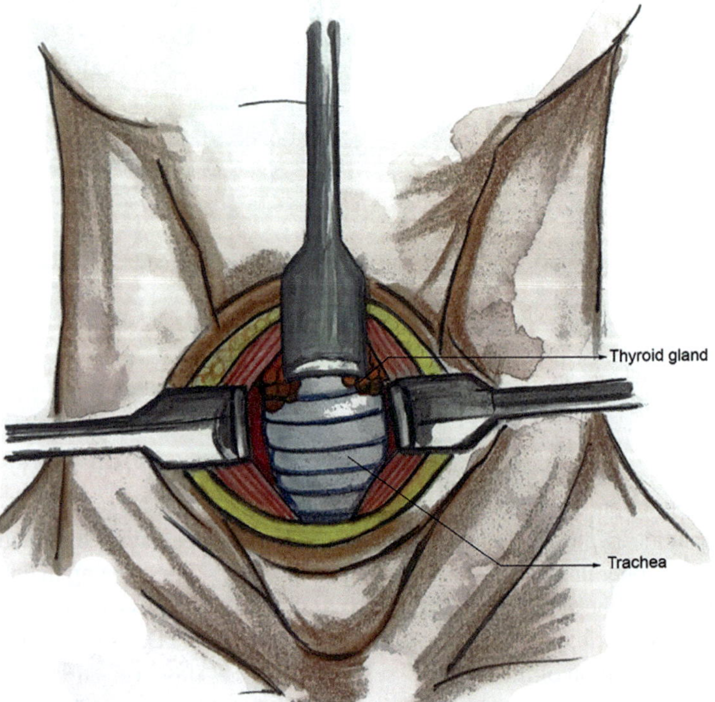

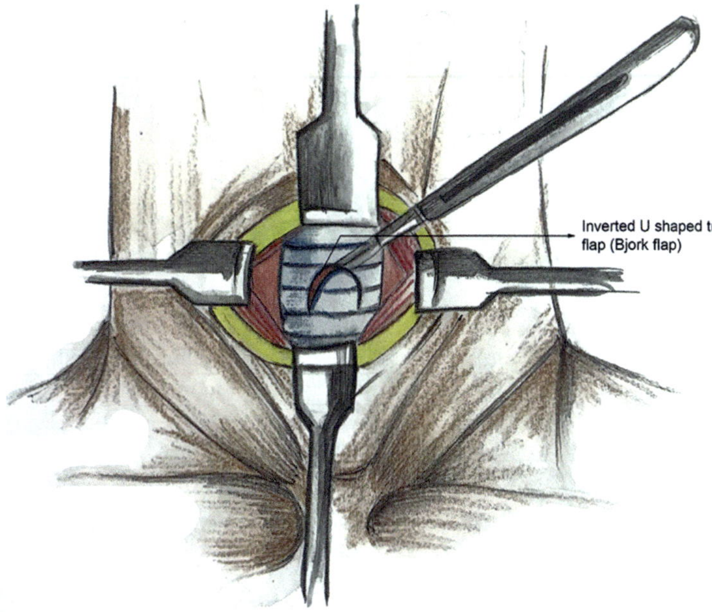

Fig. 7.7 Inverted U shaped incision on the anterior wall of trachea

After suctioning the secretions and blood clots from the trachea, the tracheostomy tube is inserted.

The endotracheal tube should be withdrawn so that its tip is just above the superior edge of the tracheostoma under direct vision if the procedure is done under GA before inserting a tracheostomy tube (Fig. 7.8).

The tracheostomy tube is then inserted, initially perpendicular to the trachea, and then rotated 90° as it is slid down into proper position.

The cuff of the tube should be inflated.

Proper placement of the tube is confirmed by direct visualization, end-tidal CO2, ease of ventilation, and adequate oxygen saturation (Figs. 7.9 and 7.10).

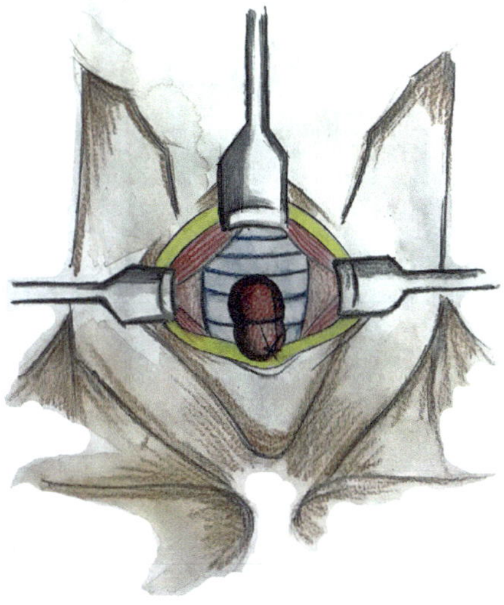

Fig. 7.8 Formation of Bjork flap

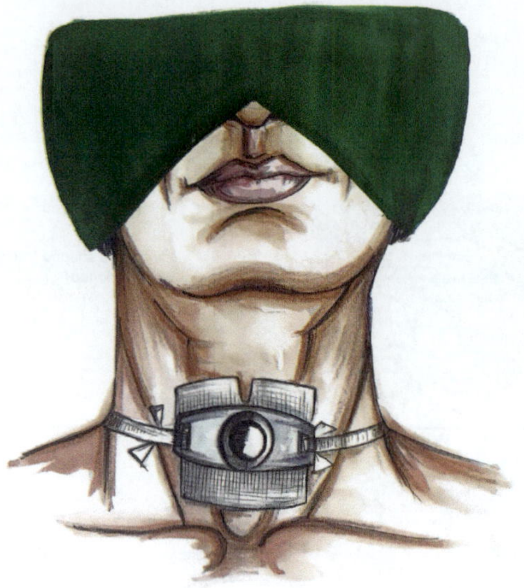

Fig. 7.9 Insertion of tracheostomy tube

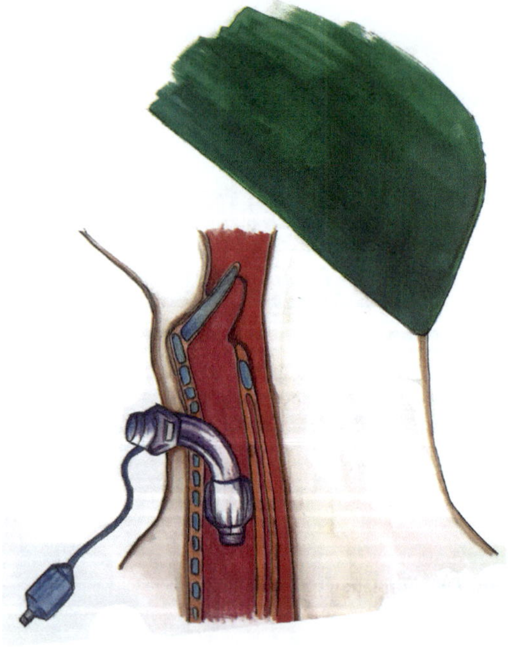

Fig. 7.10 Position of the tracheostomy tube in the lateral profile

The tracheostomy tube should be secured with sutures and tapes.

The incision should be sutured with loose ties to prevent surgical emphysema.

7.3 Postoperative Care

7.3.1 Constant Supervision

Staff in charge should be alert and aware of the situation. Blood pressure, Pulse, Respiratory rate monitoring every 15 min until the patient is awake and then every hour for the first 24 h.

7.3.2 Suctioning

As tracheostomy reduces the efficiency of coughing, the patient cannot clear secretions effectively from the tracheobronchial lumen. Therefore, regular suctioning of the tube is a must to prevent crusting and tubal occlusion. Since the tracheal suctioning is an invasive and sterile procedure, all aseptic protocols should be followed. No specific time interval can be set, and the suctioning is done when indicated.

7.3.3 Humidification

Humidification of the inspired air should be done to keep the tracheal mucosa moist, to maintain the mucociliary transport of secretions and to prevent crusting and eventual obstruction of airway. It can be achieved by keeping the wet gauze pieces on the tracheostomy tube, or by using the humidifier in the room or by delivering Oxygen or compressed air at a rate of 5–7 L/min through the reservoir containing sterile water. Sodium bicarbonate or saline should be instilled in to the trachea at a rate of 1–2 mL/h to prevent crusting.

7.3.4 Stoma Care

The tracheostomy is kept open by the tracheostomy tube, held in place by tapes. The incision site must be cleaned twice a day because tracheal secretions can easily infect it.

Bedside and Emergency Airway Equipments for Tracheostomy [8]
- Suction with catheters.
- Personal protective equipment (gloves, aprons, eye protection).
- Various sizes of Tracheostomy tubes.
- Lignocaine jelly.
- Scalpel blade or Scissors.
- Dressing.
- Tape to fix tracheostomy.
- Tracheal dilator.

Basic Airway Equipment
- Oxygen masks.
- Self-inflating bags.
- Oral and nasal airways.

Advanced Airway Equipment
- Laryngeal mask airways and laryngoscopes with appropriate tubes.
- Capnography.
- A fibreoptic scopy.

7.4 Tracheostomy Tubes

A tracheostomy tube should be selected according to the outer diameter, the inner diameter and the length of the tube, rather than the manufacturer's "size," which is not standardized. The outer diameter of the tracheostomy tube should be about 2/3 to 3/4 of the tracheal diameter. As a general rule, most adult females can accommodate a tube with an outer diameter of 10 mm, while an outer diameter of 11 mm is suitable for most adult males.

Tracheostomy tubes can be:

A. Non-metallic (Polyvinyl chloride or Silicone).
   Metallic (Jackson's and Fuller's, made of German silver /Stainless steel).
B. Uncuffed/cuffed.
C. Unfenestrated/fenestrated*.

**They include a subglottic aspiration port or speaking valve.*

- Metallic.
  - Jackson's (Fig. 7.11).
  - Fuller's (Fig. 7.12).
- Non-metallic (Fig. 7.13).

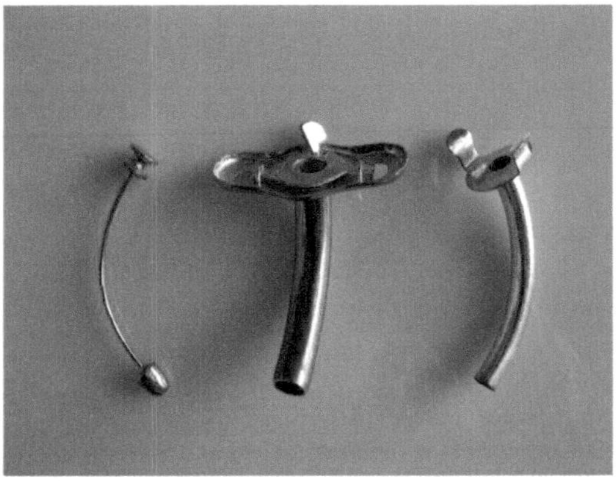

Fig. 7.11 Jackson's tracheostomy tube

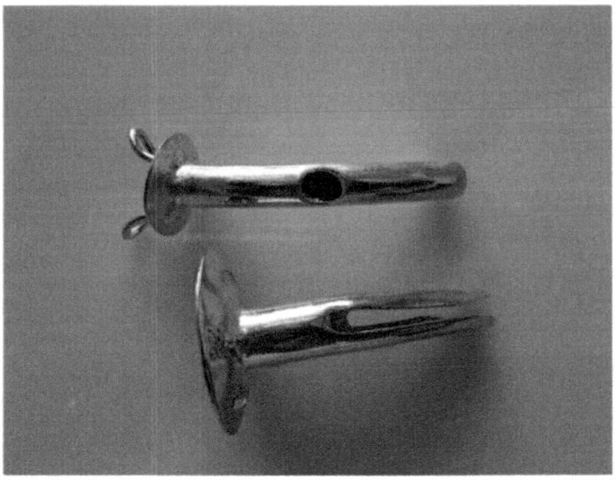

Fig. 7.12 Fuller's tracheostomy tube

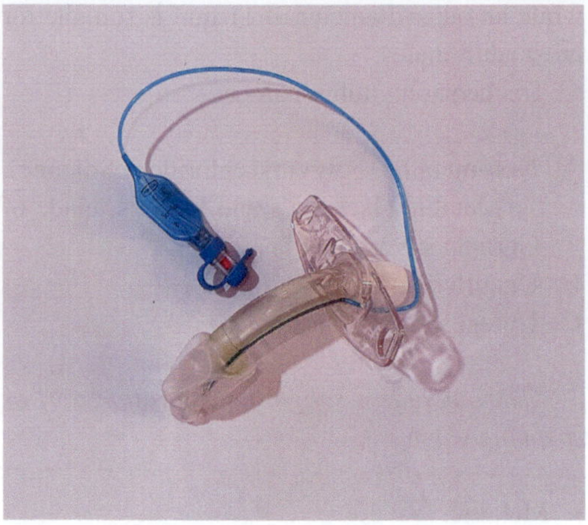

Fig. 7.13 A (non-metallic) cuffed tracheostomy tube

- Polyvinyl chloride or Silicone- cuffed/ unstuffed.
- Plastic.

Over-inflation of the cuff can cause tracheal mucosal injury and necrosis, Intra-cuff pressure should be below 20 mmHg to maintain adequate capillary perfusion.

Table listing differences between Jackson's and Fuller's tracheostomy tube

Jackson's	Fuller's
Complete outer tube	Biflanged
No opening in the shoulder	Opening present
Has obturator/pilot	No obturator
Has lock for inner tube	No lock
Phonation not possible	Phonation possible

Non—metallic (cuffed)	Metallic
Prevent aspiration	Do not prevent aspiration
Positive pressure ventilation possible	Not possible
Can be used during radiotherapy	Cannot be used
Can be used during general anesthesia	Cannot be used for GA

7.5 Outer Tube Changing

The first outer tube change usually takes place after 48–72 h, to allow for the formation of a tract. The procedure should always be carried out by two persons: one to remove the soiled tube, the other to immediately insert the clean tube, remove the introducer and tie the tapes.

7.6 Inner Tube Changing

The inner tube should be cleaned at least once daily. The soiled dressing is removed, and the wound, under the tube flanges, is cleansed using a moistened cotton wool applicator or swab. The wound is protected from tube flanges and secretions by a keyhole dressing. Gauze tapes should be tied in a reef knot at each side of the neck with the head flexed down towards the neck if possible, because the circumference of the neck is smallest at this point. After tying the tapes, check the tension and comfort level by inserting the little finger between the tapes and the neck. Clean techniques should be taught to patients for home care before discharge.

7.7 Complications

7.7.1 Procedure-Related Complications

1. **Hemorrhage**—commonly from the anterior jugular venous system, small venous tributaries and from the thyroid isthmus, which can be controlled by ligation and cauterization.
2. **Pneumothorax**—with an incidence as high as 17% in some reports. A higher incidence is seen in children due to a relatively higher position of their pleural domes.
3. **Tube/cannula misplacement**—may result in loss of airway (e. g., false passage) prolonged periods of desaturation and injury to surrounding structures (e. g., esophagus). Morbidly obese patients are at higher risk for this complication due to the increased distance from skin to trachea.
4. **Posterior tracheal perforation**—can lead to pneumomediastinum, pneumothorax, extensive subcutaneous emphysema, and respiratory distress.

5. **Thyroid injury**—Insufficient hemostasis at the time of the procedure may cause significant postoperative bleeding.
6. **Recurrent laryngeal nerve injury**—can be avoided by maintaining the midline during dissection.
7. **Subcutaneous emphysema**—may signify underlying complication such as a pneumothorax or tracheal injury.
8. **Cardiopulmonary arrest and mortality.**
9. **Airway fire caused by electrocautery**—there are several reports of airway fires caused by either laser or electrocautery during tracheostomy. This complication can be avoided by (a) Reducing inspired oxygen concentration during the procedure (b) eliminating the use of electrocautery during any work involving directly the trachea.

7.7.2 Tracheostomy Maintenance-Related Complications

1. **Tube displacement**—a life-threatening complication if occurs before the formation of the tract (i.e., within first 3 days). Though the incidence of tube displacement is low (0.35–2.6%.), it carries the highest mortality rate up to 25–100%. Risk factors for accidental decannulation include altered mental status/delirium, patient turning, a poorly secured tracheostomy tube, short neck, obese patient, large goiter obscuring normal anatomy, positive pressure ventilation with noncompliant lungs, excessive coughing, low/off midline tracheostomies, and traction on the tubing.
2. **Infectious complications**
   (a) Stoma infection—This usually occurs after the first 24 h in approximately 5% of tracheotomies. It can be prevented by aggressive and timely wound care, frequent dressing changes, regular tube changes, and humidification of inspired air.
   (b) **Necrotizing infections**—Although relatively uncommon, may lead to the dissolution of major portions of the trachea. These patients must be treated with oral intubation, 1% neomycin dressing, tracheal stenting, and eventual dedicated reconstructive procedure.
   (c) **Mediastinitis**—Rare and potentially fatal complication of an infected stoma site. Infection can track down through carotid space, paravertebral space, and retropharyngeal space into the mediastinum.
   (d) **Pneumonia.**
   (e) **Tracheitis.**
   (f) **Sternoclavicular osteomyelitis.**
   (g) **Tracheoesophageal fistula (TEF)**—May occur secondary to injury to the posterior tracheal wall during tracheostoma creation, injury to the esophagus from gastric tubing, or erosion of the tracheostomy tube cuff secondary to excessive cuff pressure.
3. Bleeding

   It can be from minimal oozing to massive bleeding from tracheostomy tube erosion into a major artery. Minimal oozing usually resolves spontaneously or with packing using adrenaline, tranexamic acid-soaked gauze packs, suture ligation, and gel foam packing.

   Massive hemorrhage due to the tubal erosion into a major artery is known to occur in less than 1–2% of patients and only 25% of patients survive this dreaded complication. The classic type described is that of a tracheo-innominate fistula. The innominate artery crosses the anterolateral surface of the trachea at the level of the ninth tracheal ring and the upper sternum. If the tracheostomy tube is placed below the third tracheal ring, the inferior portion of the cannula may damage the tracheal mucosa and eventually erode into the artery. Fistulas developing between other major arteries such as the inferior thyroid artery or an anomalous carotid artery have also been described.

7.8 Complications Seen After Decannulation

1. Tracheal stenosis—Can develop at subglottis, stoma site, or at the cuff site. 3–12% demonstrate clinically significant stenosis that ultimately requires intervention. Risk factors for the development of tracheal stenosis at the stoma site are sepsis, stomal infection, advanced age, male gender, obesity, tight-fitting or oversized tube, excessive tube motion, prolonged placement, and disproportionate excision of anterior tracheal cartilage during tracheostomy creation.

   Stenosis at the cuff site is related to pressure necrosis secondary to the associated ischemic changes. The introduction of high-volume, low-pressure cuffs has decreased the incidence by about tenfold.
2. Delayed closure of tracheostomy wound after decannulation.
3. Cosmetic deformities.
4. Tracheomalacia and tracheal granuloma—Tracheomalacia is a weakening of the tracheal wall due to ischemic injury and the destruction of tracheal cartilage. This weakening causes a collapse of the trachea during expiration, resulting in air trapping and corresponding expiratory flow limitations.

   Granulomas occur with frictional trauma from the tube, secondary infections, or stasis of secretions at the entry site of the tube.
5. Voice changes.

7.9 Pediatric Tracheostomy

The commonest indications for pediatric tracheostomy are actual or anticipated long-term ventilatory support, broncho-pulmonary secretion management, or the presence of fixed upper airway obstruction as in case of b/l choanal atresia subglottic stenosis, bilateral vocal cord paralysis, tumors, neck trauma, congenital airway malformations, and Ondine's curse.

Tracheostomy in children is more challenging than in adults because of the smaller, more pliable trachea and limited scope for extending the neck during the procedure to avoid injury to head and neck vessels and the pleura.

Differences between pediatric and adult tracheostomies:

	Paediatric	Adult
Neck extension	Minimal	Adequate
Tracheal incision	Vertical	Inverted U, cruciate, removal of circular anterior segment
"Maturation sutures"[a] For early track formation	Commonly used	Inverted U shaped flap

[a]Suturing the edge of the skin incision to the edge of the tracheal incision

Due to the small tracheal diameter, pediatric tracheostomy tubes are generally uncuffed and do not have an inner tube, to avoid reducing the internal diameter. Neonatal tracheostomy tubes are shorter in length than the pediatric tubes. Cuffed tubes are occasionally required if high ventilation pressures are needed or if there is a high risk of aspiration.

7.10 Percutaneous Tracheostomy

Percutaneous tracheostomy has become an essential procedure in the ICU setting, especially in patients who require elective tracheostomy for prolonged ventilatory support. Percutaneous tracheostomy was first described by Shelden et al. in 1957. In 1967, Toy and Weinstein described the Seldinger approach.

Preoperative Criteria

1. Ability to hyperextend the neck.
2. Presence of at least 1cm distance between the inferior border of cricoid cartilage and the suprasternal notch.
3. Patient's tolerance to transient hypercarbia and hypoxemia.

Relative Contraindications

1. Emergency airway access.
2. Difficult anatomy.
3. Morbid obesity with a short neck.
4. Limited neck movement.
5. Cervical spine injury.
6. Suspected or otherwise aberrant blood vessels.
7. Thyroid or tracheal pathology.
8. Coagulopathy.
9. Evidence of infection in the soft tissues of the neck at the insertion.

7.10.1 General Steps of the Procedure

- A small incision is made about 1 cm below the cricoid cartilage, and dissection is carried down bluntly with a hemostat.
- An assistant at the head-end advances the flexible bronchoscope till the tip of the endotracheal tube.
- Both are slowly withdrawn as a single unit until the level of the first or second tracheal ring.
- The introducer needle is advanced through the incision into the trachea.
- A guidewire is advanced, and the needle is removed while leaving the guidewire in place.
- A series of dilatations are performed over the guidewire.
- Once dilatation is done satisfactory, the tracheostomy tube is inserted over the guidewire or the dilator.
- The tracheostomy tube is then connected to the ventilator, and placement is confirmed.
- The tube is then secured in place with sutures.
- There is an option to perform the procedure without using the bronchoscope which requires more thorough dissection in order to palpate the trachea directly.

7.10.2 Techniques for Percutaneous Tracheostomy

1. Sequential dilators, Ciaglia (1985)—Multistep dilation with sequential dilators.
2. Antegrade Dilating forceps, Griggs (1990)—Dilation with specific forceps, antegrade.
3. Translaryngeal tracheostomy, Fantoni (1997)—Retrograde passage, specific cannula acts as dilator and tracheostomy tube.
4. Single-step dilator, Ciaglia Blue Rhino (1999)—Single-step dilation with a curved dilator and loading dilator, antegrade.
5. Dilating screw, Frova, and Quintel (2002)—Self-trapping screw, antegrade.
6. T-Dagger, Ambesh (2005)—Single-step dilation with curved T-shaped dilator, elliptical in cross-section, antegrade.
7. Balloon-facilitated dilational tracheostomy, Ciaglia Blue Dolphin (2005)—Single-step dilation with balloon and loading dilator assembly, antegrade.

7.11 Tracheostomy Decannulation

7.11.1 Assessment Before Decannulation

The eventual outcome and removal of the tracheostomy depend upon the original lesion. The tracheostomized patient should be regularly assessed and should follow the clinical criteria given below before they are considered for decannulation.

1. The patient should be comfortable with no signs of aspiration during eating or drinking.
2. The original condition for which the tracheostomy has been done should have been resolved or improved.

3. The comorbid factors of the patient like cardiac, pulmonary or neurologic status should have been improved or resolved.
4. The entire airway (nose, mouth, pharynx, larynx and tracheobronchial tree) should be evaluated for patency and to determine whether each part is functioning well enough to support the respiratory needs of the patient.

7.11.2 Investigations

1. Nasopharyngolaryngoscopy—Vocal cord motility is observed.
2. Rigid laryngoscope—used to confirm the findings of fiberoptic endoscopy, as well as to check sites not well assessed by fibreoptic endoscopy (e.g., valleculae, pyriform sinuses, the post-cricoid portion of the hypopharynx, laryngeal ventricles, anterior commissure, the intra-arytenoid region, and the subglottis).

7.11.3 Decannulation Procedure

The process of decannulation can be performed in two ways.

(a) The tube is removed, and the track is allowed to close down and heal.
(b) Excise the track and allow it to heal by the first intention—by suturing in layers.

In both methods, the safety of decannulation must be ensured by a prior decannulation trial. The basic principle of the trial is to carry out progressive blockage of the tube lumen. The patient should be watched carefully for any signs of respiratory distress as he carries out normal physical activities. Fuller's tube is the ideal one for the decannulation trial. If the blockade of the tube is well tolerated during the day, then it should be continued at night. Subsequently, the tube is removed, and the stoma is covered by a sterile dressing. The patient is then kept under observation for a week before discharge.

7.11.4 Surgical Decannulation

In this procedure, the tracheostomy tract is excised, and the stoma is examined under direct vision. There are several advantages to this approach:

1. It allows direct access to the tracheal stoma and permits removal of any possible obstruction under direct vision.
2. The suturing of the tracheal stoma reconstitutes the cylindrical wall of the trachea and thus increases the strength of the tracheal wall around this weakened point.
3. The removal of the fibrous track hastens healing with better cosmetic results.

7.12 Conclusion

Since the tracheostomy is a life-saving procedure, comprehensive knowledge about it is essential for all surgeons and those involved in ICU care. The complications associated with a tracheostomy may appear formidable, but this should not prevent the surgeon from performing a tracheostomy in a patient who stands to benefit from one.

Acknowledgements Dr. Sreesan PS, Junior Resident, Dept. of ENT, K S Hegde Medical Academy, Mangalore.

Dr. Gautham MK, Associate Professor, Dept. of ENT, K S Hegde Medical Academy, Mangalore.

Dr. Ahsain Kalam, Junior Resident, Dept. of ENT, K S Hegde Medical Academy, Mangalore.

Suggested Reading

1. Frost EAM. Tracing the tracheostomy. Ann Otol Rhinol Laryngol. 1976;85(5 Pt 1):618–24.
2. Stock CR. What is past is prologue: a short history of the development of tracheostomy. Ear Nose Throat J. 1987;66:166–9.
3. McClelland RMA. Tracheostomy: its management and alternatives. Proc R Soc Med. 1972;65:401–4.
4. Jackson C, et al. Laryngoscope. 1909;19:285–90.
5. Ciaglia P, Firsching R, Syniec C. Elective percutaneous dilatational tracheostomy. A new simple bedside procedure; preliminary report. Chest. 1985;87:715–9.

6. Cipriano A, Mao ML, Hon HH, Vazquez D, Stawicki SP, Sharpe RP, Evans DC. An overview of complications associated with open and percutaneous tracheostomy procedures. Int J Crit Illn Inj Sci. 2015 Jul-Sep;5(3):179–88.
7. Engels PT, Bagshaw SM, Meier M, Peter G. Brindley tracheostomy: from insertion to decannulation. Can J Surg. 2009;52(5):427.
8. McGrath BA, Bates L, Atkinson D, Moore JA. Multidisciplinary guidelines for the management of tracheostomy and laryngectomy airway emergencies. Anaesthesia. 2012;67:1025–41.
9. ICS TICS. Standards for the care of adult patients with temporary tracheostomy standards and guidelines; 2008.
10. Hess DR. Tracheostomy tubes and related appliances. Respir Care. 2005;50:497–510.
11. Greenberg JS, Sulek M, de Jong A, Friedman EM. The role of postoperative chest radiography in pediatric tracheotomy. Int J Pediatr Otorhinolaryngol. 2001;60:41–7.
12. Ahuja H, Mathai AS, Chander R, Mathew AE. Case of difficult tracheostomy tube insertion: a novel yet simple solution to the dilemma. Anesth Essays Res. 2013;7:402–4.
13. Tobler WD Jr, Mella JR, Ng J, Selvam A, Burke PA, Agarwal S. Chest X-ray after tracheostomy is not necessary unless clinically indicated. World J Surg. 2012;36:266–9.
14. Chee WK, Benumof JL. Airway fire during tracheostomy: extubation may be contraindicated. Anesthesiology. 1998;89:1576–8.
15. Wheatley TJ, Maddern GJ. Airway fire during the formation of tracheostomy. ANZ J Surg. 2002;72:157–8.
16. Dulguerov P, Gysin C, Perneger TV, Chevrolet JC. Percutaneous or surgical tracheostomy: a meta-analysis. Crit Care Med. 1999;27:1617–25.
17. Kapadia FN, Tekawade PC, Nath SS, Pachpute SS, Saverkar SS, Bhise RA, et al. A prolonged observational study of tracheal tube displacements: benchmarking an incidence <0.5–1% in a medical-surgical adult intensive care unit. Indian J Crit Care Med. 2014;18:273–7.
18. Castling B, Telfer M, Avery BS. Complications of tracheostomy in major head and neck cancer surgery; a retrospective study of 60 consecutive cases. Br J Oral Maxillofac Surg. 1994;32:3–5.
19. Massick DD, Yao S, Powell DM, Griesen D, Hobgood T, Allen JN, et al. Bedside tracheostomy in the intensive care unit: a prospective randomized trial comparing open surgical tracheostomy with endoscopically guided percutaneous dilational tracheotomy. Laryngoscope. 2001;111:494–500.
20. Goldenberg D, Ari EG, Golz A, Danino J, Netzer A, Joachims HZ. Tracheotomy complications: a retrospective study of 1130 cases. Otolaryngol Head Neck Surg. 2000;123:495–500.
21. Bernard AC, Kenady DE. Conventional surgical tracheostomy as the preferred method of airway management. J Oral Maxillofac Surg. 1999;57:310–5.
22. O'Connor HH, White AC. Tracheostomy decannulation. Respir Care. 2010;55:1076–81.
23. Hashmi A, Zerfas D, Baciewicz FA Jr. Sternoclavicular osteomyelitis: a new complication of misplaced tracheostomy tube. Ann Thorac Surg. 2011;92:2240–1.
24. Pelaez-Fernandez J, Asensio Martin MJ, Jimenez LM. Percutaneous versus standard tracheostomy. Surgery. 1997;121:112–3.
25. Wang RC, Perlman PW, Parnes SM. Near-fatal complications of tracheotomy infections and their prevention. Head Neck. 1989;11:528–33.
26. Snow N, Richardson JD, Flint LM. Management of necrotizing tracheostomy infections. J Thorac Cardiovasc Surg. 1981;82:341–4.
27. Ciaglia P, Graniero KD. Percutaneous dilatational tracheostomy. Results and long-term follow-up. Chest. 1992;101:464–7.
28. Epstein SK. Late complications of tracheostomy. Respir Care. 2005;50:542–9.
29. Heffner JE, Miller KS, Sahn SA. Tracheostomy in the intensive care unit. Part 2: complications. Chest. 1986;90:430–6.
30. Stauffer JL, Olson DE, Petty TL. Complications and consequences of endotracheal intubation and tracheotomy. A prospective study of 150 critically ill adult patients. Am J Med. 1981;70:65–76.
31. Edelson RJ, Locicero J. 3rd delayed hemorrhage from an anomalous carotid artery following tracheostomy. Am Surg. 1989;55:488–91.
32. Sue RD, Susanto I. Long-term complications of artificial airways. Clin Chest Med. 2003;24:457–71.
33. Lewis FR Jr, Schiobohm RM, Thomas AN. Prevention of complications from prolonged tracheal intubation. Am J Surg. 1978;135:452–7.
34. Weber AL, Grillo HC. Tracheal stenosis: an analysis of 151 cases. Radiol Clin North Am. 1978;16:291–308.
35. Overman AE, Liu M, Kurachek SC, et al. Tracheostomy for infants requiring prolonged mechanical ventilation: 10 years' experience. Pediatrics. 2013;131:e1491–6.
36. De Trey L, Niedermann E, Ghelfi D, Gerber A, Gysin C. Pediatric tracheotomy: a 30-year experience. J Pediatr Surg. 2013;48:1470–5.
37. Campisi P, Forte V. Pediatric tracheostomy. Semin Pediatr Surg. 2016;25:191–5.
38. Wakeham MK, Kuhn EM, Lee KJ, McCrory MC, Scanlon MC. Use of tracheostomy in the PICU among patients requiring prolonged mechanical ventilation. Intensive Care Med. 2014;40:863–70.
39. Lawrason A, Kavanagh K. Pediatric tracheotomy: are the indications changing? Int J Pediatr Otorhinolaryngol. 2013;77:922–5.
40. Shelden CH, Pudenz RH, Tichy FY. Percutaneous tracheotomy. JAMA J Am Med Assoc. 1957;165:2068–70.
41. Cheung NH, Napolitano LM. Tracheostomy: epidemiology, indications, timing, technique, and outcomes. Respir Care. 2014;59(6):895–919.
42. Cipriano A, Mao ML, David C. An overview of complications associated with open and percutaneous tracheostomy procedures. Int J Crit Ill Injury Sci. 2015;5(3):179–88.

8 Apneic Oxygenation Techniques

Indu M. Sen and Vighnesh Ashok

Key Points

- Apnoeic oxygenation refers to passive flow of oxygen into patient's alveoli in the absence of spontaneous respiration or mechanical ventilation. It prolongs safe apnea time.
- The ApOx technique demands continuous supply of oxygen for exchange of gases. Patent nasopharyngeal and/or oropharyngeal airway is a prerequisite for successful apneic oxygenation. Hemodynamics, respiratory monitoring and blood gas estimation (PaO_2, $PaCO_2$, pH) is essential. Caution is warranted for early detection of non-responders and life threatening complications.
- High Flow Nasal Oxygenation (HFNO) devices provide apneic oxygenation and additionally carbon dioxide removal.

Oxygen is a Double Edged Sword and should be used cautiously.

8.1 Introduction

Apneic oxygenation (ApOx) can be defined as passive flow of oxygen into the patient's alveoli in the absence of spontaneous respiration or mechanical ventilation. During apnea, alveolar oxygen gets absorbed into the blood but carbon dioxide gets buffered. Hence, oxygen and carbon dioxide differ in the flow rates associated with their absorption and excretion between the alveoli and bloodstream (O_2: 250 mL/min and CO_2: 8–20 mL/min). This creates a differential pressure gradient facilitating oxygen insufflation into patient's airways provided patency is maintained. Therefore, apneic oxygenation is also called mass flow ventilation. However, apnoeic oxygenation does not occur if oxygen insufflation is started after alveolar hypoxia set in; hence early intervention is the key to successful mass flow ventilation. Using this technique, sustainable oxygen levels can be maintained in critically ill patients in presence of adequate circulation and optimum gas flows.

8.2 History

1667, Hookin: Achieved oxygenation by continuous inflation of punctured canine lungs.

1946, Comroe and Dripps: Documented apnoeic oxygenation via a tracheal tube in man.

I. M. Sen (✉)
Department of Anesthesiology, PGIMER, Chandigarh, India

V. Ashok
PGIMER, Chandigarh, India

N. Gupta et al. (eds.), *Techniques in Anesthesia, Intensive Care and Emergency Medicine*,
https://doi.org/10.1007/978-981-96-1202-4_8

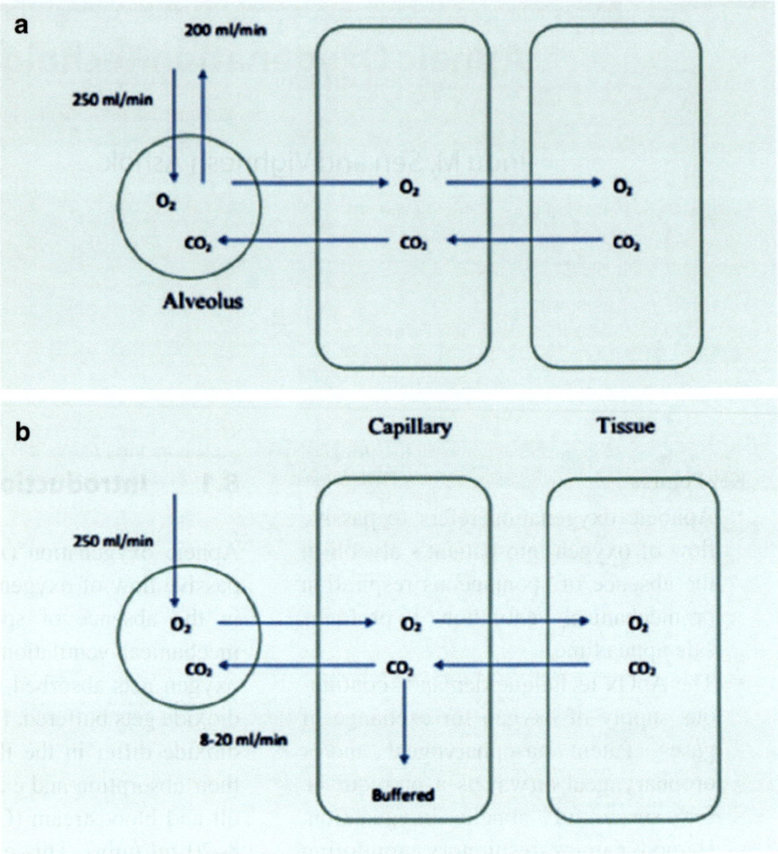

Fig. 8.1 Diagrammatic representation of gas exchange during normal breathing (**a**) and apnea (**b**)

1959, Frumin et al.: Developed apneic oxygenation technique, which delivered supplemental oxygen via nasal cannulation during surgery and anesthesia.

8.3 Physiology of Apneic Oxygenation

The uptake of oxygen from the alveoli into blood during normal breathing in a healthy adult is approximately 250 mL/min. During periods of apnea, due to differences in solubility of oxygen and carbon-di-oxide in blood, only 8–20 mL of CO_2 from blood diffuses into the alveoli per minute —the rest being buffered in blood. This creates a negative pressure gradient in the alveoli causing net airflow from the pharynx and upper airways into the lungs (Fig. 8.1). This, however, requires the presence of a patent upper airway to occur.

8.4 Techniques of Apneic Oxygenation

Apneic oxygenation can be achieved using various devices which facilitate delivery of oxygen into respiratory tract. These include

- Standard oxygenation devices (most commonly used)
  - Nasal cannulae/ prongs, nasopharyngeal catheters.
  - Buccal ApOx using RAE endotracheal tube.
  - Simple Face Masks or Venturi masks.
  - Laryngeal Oxygen Insufflation: Oxyscope, TruView, Dual Laryngoscope.
  - Transtracheal Oxygen Insufflation via jet ventilation, Tracheostomy tube.
  - Endobronchial oxygen insufflation of non-ventilated lung (during one lung ventilation).

  - Oxygen delivery through a specialized port of Fiberoptic and Rigid Bronchoscope.
- Humidified high flow nasal oxygenation systems.
  - Transnasal humidified rapid insufflation ventilator exchange (THRIVE).

1. Nasal oxygenation devices.

   Higher oxygen flow rates by nasal route extend the time of hypoxemia during apnoeic oxygenation. It has been observed that turbulent gas flows reach more distally into the airways resulting in improved gas exchange. Different techniques used are nasal cannula, nasopharyngeal catheter, supraglottic airway device, rigid bronchoscope, tracheal tube, and front-of-neck catheter.

   NODESAT (Nasal Oxygen During Efforts Securing A Tube) is a special application of apneic oxygenation delivered via the nasal route at flows of 5–15 L/min after the induction of general anaesthesia. This was first described by Weingard and Levitan in 2012. The technique helps to splint the upper airway in effect creating a pharyngeal oxygen reservoir leading to delivery of oxygen down the airways by apneic mass movement and takes part in exchange of gases at the alveolar level. Additionally, the supplemental oxygen flow can compensate for room air entrainment which would otherwise impede the provision of increased FiO_2 concentrations. This has been demonstrated to extend the duration of apnea without desaturation upto 10 min.

   A nasal cannula with cold dry oxygen flow up to 15 L/min is used to delay critical desaturation during rapid-sequence induction of anaesthesia. Two different oxygen sources are needed to practice NODESAT, one for nasal cannula and second for face mask ventilation. Most of the anesthesia work station have an auxillary oxygen port which can be used for this purpose. However, prolonged use of cold dry nasal oxygen >10 L/min of can cause mucosal trauma.

2. Transnasal humidified rapid insufflation ventilatory exchange (THRIVE).

   THRIVE uses rapidly insufflated, heated, humidified gases administered via high flow nasal cannula (HFNC) to achieve apneic oxygenation and ventilation. The non-invasive nasal route provides ventilation which can be continued in between efforts to secure an airway.

   Delivery of upto 70–90 L/min nasal oxygen creates a highly turbulent "primary supraglottic vortex" which constantly replenishes the pharynx with oxygen and prevents entrainment of room air. The vortex effectively bypasses the upper airways responsible for approximately 50% of the resistance of the entire respiratory system to airflow. Moreover, it can be used for preoxygenation, without the need for an occlusive face mask. The high flow rates used in THRIVE can help generate a continuous positive airway pressure (CPAP) of up to 7 cmH_2O. The CPAP effect prevents collapse of upper airways by a splint opening mechanism and reduces distal airway atelectasis and shunting. Additionally, in addition to maintaining oxygenation, THRIVE also allows for some CO_2 clearance through CPAP and flow-dependent airway flushing.

   A physiological study of apnoeic oxygenation using THRIVE during laryngeal surgery showed that this technique can keep patients with mild systemic disease and a BMI < 30 well oxygenated for up to 30 min. Warm humidified air is safe for nasal mucosa and does not impair ciliary function. THRIVE, however, requires dedicated equipment. This includes a corrugated tubing, nasal cannulae and a fixation device.

   THRIVE has been shown to have valuable application in anticipated difficult airways, rapid sequence intubations particularly in obese, procedural sedations and intensive care.

3. Buccal apneic oxygenation.

   This technique provides supplementary oxygen flow via the oropharyngeal route using a preformed oral RAE (Ring-Adair-Elwyn) endotracheal tube. This is usually secured in the left buccal space and fixed over the left cheek. The technique is useful when the nasal route is contraindicated. Oxygen delivery by buccal route bypasses the obstruction of naso-pharynx caused by tongue/soft palate. It offers additional protection against baro/volutrauma. Due to venting of excess gases via oral cavity. Oxygen flow needed for this technique is around 10 L/ min, i.e., two third of the flow needed for nasal oxygenation.

In obese patients, apneic oxygenation using a buccal oxygenation at 10 L/min has been demonstrated to significantly reduce the risk of desaturation during apnoeic episodes in excess of 12 min. The technique provides a high pharyngeal oxygen concentration during apnea allowing apneic oxygenation. But there is negligible CPAP and buccal apneic oxygenation does not produce the apneic ventilation phenomenon and CO_2 clearance that is seen in THRIVE.

4. Endobronchial catheters.

   Studies done with catheters inserted into either or both mainstem bronchii with oxygen flowrates of 0.6–0.7 L/min in elective surgical patients have shown to significantly prolong durations of safe apnea. However, there are very limited clinical applications of this technique. As such, insufflation of oxygen through a suction catheter inserted into the main bronchi of the deflated lung, has shown to be an acceptable and clinically relevant technique to improve oxygenation and prevent/treat desaturation during one lung ventilation with a double lumen tube in-situ.

8.5 Clinical Applications of Apneic Oxygenation

Apneic oxygenation technique involves choosing the appropriate patient, a good understanding of optimal oxygen flow and proper size of cannula for insufflation. The success of apneic oxygenation depends on three important factors:

- Maintenance of a patent air passage between nasal-oral-pharyngeal airspaces and the lung alveoli.
- Continuous supply of oxygen to the nasopharyngeal and oropharyngeal reservoirs.
- Monitoring and documentation of hemodynamic, respiratory and blood gas parameters (PaO_2, $PaCO_2$, pH) to follow the course and for early management of desaturation.

8.5.1 Critical Care

- During transport of hypoxemic patients and/or those with low GCS by emergency medical care team.
- Transport of witnessed out-of-hospital cardiac arrest victim. Oxygen insufflation during compression only CPR using oral oxygen delivery device.
- Before emergency endotracheal intubation in acute respiratory failure (as part of pre-oxygenation).
- Ultra protective lung ventilation. (combination of Apneic Oxygenation and Extracorporeal Carbon Dioxide Removal, i.e., $ECCO_2R$, to reduce systemic and pulmonary inflammatory mediators in acute respiratory distress syndrome vis a vis conventional lung-protective ventilation strategies).
- Diagnosis of Brain Death: absence of any respiratory efforts despite an increase in arterial carbon dioxide is consistent with brainstem death. Hypoxemia during the apnea test is prevented by oxygen delivered via the airway conduit during the time of testing.

8.5.2 Perioperative Settings

- During apneic period of rapid sequence induction and intubation using conventional laryn-

goscopic or videolaryngoscope-assisted endotracheal intubations.
- Tube-less anesthesia for vocal cord biopsies, thyroplasty, balloon dilatation for sub-glotic stenosis and other airway surgeries.
- One lung ventilation: apneic oxygenation of deflated lung using either endobronchial catheter or by surgically placed suction catheter distal to anastomosis.
- Anticipated difficult airway scenarios to provide a favorable apneic window to facilitate securement of the airway in an unpressurised environment.

8.5.3 Special Patient Groups

- **Pediatrics:** The low functional residual capacity and high oxygen requirements makes pediatric patients an "at-risk" patient group for significant hypoxemia with reduced apneic times. High flow nasal oxygen at 1–2 L/kg/min has been used successfully to reduce the incidence of desaturation during induction of general anaesthesia in children. Same cannula can be used at the completion of surgery and before extubation criteria are met. Utilization of higher flow rates can help achieve a CPAP of up to 4 cmH_2O.

- All routes of oxygen administration can be used in children. However, cannula size and oxygen flow rate are chosen according to age and the child's inspiratory demand. Besides, the cannula size also varies according to age and body weight. It has been recommended that the outer diameter of the cannula should be less than two-third of the patient's nares. Otherwise, there is an unexpected risk of elevations in airway pressure and resultant barotrauma. There are wide range of cannulas available from extra small to extra large (XS, S, M, L XL) to meet the requirements of various age groups from neonate to near-adults.
- **Obstetrics:** With their reduced functional residual capacity and physiological airway changes, parturients represent another "at-risk" patient group that could benefit from the longer and safer apneic times that apneic oxygenation can provide. Difficult airway societies recommend application of apneic oxygenation in the management of a difficult obstetric airway. Non labouring parturient models have been studied with various FiO_2 levels used for apnoeic oxygenation before rapid sequence intubation with favourable results.
- **Obese:** Obese patients are another important group of patients that are at a significant risk of desaturation and hypoxemia during the apneic period of airway management. Studies have shown that obese patients benefit from application of apneic oxygenation in both perioperative and critical care settings.

8.6 Cautionary Warning

- Nasal cannula can interfere with the face-mask seal causing leakage of gases. Hence, oxygen tubing should be secured on both sides in front of the tragus and a well-fitting mask with air cushion should be used for ventilation.
- Cold dry gases can cause drying of nasal and respiratory mucosa causing sinus pain, mucosal dehiscence and epistaxis.
- The gradient between $PaCO_2$ and end-tidal carbon dioxide ($ETCO_2$) increases with apnea duration. According to Bohr's hypothesis, this divergence is caused by atelectasis and ventilation–perfusion mismatch. The implication

of this phenomenon is progressive underestimation of hypercarbia using $ETCO_2$ measurements. Persistent carbon dioxide retention leads to reduction in pH values and respiratory acidosis. If profound academia occurs, i.e., pH < 7.0, it can lead to lethal arrhythmias.

- Apneic oxygenation is not the technique of choice in persistent obstruction of the airway due to congenital malformations, airway malignancies with significantly obstructed nares/nasopharynx or severe maxillofacial/ base of skull trauma requiring urgent oral endotracheal intubation.
- Apneic oxygenation does not help deliver volatile anaesthetic agent during general anaesthesia. Hence, an alternate technique such as total intravenous anesthesia (TIVA) needs to be used to prevent awareness during airway management and surgery.
- Apneic oxygenation does not lead to aerosol delivery in nebulized gases.
- Laser procedures using high flow apneic oxygenation or long bursts of diathermy can cause airway fires.
- Barotrauma in the form of pneumothorax, pneumomediastinum, pneumocephalus, pneumoorbitus, esophageal and gastric rupture can occur, especially if there is no clear route for egress of gases during apneic oxygenation, particularly in pediatric patients.

Apneic oxygenation techniques

Do's	Don't
Make sure that the airway is patent	Don't provide high flows of oxygen in a patient with obstructed and profusely bleeding upper airway
Use warm humidified oxygen in optimum concentration and volume	Don't use very high flow in pediatric patient. Can lead to barotrauma and worsen the situation
Monitor ventilation with serial blood gases or percutaneous CO_2 measurement, when apneic oxygenation is used	Don't base your observations on end tidal carbon-di-oxide measurements. This is not reliable during apneic oxygenation
Do keep on looking for underlying causes of apnea and try to trouble shoot wherever feasible	Don't consider ApOx as panacea for definitive management

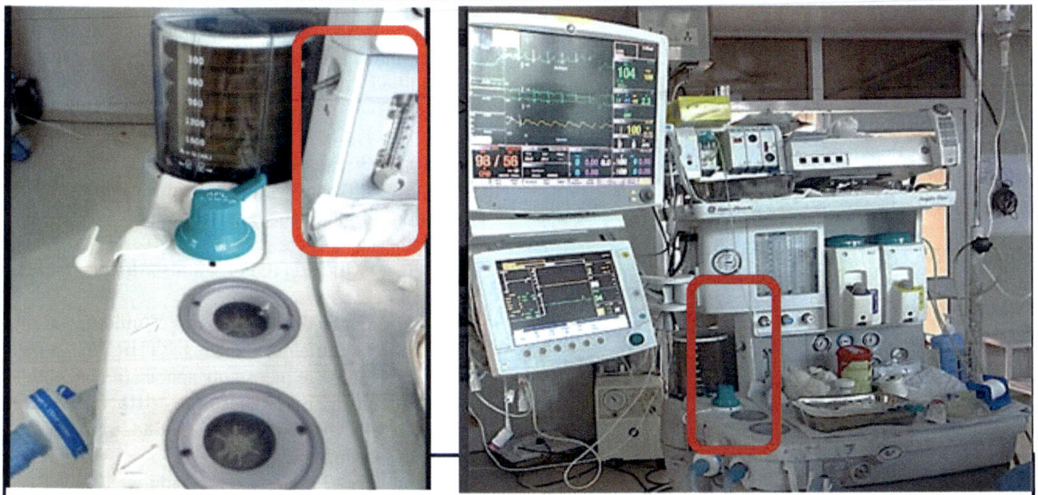

Anaesthesia work station with extra port for oxygen

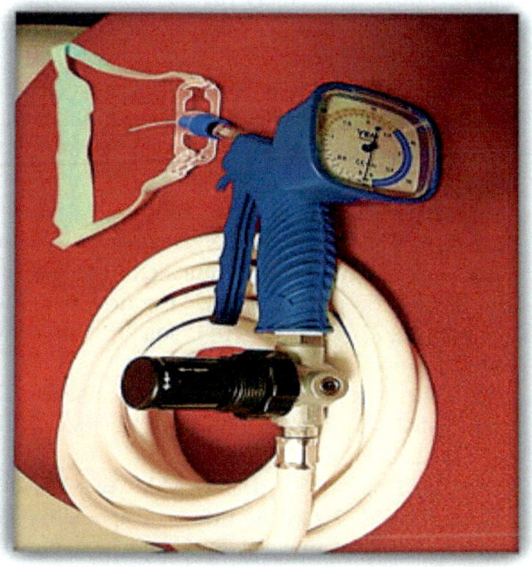

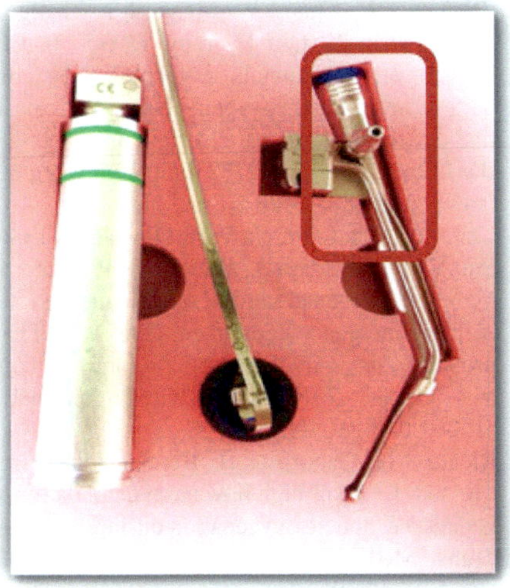

Transtracheal Jet Ventilation True-view VDL Oxygen port

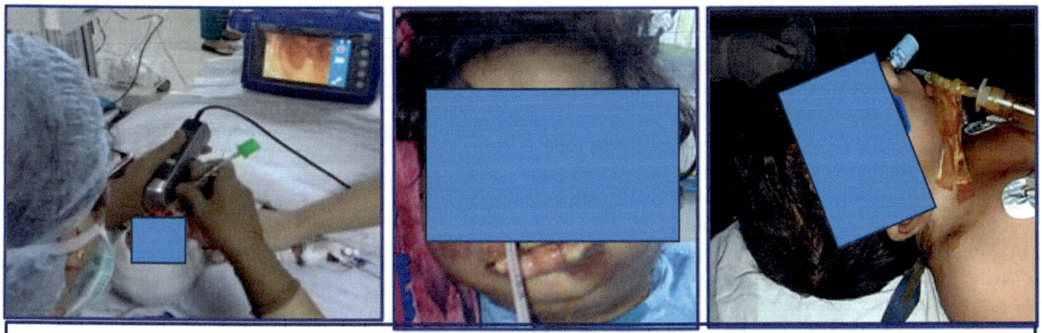

Para-oxygenation with Nasal Prongs & Nasal Airway

Suggested Reading

1. Frumin MJ, Epstein Robert M, Cohen G. Apneic oxygenation in man. Anesthesiology. 1959;20:789–98.
2. Jhou H-J, Chen P-H, Lin C, Yang L-Y, Lee C-H, Peng C-K. High-flow nasal cannula therapy as apneic oxygenation during endotracheal intubation in critically ill patients in the intensive care unit: a systematic review and meta analysis. Sci Rep. 2020;10:3541. https://doi.org/10.1038/s41598-020-60636-9.
3. Liua Q, Zhua C, Lana C, Chen R. High-flow nasal cannula versus conventional oxygen therapy in patients with dyspnea and hypoxemia before hospitalization. Expert Rev Respir Med. 2020;14:425. https://doi.org/10.1080/17476348.2020.1722642.
4. Huang C-C, Lan H-M, Li C-J, Lee T-H, Chen W-L, Lei W-Y, Hsieh P-Y, Yang M-C, Chou C-C, Wu H-P, Syue Y-J. Use high-flow nasal cannula for acute respiratory failure patients in the emergency department: a meta-analysis study. Emerg Med Int. 2019;2019:2130935. https://doi.org/10.1155/2019/2130935.
5. Zhonghua L, Chang W, Meng S-S, Zhang X, Xie J, Jing-Yuan X, Qiu H, Yang Y, Guo F. Effect of high-flow nasal cannula oxygen therapy compared with conventional oxygen therapy in postoperative patients: a systematic review and meta-analysis. BMJ Open. 2019;9:e027523. https://doi.org/10.1136/bmjopen-2018-027523.
6. Chua MT, Khan FA, Ng WM, Qingshu L, Low MJW, Yau YW, Punyadasa A, Kuan WS. Pre- and apnoeic high flow oxygenation for RApid sequence intubation in The Emergency department (Pre-AeRATE): study protocol for a multicentre, randomised controlled trial. Trials. 2019;20:195. https://doi.org/10.1186/s13063-019-3305-8.
7. Ricard J-D, Gaborieau B, Bernier J, Le Breton C, Messika J. Use of high flow nasal cannula for preoxygenation & apneic oxygenation duringintubation. Ann Transl Med. 2019;7:S380. https://doi.org/10.21037/atm.2019.12.106.
8. Humphreys S, Lee-Archer P, Reyne G, et al. Transnasal humidified rapid-insufflation ventilatory exchange (THRIVE) in children: a randomized controlled trial. Br J Anaesth. 2017;118:232–8.
9. Lyons C, Callaghan M. Uses and mechanisms of apneic oxygenation: a narrative review. Anaesthesia. 2019;74:497–507. https://doi.org/10.1111/anae.14565.
10. Sohn L, Hajduk J, Jagannathan N. Apneic oxygenation as a standard of care in children: how do we get there? Anesth Analg. 2020;130(4):828–30. https://doi.org/10.1213/ANE.0000000000004483.
11. Lyons C, Callaghan M. Apnoeic oxygenation with high-flow nasal oxygen for laryngeal surgery: a case series. Anaesthesia. 2017;72:1379–87. PMID:29047136. https://doi.org/10.1111/anae.14036.
12. Gustafsson IM, Lodenius Å, Tunelli J, Ullman J, Jonsson Fagerlund M. Apnoeic oxygenation in adults under general anaesthesia using transnasal humidified rapid-insufflation ventilatory exchange (THRIVE)—a physiological study. Br J Anaesth. 2017;118(4):610–7. PMID:28403407. https://doi.org/10.1093/bja/aex036.
13. Pillai A, Chikhani M, Hardman JG. Apnoeic oxygenation in pregnancy: a modelling investigation. Anaesthesia. 2016;71(9):1077–80. Epub 2016 Jul 20. PMID:27440389. https://doi.org/10.1111/anae.13563.
14. Patel A, Nouraei SA. Transnasal Humidified Rapid-Insufflation Ventilatory Exchange (THRIVE): a physiological method of increasing apnoea time in patients with difficult airways. Anaesthesia. 2015;70(3):323–9. Epub 2014 Nov 10. PMID:25388828. https://doi.org/10.1111/anae.12923.
15. Mitterlechner T, Herff H, Hammel CW, Braun P, Paal P, Wenzel V, Benzer A. A dual-use laryngoscope to facilitate apneic oxygenation. J Emerg Med. 2015;48(1):103–7. Epub 2014 Oct 11. PMID: 25308899. https://doi.org/10.1016/j.jemermed.2014.06.061.
16. Rudlof B, Hohenhorst W. Use of apneic oxygenation for the performance of pan-endoscopy. Otolaryngol Head Neck Surg. 2013;149(2):235–9. https://doi.org/10.1177/0194599813486248.
17. Sanchez-Lorente D, Gómez-Caro A, Jimenez MJ, Molins L. Apnoeic oxygenation on one-lung ventilation in functionally impaired patients during sleeve lobectomy. Eur J Cardiothorac Surg. 2011;39(4):e77–9. Epub 2011 Jan 12. https://doi.org/10.1016/j.ejcts.2010.11.056.
18. Christopher KL. Transtracheal oxygen catheters. Clin Chest Med. 2003;24(3):489–510. Review. PMID: 14535222.
19. Toner AJ, Douglas SG, Bailey MA, Avis HJ, Pillai AV, Phillips M, Heard A. Effect of apneic oxygenation on tracheal oxygen levels, tracheal pressure, and carbon dioxide accumulation: a randomized, controlled trial of buccal oxygen administration. Anesth Analg. 2019;128(6):1154–9. https://doi.org/10.1213/ANE.0000000000003810.
20. Lodenius Å, Piehl J, Östlund A, Ullman J, Jonsson FM. Transnasal humidified rapid-insufflation ventilatory exchange (THRIVE) vs. facemask breathing pre-oxygenation for rapid sequence induction in adults: a prospective randomised non-blinded clinical trial. Anaesthesia. 2018;73(5):564–71. https://doi.org/10.1111/anae.14215.
21. Patel A, Nouraei SAR. Transnasal humidified rapid-insufflation ventilatory exchange (THRIVE): a physiological method of increasing apnoea time in patients with difficult airways. Anaesthesia. 2015;70:323–9.

Ultrasound of the Airway

9

Debendra Kumar Tripathy

Key Points

- Airway ultrasound is a rapidly evolving field that is becoming increasingly important in emergency and critical care medicine.
- Advances in ultrasound technology have enabled improved visualization of airway structures, leading to greater accuracy and precision in airway management.
- Airway ultrasound can be performed quickly and easily at the bedside, making it a useful tool for assessing and managing the airway, with applications in intubation, ventilation, emergency airway access, and monitoring airway anatomy and function.
- A systematic approach, proper training, and experience are essential for the accurate interpretation of airway ultrasound images.

9.1 Introduction

Airway ultrasound is a medical imaging technique that uses high-frequency sound waves to visualize the airways and surrounding structures. It is a non-invasive and real-time method that allows clinicians to obtain detailed images of the airways, including the trachea, bronchi, and lungs.

The main advantage of airway ultrasound is its ability to provide real-time visual information about the airways and surrounding tissues. It can be very useful in emergency and critical care settings where a quick and accurate assessment of the airways is essential. For example, it can be used to evaluate the patient's position and level of consciousness, assess for potential airway obstruction, and determine the best approach for airway management.

Airway ultrasound is performed using a handheld ultrasound probe placed over the patient's neck or chest. The sound waves produced by the probe are reflected back to the probe and captured to create images of the airways and surrounding tissues.

9.2 Indications

Airway ultrasound is a valuable tool for evaluating the airway and surrounding structures, providing real-time, non-invasive visual information that can aid in managing critically ill or injured

D. K. Tripathy (✉)
Professor and Head, Department of Trauma & Emergency, AIIMS Raipur,
Raipur, Chhattisgarh, India
e-mail: debendra.anaes@aiimsrishikesh.edu.in

N. Gupta et al. (eds.), *Techniques in Anesthesia, Intensive Care and Emergency Medicine*,
https://doi.org/10.1007/978-981-96-1202-4_9

Table 9.1 Indications for airway ultrasound

Indication	Description
Evaluation of vocal cords	Airway ultrasound can be used to evaluate the position and movement of the vocal cords, which can be helpful in assessing for conditions such as vocal cord paralysis or laryngospasm or paradoxical vocal cord motion
Detection of endotracheal tube placement	Ultrasound can confirm proper placement of an endotracheal tube in the trachea, as well as detect complications such as endobronchial intubation or esophageal intubation
Prediction of difficult airway	Airway ultrasound can be a useful tool for predicting difficult airway management and guiding airway management decisions in patients who may have a difficult airway. However, it should be used in conjunction with other clinical assessments and tools, and its limitations and potential pitfalls should be recognized
Assessment of airway edema	Airway ultrasound can detect the presence of airway edema, which may be caused by conditions such as angioedema or anaphylaxis
Evaluation of foreign bodies	Ultrasound can be used to detect foreign bodies in the airway, which may be helpful in diagnosing choking or aspiration
Assessment of neck masses	Airway ultrasound can evaluate the size and characteristics of neck masses that may be impinging on the airway or causing airway obstruction
Evaluation of tracheal stenosis	Airway ultrasound can be used to assess the degree of narrowing or stenosis in the trachea, which can be caused by conditions such as tracheal tumors or scarring
Evaluation of tracheal deviation	Airway ultrasound can assess the degree of tracheal deviation, which may be caused by conditions such as mediastinal tumors or pneumothorax
Assessment of upper airway obstruction	Airway ultrasound can be used to evaluate the presence and location of upper airway obstruction, which may be caused by conditions such as epiglottitis or croup
Diagnosis of vocal cord nodules/polyps	Airway ultrasound can detect vocal cord nodules or polyps, which may be causing hoarseness or other voice changes
Monitoring of endotracheal cuff pressure	Airway ultrasound can be used to monitor endotracheal cuff pressure, which can help prevent complications such as tracheal injury or aspiration
Diagnosis of subglottic stenosis	Airway ultrasound can detect narrowing of the subglottic area, which may be caused by conditions such as acquired subglottic stenosis or congenital anomalies
Prediction of the appropriate diameter of endotracheal, tracheostomy tubes and cuff placement	Airway ultrasound can assess the size, location, and characteristics of the endotracheal and tracheostomy tubes
Tracheostomy and percutaneous tracheostomy	Airway ultrasound is used for the localisation of tracheal cartilages, interspaces and vessels. It is also used for real-time needle guidance and the detection of subcutaneous vessels
Assessment of airway trauma	Airway ultrasound can evaluate the extent and location of airway trauma, which may be caused by blunt or penetrating trauma
Monitoring of extubation readiness	Airway ultrasound can help determine if a patient is ready for extubation by evaluating airway patency, vocal cord movement, and other factors.
Airway related nerve blocks	Ultrasound-guided nerve blocks can be useful in managing airway-related pain and discomfort. Ultrasound also allows real-time visualization of the spread of local anesthetic, ensuring that the target nerve is adequately anesthetized
Dynamic assessment of airway	Airway ultrasound can detect change of tracheal diameter with external manipulation
Monitoring of airway resistance	Airway ultrasound can detect changes in airway resistance, which may be useful in monitoring the progress of conditions such as asthma or chronic obstructive pulmonary disease (COPD)

patients. Literature has reported various use (Table 9.1), and there may be additional indications for airway ultrasound depending on the individual patient and clinical scenario.

9.3 Airway Ultrasound Basics

Echogenicity refers to how well tissues reflect an ultrasound wave. When a tissue is hyper-echoic, it reflects more sound waves than the surrounding tissue, while an-echoic tissue doesn't reflect any echoes. In ultrasonography, air is a poor medium for visualizing deeper structures, and intraluminal air can produce both comet tail and reverberation artifacts. Linear structures such as the mentum, mandible rami, hyoid bone, and sternum appear as light hyperechoic structures with hypoechoic acoustic shadows underneath. The thyroid and cricoid cartilage are homogeneous, hypoechoic cartilage structures. Muscle and connective tissue display a striated, hypoechoic, and heterogeneous appearance. The echogenicity of fat and glandular structures depends on the glandular parenchyma's fat content, with both appearing slightly to strongly hyperechoic compared to neighboring soft tissues. The Air-Mucosa (A-M) contact appears hyperechoic and linear (Fig. 9.2).

9.4 Systematic Airway Scan

A systematic airway ultrasound scan is a standardized approach to using ultrasound to evaluate the airway. It involves scanning specific landmarks and structures to assess their anatomy and function to identify any potential issues that may affect airway management.

The airway ultrasound can be divided into two areas, neck or infra-hyoid scan (Fig. 9.1A, B, a, b) and oral cavity or suprahyoid scan (Fig. 9.1C, D, c, d). The neck scan is typically performed using a high-frequency linear probe (5–15 MHz), and a curvilinear probe (1–5 MHz) is used for the oral cavity scan, allowing for detailed airway structure imaging. However, a curvilinear probe can be used for both the oral cavity and neck ultrasound.

The patient should be positioned in a semi-upright position with the head tilted back, and the neck extended. The transducer is placed on the skin over the anterior neck, and the ultrasound beam is directed towards the trachea and adjacent structures. Transverse, sagittal, and parasagittal scanning is to be done in each areas (neck and oral cavity) at various levels for complete evaluation of the airway (Fig. 9.1).

During the scan, various measurements may be taken of specific structures, such as the hyomental distance and the subglottic diameter. The scan results are then used to help guide airway management decisions, such as the choice of

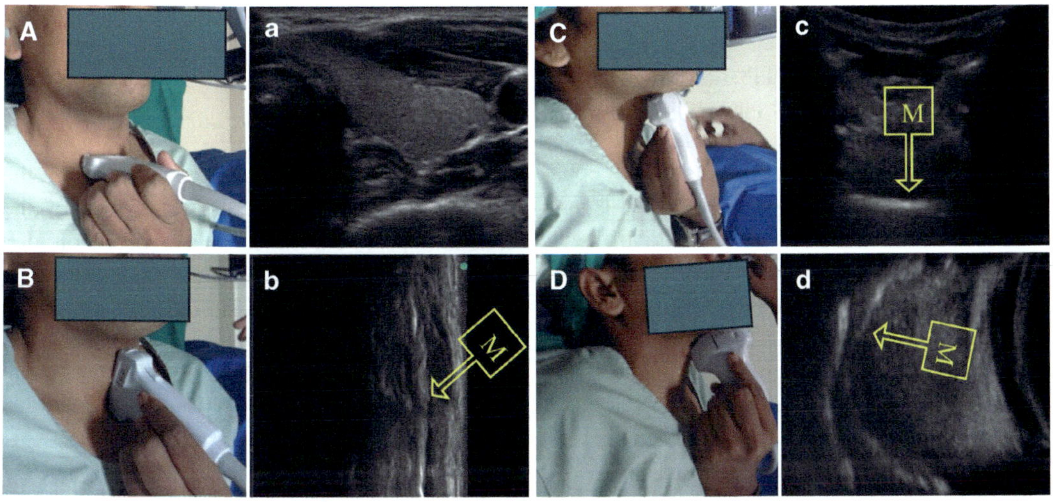

Fig. 9.1 (**A**) Linear probe placement for transverse scan at the level of suprasternal notch, (**a**) corresponding ultrasound image, (**B**) Linear probe placement for sagittal view of neck, (**b**) corresponding ultrasound image, (**C**) Curvilinear probe placement for transverse scan of oral cavity, (**c**) corresponding ultrasound image, (**D**) Curvilinear probe placement for sagittal scan of oral cavity, (**d**) corresponding ultrasound image, *M* Air-Mucosa (AM) lines

Table 9.2 Scanning areas and airway structures visible

Scanning areas	Airway structure visible
Neck or infrahyoid area (sagittal and para sagittal view)	Tracheal cartilage, cricoid cartilage, thyroid cartilage, crico-thyroid membrane, hyoid bone, annular ligament, arytenoid cartilage, epiglottis and oesophagus
Neck or infrahyoid area (transverse view at various level)	Tracheal cartilage, cricoid cartilage, thyroid cartilage, crico-thyroid membrane, hyoid bone, annular ligament, arytenoid cartilage, true and false vocal cords, epiglottis and esophagus
Oral cavity or suprahyoid area (sagittal and para sagittal view)	Mandible, hyoid bone, mylohyoid muscle, epiglottis, thyroid cartilage, peri epiglottis space, genioglossus muscle, geniohyoid muscle, hard and soft palate, tonsils, submandibular and sublingual glands, tongue, tongue surface, hard and soft palate
Oral cavity or suprahyoid area (transverse view at various level)	Hyoid bone, mandible, mylohyoid muscle, epiglottis, thyroid cartilage, peri epiglottis space, genioglossus muscle, geniohyoid muscle, hard and soft palate, tonsils, submandibular and sublingual glands, tongue, tongue surface, hard and soft palate

intubation technique or the need for a surgical airway.

A systematic airway ultrasound scan can provide valuable information (Table 9.2) about the anatomy and function of the airway and can help identify potential issues that may affect airway management.

9.5 Ultrasound Description of Various Airway Structures

9.5.1 Cricoid, Thyroid, and Tracheal Cartilages

The cricoid cartilage appears as an oval, hypoechoic structure in the parasagittal view and as a hump in the transverse view. The cricoid cartilage is best viewed by shifting the probe cephalad. It appears as a C-shaped mixed-echoic structure, thicker than the tracheal cartilages, with a hyperechoic A-M interface directly under it. The cricothyroid membrane appears as a hyperechoic ribbon linking the thyroid and cricoid cartilage in the sagittal and parasagittal views The cricothyroid membrane appears as a hyperechoic strip line wedged between the cricoid and thyroid cartilage on the transverse view. The tracheal ring appears as a hyperechoic "string of beads" in the sagittal and parasagittal views and an inverted "U" in the transverse view (Figs. 9.2 and 9.3).

9.5.2 Thyroid and Esophagus

In the transverse view, the thyroid gland can be recognized as two lobes and an isthmus at the suprasternal notch level. It appears homogenous and echogenic, with a more hyperechoic appearance than the neighbouring strap muscle. Other associated structures, such as the esophagus, vertebral body, and internal carotid artery, can also be detected on the thyroid gland's side in the oblique transverse view. The oesophagus is easily located when the patient swallows, resulting in a prominent peristaltic movement of the esophagal lumen (Fig. 9.2).

9.5.3 Tongue

The tongue can be seen more deeply within the floor of the mouth. The dorsal surface of the tongue appears curvilinear and hyperechoic due to the A-M interface. The inner musculature of the tongue gives it a striated appearance on sonography, with the genioglossus and hyoglossus muscles running fanlike towards the dorsal surface of the tongue (Figs. 9.4 and 9.5).

9.5.4 Epiglottis

Using a linear or curvilinear transducer, with varying cephalad or caudad angulation allows

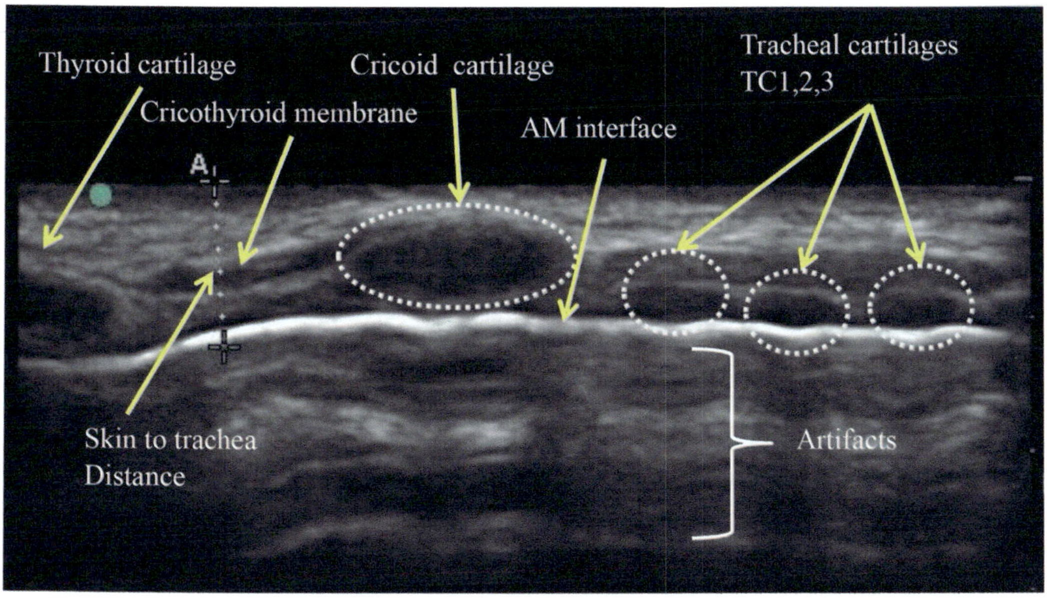

Fig. 9.2 Sagittal view of neck with a linear probe showing airway structures

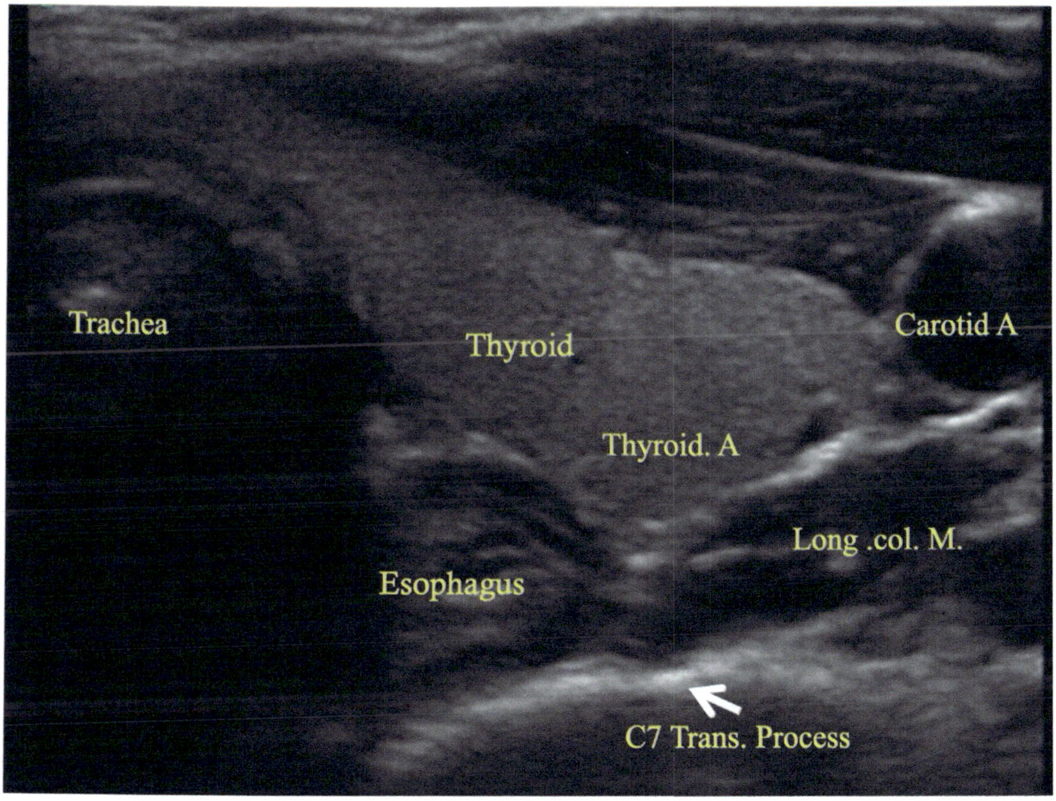

Fig. 9.3 Transverse view of neck with a linear probe at the level of suprasternal notch showing airway structures

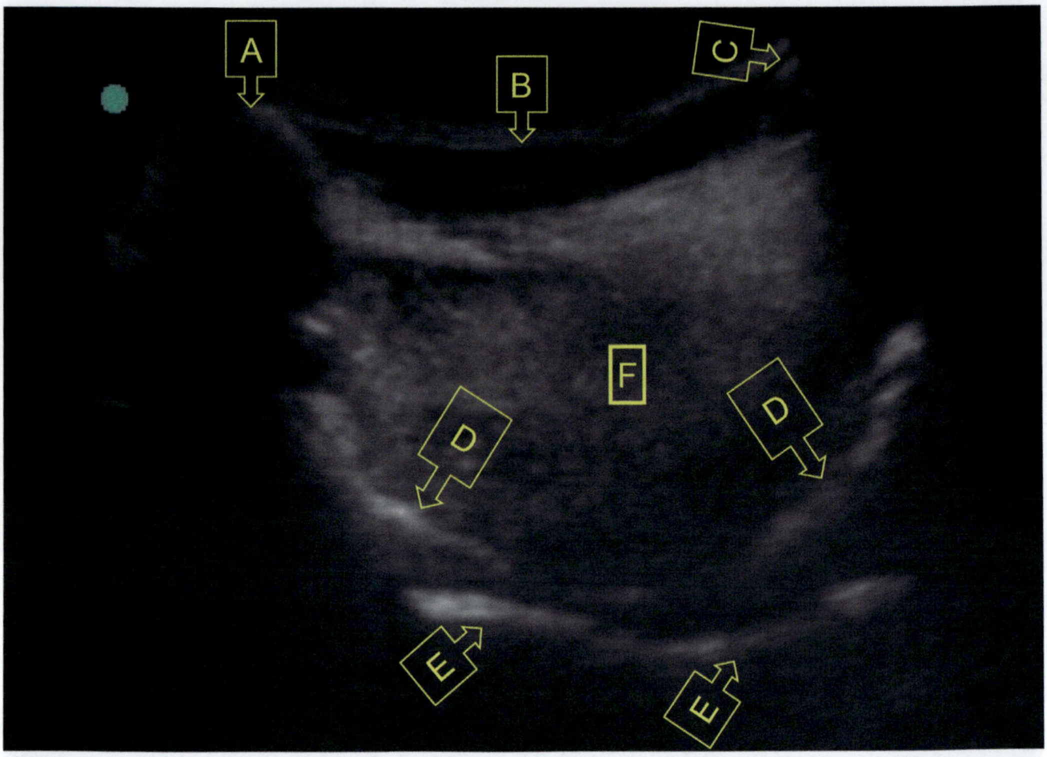

Fig. 9.4 Sagittal view of oral cavity with a curvilinear probe. *A* mentum, *B* mylohyoid muscle, *C* hyoid bone, *D* dorsal surface of tongue, *E* hard palate

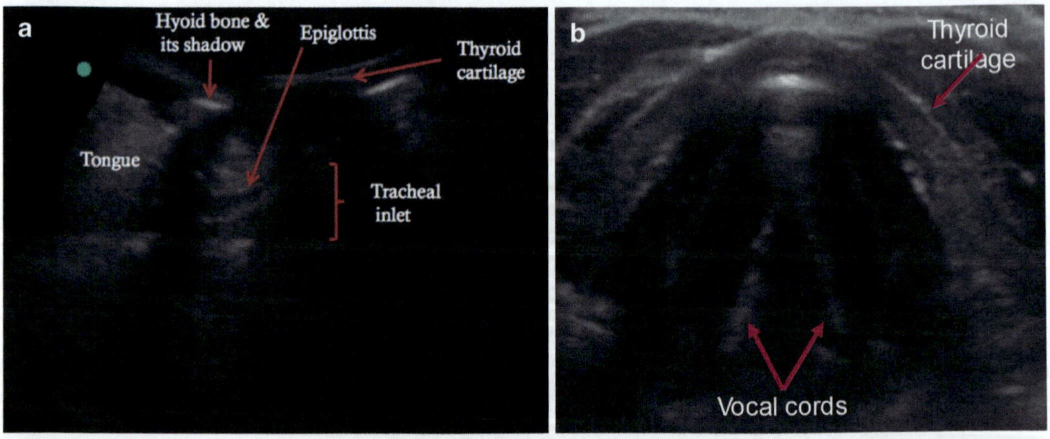

Fig. 9.5 (**a**) Sagittal view of glottic opening with a curvilinear probe, (**b**) Transverse view of vocal cords with linear probe

easy identification of the epiglottis in the transverse plane of virtually all adults. The epiglottis is a visible structure in the throat that appears as a curvilinear, hypoechoic object. It is bounded anteriorly by the hyperechoic pre-epiglottic space and posteriorly by the bright, linear A-M interface. The parasagittal view is not ideal for visualizing the epiglottis due to the acoustic shadowing of the hyoid bone. However, a comprehensive submandibular sagittal view using a curved transducer may be helpful. Protrusion and swallowing of the tongue can also aid in identifying the epiglottis, which appears as a discrete, movable structure beneath the base of the tongue (Fig. 9.5a).

9.5.5 Vocal Cord

To visualize the vocal cords, the transverse view at the level of the thyroid cartilage provides the best window. The vocal cords are an isosceles triangle with a tracheal shadow in the centre. Hyperechoic vocal ligaments separate the vocal cords on the medial side, while false vocal cords are more hyperechoic and parallel to the true vocal cords. A 3D probe with a fluid interface is the best way to observe vocal cord movement (Fig. 9.5b).

9.6 Difficult Airway Parameters

These ultrasound measurements can be used with other clinical assessment tools to predict difficult airway management and guide airway management decisions. It is important to note that ultrasound measurements alone are not sufficient to predict difficult airway management and should be used as part of a comprehensive evaluation (Figs. 9.4, 9.5, 9.6, and 9.7). Various measurements and their relevance is enumerated in Table 9.3, and the list is ever-expanding with newer evidence.

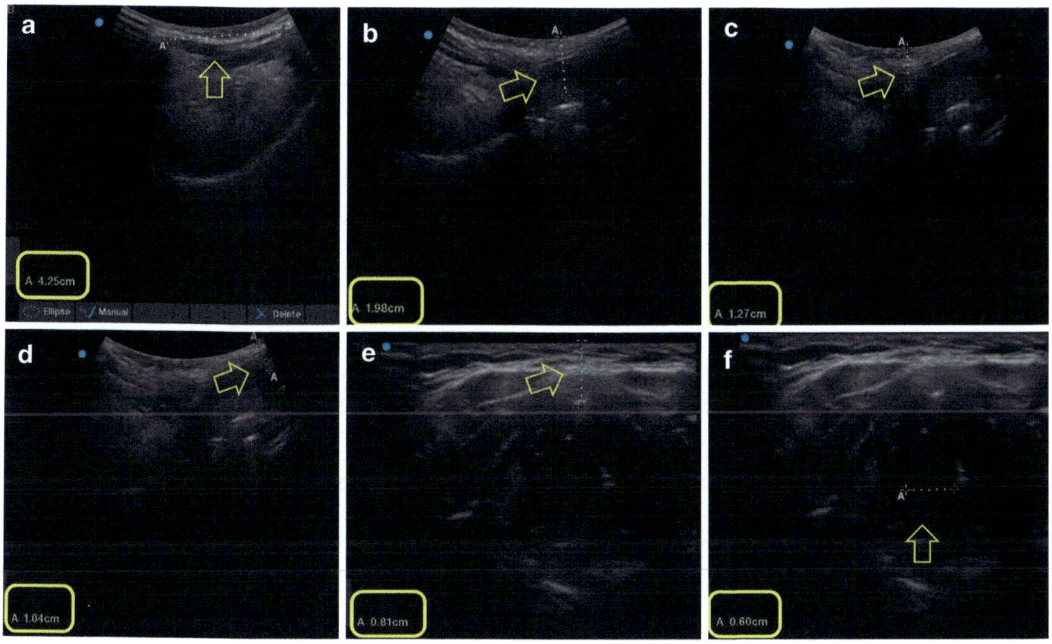

Fig. 9.6 Various airway measurements, Yellow area pointing at the measurement area. (**a**) Hyomental distance, (**b**) Skin to epiglottis distance, (**c**) Skin to hyoid distance, (**d**) Skin to thyroid distance, (**e**) Skin to anterior commissure distance, (**f**) Vocal cord opening

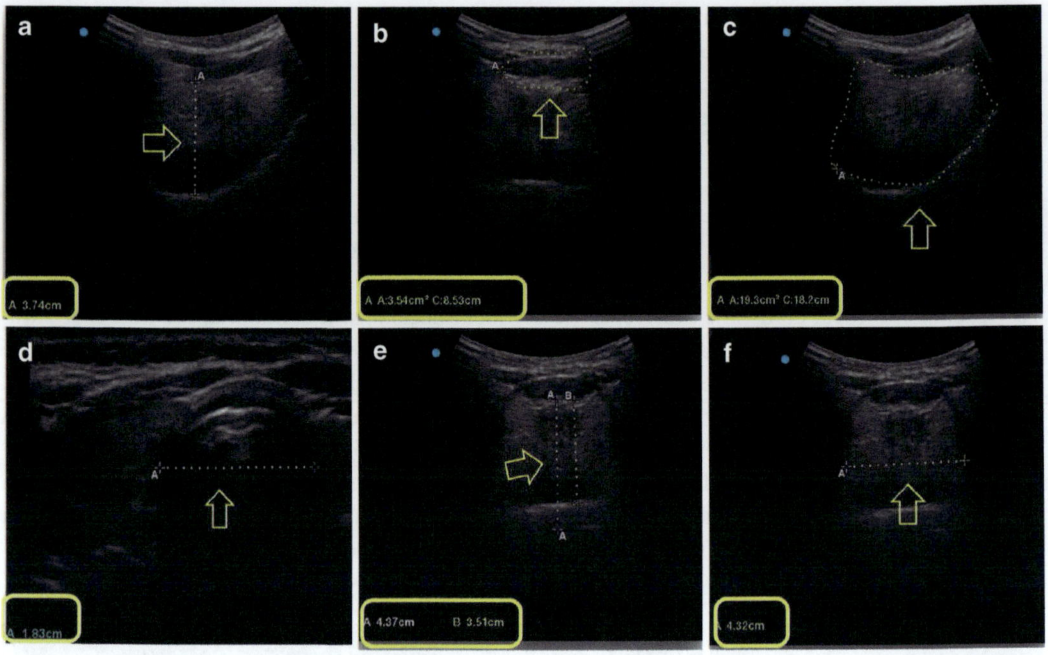

Fig. 9.7 Various airway measurements, Yellow area pointing at the measurement area. (**a**) Tongue thickness, (**b**) Cross sectional area of floor of oral cavity, (**c**) Cross sectional area of tongue, (**d**) Measurement of tracheal diameter, (**e**) Tongue and oral cavity height, (**f**) Tongue width

Table 9.3 Various ultrasound parameters used for difficult airway assessment

Measurement	Description	Significance in difficult airway
Hyomental distance	The distance between the hyoid bone and the mentum (lower jaw)	Shorter distance is associated with difficult airway management
Thyromental distance	The distance between the thyroid cartilage and the mentum	Shorter distance is associated with difficult airway management
Retrognathia	The degree of posterior displacement of the mandible	Increased degree of retrognathia is associated with difficult airway management
Epiglottic angle	The angle between the base of the tongue and the epiglottis	Smaller angle is associated with difficult airway management
Subglottic diameter	The diameter of the subglottic region	Narrower diameter is associated with difficult airway management
Vocal cord mobility and thickness	The degree of vocal cord movement and the thickness of the vocal cords	Reduced mobility or thicker vocal cords are associated with difficult airway management
Cricothyroid membrane thickness	The thickness of the cricothyroid membrane	Thicker membrane is associated with difficult cricothyrotomy
Thyroid cartilage notch depth	The depth of the thyroid cartilage notch	Shallow notch depth is associated with difficult airway management
Anterior neck soft tissue thickness at various level	The thickness of the soft tissues in the anterior neck	Increased thickness is associated with difficult airway management
Tongue size and position	The size and position of the tongue	Enlarged or posterior displacement of tongue is associated with difficult airway management
Tracheal deviation	Deviation of the trachea from the midline	Deviation is associated with difficult airway management

9.7 Conclusion

Airway ultrasonography is a valuable technique that can be used to visualize airway structures, detect abnormalities, and guide airway management interventions. It is a non-invasive and safe method that can be used in various clinical settings. However, performing and interpreting the images accurately requires appropriate training and experience.

Suggested Reading

1. Ji C, Ni Q, Chen W. Diagnostic accuracy of radiology (CT, X-ray, US) for predicting difficult intubation in adults: a meta-analysis. J Clin Anesth. 2018;45:79–87.
2. Kundra P, Mishra SK, Ramesh A. Ultrasound of the airway. Indian J Anaesth. 2011;55(5):456–62.
3. Osman A, Sum KM. Role of upper airway ultrasound in airway management. J Intensive Care. 2016;4:52.
4. Lakhal K, Delplace X, Cottier JP, et al. The feasibility of ultrasound to assess subglottic diameter. Anesth Analg. 2007;104:611–4.
5. Tripathy DK, Gupta B. Imaging of the airway. In: Ubaradka RS, Gupta N, Bidkar PU, Tripathy DK, Gupta A, editors. The airway manual. Singapore: Springer; 2023. https://doi.org/10.1007/978-981-19-4747-6_4.
6. Sustić A, Miletić D, Protić A, et al. Can ultrasound be useful for predicting the size of a left double-lumen bronchial tube? Tracheal width as measured by ultrasonography versus computed tomography. J Clin Anesth. 2008;20:247–52.
7. Shibasaki M, Nakajima Y, Ishii S, et al. Prediction of pediatric endotracheal tube size by ultrasonography. Anesthesiology. 2010;113:819–24.
8. Hui CM, Tsui BC. Sublingual ultrasound as an assessment method for predicting difficult intubation: a pilot study. Anaesthesia. 2014;69:314–9.
9. Adhikari S, Zeger W, Schmier C, et al. Pilot study to determine the utility of point-of-care ultrasound in the assessment of difficult laryngoscopy. Acad Emerg Med. 2011;18:754–8.
10. Adi O, Kok MS, Abdull Wahab SF. Focused airway ultrasound: an armamentarium in future airway management. J Emerg Crit Care Med. 2019;3:31.
11. Chou HC, Chong KM, Sim SS, et al. Real-time tracheal ultrasonography for confirmation of endotracheal tube placement during cardiopulmonary resuscitation. Resuscitation. 2013;84:1708–12.
12. Das SK, Choupoo NS, Haldar R, et al. Transtracheal ultrasound for verification of endotracheal tube placement: a systematic review and meta-analysis. Can J Anaesth. 2015;62:413–23.
13. Uya A, Spear D, Patel K, et al. Can novice sonographers accurately locate an endotracheal tube with a saline-filled cuff in a cadaver model? A pilot study. Acad Emerg Med. 2012;19:361–4.
14. Kim J, Kim JY, Kim WO, et al. An ultrasound evaluation of laryngeal mask airway position in pediatric patients: an observational study. Anesth Analg. 2015;120:427–32.
15. Rajajee V, Fletcher JJ, Rochlen LR, et al. Real-time ultrasound-guided percutaneous dilatational tracheostomy: a feasibility study. Crit Care. 2011;15:R67.
16. Gobatto ALN, Besen BAMP, Tierno PFGMM, et al. Ultrasound-guided percutaneous dilational tracheostomy versus bronchoscopy-guided percutaneous dilational tracheostomy in critically ill patients (TRACHUS): a randomized noninferiority controlled trial. Intensive Care Med. 2016;42:342–51.
17. Sawka A, Tang R, Vaghadia H. Sonographically guided superior laryngeal nerve block during awake fiberoptic intubation. A A Case Rep. 2015;4:107–10.
18. Tripathy DK, Bhat RR, Dhanger S. Airway ultrasound to detect endotracheal tube cuff herniation. Indian J Anaesth. 2017;61(6):511.
19. Ding LW, Wang HC, Wu HD, et al. Laryngeal ultrasound: a useful method in predicting post-extubation stridor. A pilot study. Eur Respir J. 2006;27:384–9.
20. Tripathy DK, Gupta B, Patil AG, Khan A. Dynamic ultrasound assessment of airway: a novel approach in a patient with goitre. Airway. 2019;2(2):93.
21. Tripathy DK, Gupta B, Jadhav RV, Hareesh P. Real-time point-of-care ultrasound for accurate endotracheal tube positioning in a neonate with type C tracheoesophageal fistula. Saudi J Anaesth. 2022;16(4):510.
22. Wojtczak JA. Submandibular sonography: assessment of hyomental distances and ratio, tongue size, and floor of the mouth musculature using portable sonography. J Ultrasound Med. 2012;31:523–8.
23. Ezri T, Gewürtz G, Sessler DI, et al. Prediction of difficult laryngoscopy in obese patients by ultrasound quantification of anterior neck soft tissue. Anaesthesia. 2003;58:1111–4.
24. Komatsu R, Sengupta P, Wadhwa A, et al. Ultrasound quantification of anterior soft tissue thickness fails to predict difficult laryngoscopy in obese patients. Anaesth Intensive Care. 2007;35:32–7.
25. Yao W, Bin W. Can tongue thickness measured by ultrasonography predict difficult tracheal intubation? Br J Anaesth. 2017;118(4):601–9.
26. Pinto J, Cordeiro L, Pereira C, et al. Predicting difficult laryngoscopy using ultrasound measurement of distance from skin to epiglottis. J Crit Care. 2016;33:26–31.
27. Yao W, Wang B. Can tongue thickness measured by ultrasonography predict difficult tracheal intubation? Br J Anaesth. 2017;118:601–9.

Jet Ventilation

10

Anju Gupta and Preeti Yadav

Key Points

- Jet ventilation is highly versatile; gas delivery is possible at various points along the airway.
- High driving pressures of gas are used and barotrauma will occur if there is inadequate egress of air at the time of expiration.
- LFJV can be used for CICV situation and in paediatric patients.
- Modern high-frequency jet ventilators monitor airway pressures and can warm and humidify the inspired gas.
- High-frequency jet ventilation requires large minute volumes to ensure adequate CO_2 removal.
- HFJV is a safe and effective technique with ever growing indications for elective and emergency use.
- HFOV and SHFJV both can be used for specific paediatric populations.

A. Gupta (✉) · P. Yadav
Anesthesiology, Pain Medicine, Critical Care, All India Institute of Medical Sciences, New Delhi, Delhi, India

10.1 History and Background

Ventilating bronchoscopes are in use since the 1950s; these instruments have allowed ventilation through a side arm by occlusion of the proximal end of the bronchoscope by the surgeon's thumb or a glass window, but these maneuvers required withdrawal of instruments and temporary cessation of surgery. To overcome these drawbacks, jet ventilation was developed in the late 1960s.

Douglas Sanders formulated a technique to allow uninterrupted patient ventilation as well as unhindered surgical access through an open, rigid bronchoscope. The technique involved oxygen being delivered at the supply pressure of 50 lb in^{-} in a jet through a 0.035-in. diameter nozzle inside the lumen of the bronchoscope via an adapter attached to proximal end of the bronchoscope. There was entrainment of air with each jet of air which contributed to the tidal volume. The pause between each jet delivery allowed passive expiration. Further research allowed major changes which included the development of narrow, non-distensible catheters that could be used in multiple settings which included rigid bronchoscopes, laryngoscopes and tracheal tubes.

In 1977, Klain and Smith developed a fluidic logic controlled ventilator with the capability of delivering jets at rates of 60–100/min. Its use was described in fiberoptic bronchoscopy. Babinski and colleagues [3] used high-frequency jet ventilation (HFJV) via a narrow-bore, rigid, tracheal

N. Gupta et al. (eds.), *Techniques in Anesthesia, Intensive Care and Emergency Medicine*,
https://doi.org/10.1007/978-981-96-1202-4_10

catheter in patients undergoing laryngoscopy. One disadvantage was that it allowed superimposed resumption of spontaneous respiration during emergence.

10.2 Mechanism of Jet Ventilation

The mechanism of gas exchange via low-frequency jet ventilation (LFJV) is convective ventilation or bulk flow, (i.e., the mass flow of gases into and out of the lung) similar to spontaneous respiration. HFJV utilizes tidal volumes that are smaller than anatomical plus equipment dead space combined. Consequently, normal physiological principles cannot be used. A small number of alveoli are close to the conducting airways and some gas may enter during HFJV by bulk flow even, but inadequate to support effective gas exchange (Fig. 10.1).

Laminar flow occurs in small airways: air closest to the wall has lower velocity than air in the center of the airway. The other mechanisms of ventilation with jet ventilation are as follows:

- Pendelluft.
- Convective streaming or Taylor dispersion.
- Cardiogenic mixing.
- Bulk flow.

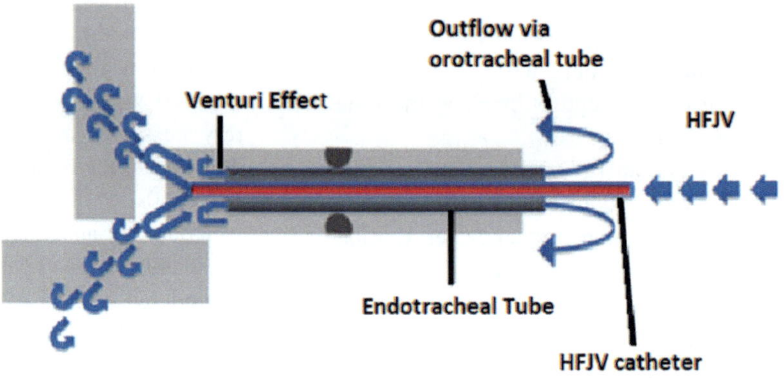

Fig. 10.1 Mechanism of HFJV

10.3 Types of Jet Ventilation

Jet ventilation can be high or low frequency. The principles of these methods are the same: jet-streams originating from high-pressure sources interrupted by pneumatic or electronically controlled devices; the tidal volume generated is supplemented by entrainment of gases at the nozzle of the jet. Expiration is passive and is dependent on chest-wall recoil (Table 10.1).

10.3.1 Low-Frequency Jet Ventilation

10.3.1.1 Indications

LFJV can be used in investigative procedures such as laryngoscopy or bronchoscopy, management of a difficult airway or a CICV (cricothyroidotomy cannula).

10.3.1.2 Equipment

Cannulae: short, narrow-bore and non-compliant and integrated to devices such as the rigid bronchoscope or laryngoscope.

Primary gas source: high-pressure wall-piped oxygen (4 bar).

Safety features: Pressure valve and regulator.

10.3.1.3 Technique

A Luer-Lock connection is used to secure the cannula and the handset. A jet frequency of about 10/min allows adequate time for exhalation and prevent air-trapping and barotrauma. The effective FiO_2 in the trachea is 0.8–0.9 when 100% oxygen is used as the jet gas (dilution by entrainment of air). A side-arm attachment to a bronchoscope or laryngoscope can prevent the ambient air entrainment.

Do's	Don'ts
Short narrow bore cannulae Align cannulae along airway axis Use total intravenous anesthesia (TIVA)	High frequency-inadequate exhalation

10.3.2 High-Frequency Jet Ventilation

HFJV is a versatile, safe and effective technique with ever growing indications for elective and emergency use. This form of jet ventilation is most commonly used in clinical settings. Thus though this chapter will mostly be dealing with HFJV, most of the parameters can be extended to other forms jet ventilation.

10.3.2.1 Working Principle

HFJV is characterized by delivery of small tidal volumes (1–3 mL/kg) from a high pressure jet at high frequencies (1–10 Hz), made into square wave pressures by a high-frequency flow interrupter, e.g., electrical solenoid valve, followed by passive expiration. Other options available are fluidic or rotating cylinder valve. The criteria mentioned below can be modified to fit to a particular patient and situation:

- Driving-pressure.
- Frequency.
- Inspiratory time composition of the jet gas.

High pressure safety devices need to be instituted in these ventilators. Jet catheters can be inserted via tracheal tubes or can be used alone.

Table 10.1 Types of jet ventilation with the specialized ventilators/equipment for facilitating gas exchange

Ventilation type	Gas exchange equipment	Examples
LFJV	Hand triggered devices	Sanders injector and Manujet III (VBM, Germany)
HFJV	HFJV ventilators	Mistral/monsoon jet ventilators
SHFJV	Jet ventilators	Bronchotron respirator, laryngojet

Various modifications can be made in HFJV by using trans tracheal jet cannulae, various catheter design, different catheter material and number of lumens. CO_2 sampling and intra-tracheal pressure monitoring can be done with the help of extra lumens. The catheter tip position can be either above or below the vocal cords.

Do's	Don'ts
Humidification	Rapid increase in set ventilator parameters

10.3.2.2 Indications

HFJV is indicated when it offers advantages over conventional ventilation. These indications fall into two categories; to facilitate surgical access and to optimize pulmonary function (Tables 10.2 and 10.3).

10.3.2.3 Precautions

Humidification is needed to prevent drying of airways and heat loss. Rapid increase in set ventilatory parameters should be avoided (Tables 10.4 and 10.5).

> **Tip** The combination of PCV and HFJV is beneficial in cases of ARDS complicated by BPF.

10.3.3 Superimposed High Frequency Jet Ventilation

10.3.3.1 Definition

A combination of HFJV and LFJV is called superimposed high frequency jet ventilation (SHFJV) and is a double-jet technique.

10.3.3.2 Working Principle

SHFJV enables enhanced convection from normal frequency jet ventilation with enhanced diffusion and alveolar mixing from HFJV which produces more effective gas exchange in the presence of a tracheal stenosis. Two jet streams with different frequencies are applied at the same time. The continuous high-frequency jet stream is superimposed during the inspiratory and expiratory phases of the low-frequency jet ventilation.

The low-frequency jet stream results in phased airway pressure changes similar to conventional ventilation with a frequency of 0.2–0.3 Hz, and provided the upper pressure level. The high-frequency jet stream with a frequency of 1.5–15 Hz generates the lower pressure level (PEEP).

Table 10.2 Indications for HFJV

Improving surgical access	Optimize pulmonary function
1. ENT Diagnostic laryngoscopy—delivery of small tidal volumes—less vocal cord movement whilst high-pressure ventilation permits the use of narrow bore jet ventilation catheters (constructed from non-flammable, fluoroplastic material—can be used in laser surgery)	1. Thoracic surgery Anastomosis of a major conducting airway (airtight connection between airway and breathing system not needed) Selective HFJV of non-dependent lung (minimizing shunt by increasing MAWP, aiding perfusion and allowing carbon dioxide removal. Major bronchopleural fistulae and tracheobronchial disruptions (smaller gas leak through pathological low-resistance pathways-minimal mediastinal and interstitial emphysema)
2. Radiofrequency ablation (RFA) Liver tumours—reduced breathing-related liver motion (12 mm to 2 mm) RFA of the left atrium—more stable left atrial environment with less variation in left atrium volume and fewer ablations required Lithotripsy-elimination of diaphragmatic excursion for use in extra-corporeal shock wave lithotripsy—reduced urinary calculus movement and less patient exposure to tissue trauma	2. Critical care HFJV is well suited for lung protective ventilation strategies for patients with acute lung injury or ARDS. Low tidal volumes reduce the risk of over-distension and volutrauma. The shear stresses associated with repeated opening and closing of terminal airways is much less as compared to conventional ventilation strategies. Reduced pressure swings during the ventilatory cycle and increased MAWP optimize end-expiratory lung volume, preventing collapse and cyclic atelectatrauma

Table 10.3 Adjustments of HFJV components in cases of hypoxemia and hypercapnia

Adjustments of HFJV components		
	Hypoxemia	Hypercapnia
F (frequency)	—	↓
FiO_2	↑	↑
IT (%) {inspiratory time}	↑	↑
DP (driving pressures) Bar	↑	↑

Table 10.4 Contraindications of HFJV

Absolute	Relative
Pneumonia Active asthma	Morbid obesity (poor basal oxygenation) Uncontrolled coagulopathy Tracheal obstruction

Table 10.5 Advantages and disadvantages of HFJV

Advantages	Disadvantages
1. Decreased peak airway pressure	1. Risk of barotrauma
2. Less hemodynamic compromise	2. Cooling and drying of gases
3. Less fluid retention	3. Less predictable gas exchange
4. Better surgical access	4. Increase in dead space due to pendelluft
5. Less chances of airway fires	5. Lower airway soiling can occur
6. Good in low resistance and large volume leaks	6. Contamination of expired gases by surgical debris
7. Versatile	7. High gas flow is required
	8. CO_2 measurement is difficult
	9. Inhalational agents cannot be used

10.3.3.3 Indications

SHFJV is mainly reserved for micro laryngeal surgeries and laryngeal LASER surgeries with severe tracheal stenosis. It is very useful in paediatric patients as it is less invasive and provides supraglottic access to surgical field. It can also be used to tracheal and bronchial stents.

10.3.3.4 Advantages

SHFJV produces more effective gas exchange as compared to HFJV alone over a wide range of frequencies. Both HFJV and SHFJV generate high auto-PEEP distal to any form of tracheal stenosis. The risk of barotrauma is less as compared to other forms of jet ventilation.

10.3.4 High-Frequency Oscillatory Ventilation (HFOV)

10.3.4.1 Working Principle

In HFOV both inspiration and expiration are active, i.e., the oscillatory flow is generated by a piston or a diaphragm of a pump or a similar device at the airway opening with a tracheal tube. HFO can also be generated by rapid thoracic or whole body surface compressions (Table 10.6).

10.3.4.2 Indications

It has been mainly used in the neonatal intensive care setting, but can be used in any age group. Ventilator frequencies of 10–15 Hz are used. This type of ventilation can be superimposed on top of conventional ventilation to improve oxygenation and reduce ventilator-associated lung injury. In case surgical procedures in pediatric patients with abdominal wall defects and diaphragmatic hernia, conventional ventilation cannot provide adequate oxygenation without using high FiO_2 and high infiltrating pressures.

10.3.4.3 Advantages

There are less chances of lung injury and retrolental fibroplasia in premature infants with HFOV. It can be used in infants with abnormal lung compliance.

Table 10.6 Approaches for jet ventilation

Technique	Advantages	Disadvantages
Supraglotic	Tubeless field	Rapid increase in airway pressure Reliance on surgeons for adequate ventilation No PAWP/PETCO$_2$ monitoring Vocal cord movement No control of FiO$_2$
Trans tracheal	Tubeless field Control FiO$_2$	Incomplete control of ventilation Contraindicated in tight stenosis No PAWP/PETCO$_2$ monitoring
Subglottic	Minimal increase in airway pressure Controls FiO$_2$ PAWP/ETCO$_2$ monitoring	Catheter in surgical field

10.3.4.4 Disadvantages

This mode cannot be used for transporting a patient between the ICU and operation theatre. Also routine capnography is not possible with this mode of ventilation. There is very little experience in this mode among the anesthesiologists which is a major limitation.

10.4 Approaches and Techniques of Jet Ventilation (Table 10.7)

10.4.1 Supraglotic Technique (Fig. 10.2)

- It does not require an expiration valve.
- When the pre-set value is reached, the alarm is activated, and further inspiration is suspended (end-expiratory pressure or high limit for PEEP). Jiang and Kacmarek suggest a value of less than 10 cmH$_2$O, especially in the case of moderate-to-severe tracheal stenosis where high auto-PEEP can drastically increase due to compromised expiration.
- The pre-set *bypass* allows a fresh gas flow between 0 and 70 L/min.

10.4.2 Trans Tracheal Approach

Trans tracheal jet ventilation (TTJV) is the introduction of pressurized oxygen usually through a narrow bore cannula cricothyrodotomy. Narrow bore cannula has been defined as <4 mm or <2 mm. Scalpel cricothyrodotomy is usually preferred as it gives better access. In case of CICV situation, an angiocath can be directly inserted in to the trachea. The non-dominant hand is used to stabilize the trachea and palpate the cricothyroid membrane. The tip of the angiocath needle attached to a 10 cm syringe with 5 mL of saline in is inserted in to the cricothyroid membrane. Free return of air confirms the intraluminal position. Angiocath is then advanced over the needle. The hub is connected to a hand operated valve which in turn is connected to the wall mounted oxygen supply at a pressure of 50 psi.

10.4.3 Subglottic Approach

In this approach, the patient is induced after adequate pre-oxygenation. A subglottic catheter is inserted (Hunsaker tube). The tip is placed infraglottically while aiming not to touch the tracheal walls with the aid of laryngoscope, Magill's forceps. In case of CO$_2$ laser surgery laser resistant catheters are used. One lumen or multiple lumen catheters can be used. After a proper fixation, the surgical procedure can be started immediately or a LMA can be inserted for ventilation. CO$_2$ can be monitored from the side port.

The subglottic technique causes less obstruction to expiration as compared to supraglottic technique. The reasons for this are as follows:

- Venturi Effect—gas flow at a constriction speeds up causing a pressure drop and entrain-

Table 10.7 Important features of various jet ventilation approaches

	Supraglottic	Trans tracheal	Subglottic
Uses	Induction (bronchoscopy, ENT procedures) Procedural ventilation (positive pressure ventilation) Laser procedures (FiO_2–0.4) BPF	Complete upper airway obstruction CICV	Reducing expiratory impedance, gas trapping ENT procedures
Humidification	0–100% Sterile water Prewarmed fresh gas	0–100% Sterile water	0–100% Sterile water
Safety features	Alarms—pause pressure (*PP*) High peak inspiratory pressure (*PIP*)	PP and PIP	
Surgical access	Full surgical access Tubeless	Full surgical access	Partial surgical access

Do's	Don'ts
• Set parameters at lower values initially and increase as per need later • Increase according to $EtCO_2$/$PaCO_2$/clinical parameters	• Saline for humidification

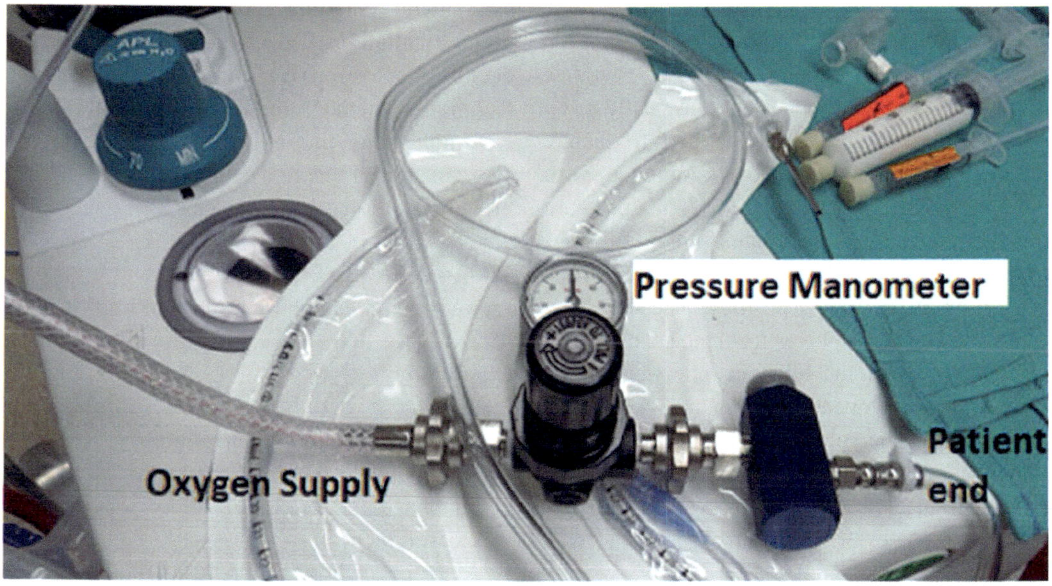

Fig. 10.2 Transoral jet ventilation set up

ment. Supraglottic jet ventilation is a true Venturi type of ventilation and the tidal volume is the sum of injected and entrained air.

- Flow characteristics in conducting airways—turbulent flow exists in the conducting airways, with primarily laminar flow in distal airways and alveoli. A supraglottic point of injection creates a greater column of turbulent flow causing a greater resistance to expiratory flow and gas trapping.
- Double jetting—when a supraglottic jet is applied, some gas is reflected from the glottis/stenosis thereby increasing supraglottic pressure. This acts as a second high pressure

jet source directing gas beyond the stenosis as well as creating an unfavourable pressure gradient for exhaust gases, thus impeding expiratory flow and increasing gas trapping.
- Expiratory impedance—exhaust gas must be expired through the glottis/stenosis, which is only open during the expiratory phase of the cycle with supraglottic techniques. Expiratory impedance therefore depends on the inspiratory: expiratory (I:E) ratio and the area of the stenosis aperture.

> **Tip** On emergence from anesthesia, small V_T values and low peak and mean airway pressures associated with subglottic HFJV enable the patient to breathe spontaneously, facilitating a transition to adequate spontaneous ventilation.

10.4.4 Equipment

The Mistral jet ventilator is an electrically powered, solenoid cycled, automatic, high frequency jet ventilator. The ventilator is supplied with compressed air. After passing through a pressure regulator, the gas reaches a manifold of four electromagnetic solenoid valves in parallel, which are closed in the resting position. The supply of oxygen is at 4 atmospheres from the hospital supply system. When the solenoids are excited, one or more valves open, and generate a discrete pulse of gas. The volume of each pulse is determined by setting the respiratory frequency, I:E ratio, and DP. The output of the ventilator is not influenced by external factors such as airway resistance or lung compliance.

This limit is set as the pause pressure (PP), which is the pressure inside the airway and is measured from the tip of the jet ventilation catheter between each jet. The PP approximates the mean airway pressure.

10.4.4.1 Oxygen Delivery

FiO_2 depends on the degree of air entrainment. A decrease in chest wall or lung compliance will result in a reduction in minute ventilation as pressure HFJV is a time-cycled, pressure-limited ventilation. End-expiratory pressure can be measured through the injector placed at the end of insufflation but there can be regional variations that are exaggerated at high frequencies. Modern jet ventilators are equipped with a second airway measurement line, which monitors the airway pressure continuously and independently of the jet insufflation line. Despite a frequency-dependent positive end-expiratory pressure is usually present, the resulting mean and peak airway pressures are much lower than during conventional ventilation. Some modern jet ventilators ex. the Monsoon, Acutronic Medical Systems AG, Baar, Switzerland allow FiO_2 selection.

10.4.4.2 Carbon Dioxide Measurement

Carbon dioxide measurement is difficult in such an open breathing system utilizing high gas flow; it requires temporary cessation of respiration for side-stream sampling following standard, tidal volume inflation. The driving pressure is the deciding factor for CO_2 elimination. Alternative techniques include trans-cutaneous continuous CO_2 monitoring, intermittent blood gas sampling from an arterial line or a continuous intra-arterial blood-gas measurement device.

10.4.4.3 Safety Equipment

Jet ventilation can cause rapid build-up of pressure in case of inadequate egress of air during expiration.

- A ventilator high pressure alarm.
- An automatic shutdown facility.
- Esophageal or intra-pleural pressure measurement.
- A PP exceeding the pre-set value results in activation of an alarm and suspension of further ventilation.

10.4.4.4 Jet Ventilation Catheters

Supraglottic

This techniques employ "tubeless" HFJV, with jet ventilation catheters used for trans tracheal and subglottic approaches.

Subglottic Catheters (Fig. 10.3)

The Hunsaker Mon-Jet and LaserJet catheters are double lumen catheters designed for subglottic HFJV. They have a metal stylet to aid intubation and are made of non-flammable, laser-resistant material. The LaserJet Catheter comes in two lengths—40 or 70 cm. They have an external diameter of 3.4 mm. they have two lumens, one for delivering gas and the other for monitoring airway pressure and $ETCO_2$. Tube length can be decided by approximating the length from the lips to the glottis by placing the tube along the patient's airway before insertion. The red cuff surrounding the tube is then positioned at the correct point.

Trans Tracheal Catheters

These are available in a large variety. Most commonly used is the Ravussin jet ventilation catheter, which is available in three sizes: 13 G, 14 G and 16 G for adults, children and infants respectively. They are kink resistant and are also used in manual jet ventilation (Fig. 10.4).

10.4.5 Parameters and Settings

Variables for clinical use are—rate/frequency, driving pressure, DP; inspiratory time, I-time (% ventilatory cycle); and inspired oxygen fraction, FiO_2. The tidal volume is a function of entrainment volume, driving pressure, inspiratory time, cannula resistance, and impedance of the respiratory system. Increasing the frequency can induce hypercapnia by reducing the tidal volume if DP and I-time are kept constant. Intrinsic PEEP is an important component of HFJV; it is inversely related to expiratory time and increases with the frequency. It is most likely to exceed safe values in lung units with long time-constants. Increasing DP leads to increased VT and airway pressure and a reduced PCO_2. However, large increases in DP may lead to CO_2 retention if the set frequency is too high to allow time for adequate expiration as the respiratory cycle has been shortened. In cases of bronchopleural fistula (BPF), these settings are most commonly used-rate > 200/min, DP at 1.5 bar or less, and an injection time around 40%. The complications of jet ventilation are summarized in Table 10.8.

> **Tip** Total outflow obstruction with resultant barotrauma during subglottic HFJV can be quickly precipitated by surgical instrumentation, glottic edema, laryngospasm, or closure of the vocal cords due to inadequate

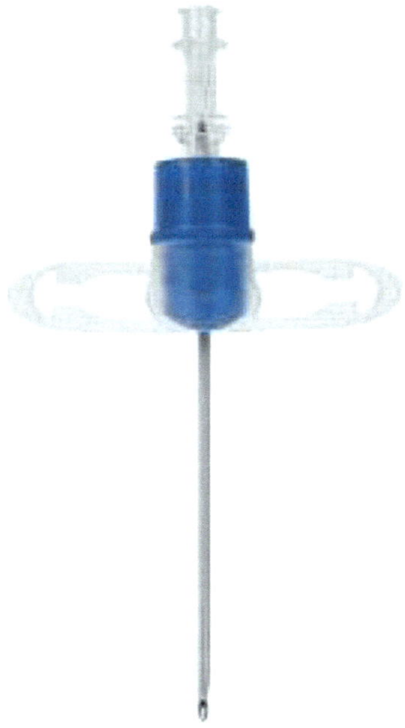

Fig. 10.4 Transtracheal catheter

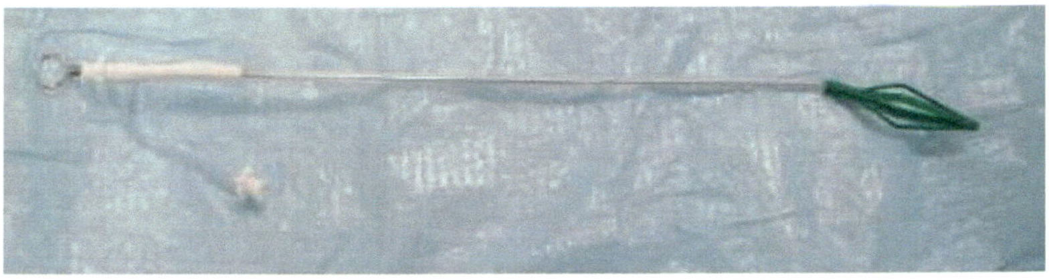

Fig. 10.3 Subglottic jet ventilation catheter

Table 10.8 Complications of jet ventilation

Barotrauma	Faulty ventilation	Dry gas
Pneumothorax Pneumopercardium Subcutaneous emphysema Hypotension Pneumomediastinum Right ventricular failure	Hypoxia Hypercapnia Airway contamination	Mucosal trauma Tracheal necrosis Atelectasis

depth of anesthesia or inadequate muscle relaxation. Hence adequate plane of anaesthesia/muscle relaxation should be maintained during HFJV.

10.4.6 Recent Advances

Jet ventilation is being used in various fields and situations. Its use is no longer limited to bronchoscopy and ENT surgeries. Recent study showed better results in atrial ablation with HFJV.

There is rigorous research regarding its use in premature infants. Its use is also being explored in out of OT procedures, for example colonoscopy. Despite all this, it cannot be denied that jet ventilation requires expensive equipment and manpower training. For it to become a general practice, extensive research showing positive results in comparison to other conventional methods of ventilation will be required.

Suggested Reading

1. Ravussin P, Freeman J. A new transtracheal catheter for ventilation and resuscitation. Can Anaesth Soc J. 1985;32(1):60–4. https://doi.org/10.1007/BF03008540.
2. Klain M, Smith RB. High frequency percutaneous transtracheal jet ventilation. Crit Care Med. 1977;5(6):280–7. https://doi.org/10.1097/00003246-197711000-00007.
3. Babinski M, Smith RB, Klain M. High-frequency jet ventilation for laryngoscopy. Anesthesiology. 1980;52(2):178–80.
4. Brice JW, Davis WB. High frequency ventilation in the adult. Clin Pulm Med. 2004;11(2):101–6. https://doi.org/10.1097/01.cpm.0000117768.13803.be.
5. Abe K, Oka J, Takahashi H, Funatsu T, Fukuda H, Miyamoto Y. Effect of high-frequency jet ventilation on oxygenation during one-lung ventilation in patients undergoing thoracic aneurysm surgery. J Anesth. 2006;20(1):1–5. https://doi.org/10.1007/s00540-005-0352-y.
6. Biro P, Spahn DR, Pfammatter T. High-frequency jet ventilation for minimizing breathing-related liver motion during percutaneous radiofrequency ablation of multiple hepatic tumours. Br J Anaesth. 2009;102(5):650–3. https://doi.org/10.1093/bja/aep051.
7. Canty DJ, Dhara SS. High frequency jet ventilation through a supraglottic airway device: a case series of patients undergoing extra-corporeal shock wave lithotripsy. Anaesthesia. 2009;64(12):1295–8. https://doi.org/10.1111/j.1365-2044.2009.06079.x.
8. Ethawi YH, Abou Mehrem A, Minski J, Ruth CA, Davis PG. High frequency jet ventilation versus high frequency oscillatory ventilation for pulmonary dysfunction in preterm infants. Cochrane Database Syst Rev. 2016;5:CD010548. https://doi.org/10.1002/14651858.CD010548.pub2.
9. Herridge MS, Slutsky AS, Colditz GA. Has high-frequency ventilation been inappropriately discarded in adult acute respiratory distress syndrome? Crit Care Med. 1998;26(12):2073–7. https://doi.org/10.1097/00003246-199812000-00044.
10. Courtney SE, Durand DJ, Asselin JM, Eichenwald EC, Stark AR. Pro/con clinical debate: high-frequency oscillatory ventilation is better than conventional ventilation for premature infants. Crit Care. 2003;7(6):423–6. https://doi.org/10.1186/cc2178.
11. Yang Z-Y, Meng Q, Xu Y-H, Wang J-W, Yu D-S, Wei H-F. Supraglottic jet oxygenation and ventilation during colonoscopy under monitored anesthesia care: a controlled randomized clinical trial. Eur Rev Med Pharmacol Sci. 2016;20(6):1168–73.

11 Central Venous Catheter

Mayur Rama Krishna Chillal

Key Points

- A central venous catheter (CVC) is a catheter placed into a large vein in the body located in the neck, chest, or groin. It is used for a variety of medical purposes, including administering medications, fluids, and nutrition.
- Complications associated with CVC include infection, bleeding, and damage to the surrounding structures.
- The site and number of lumens used should be selected carefully.
- CVC must be cared regularly to reduce the risk of infection and other complications.

11.1 Definition of CV Access

A central venous catheter (CVC) is an indwelling device that is inserted into a large, central vein (most commonly the subclavian, internal jugular, or femoral), and advanced until the distal orifice resides within the inferior vena cava (IVC), superior vena cava (SVC), aortocaval junction, right atrium (RA), or the brachiocephalic vein. Most often, the desired position of the distal tip of the central line is the SVC or more specifically aortocaval junction. The term peripherally inserted central catheter (PICC) is used when the CVC is inserted into the central compartment via a peripheral vein.

11.2 History of CVC

It was in 1929 when the placement of a CVC was first described. Following this, central venous access has rapidly developed into an experimental instrument for studying cardiac physiology and an indispensable clinical tool in treating many disease processes. The procedure has remained relatively unchanged since the advent of the Seldinger technique in the 1960s. However, a notable exception is the supplementation of ultrasound guidance, which has recently become the standard of care for CVCs placed in the internal jugular vein, resulting in decreased complications, and increased first-pass success (Fig. 11.1).

Indications

1. For hemodynamic monitoring.
2. Transfusion of products, that may be incompatible with peripheral intravenous access, such as vasopressors, total parenteral nutrition, chemotherapy, and other medications that are irritable to the peripheral veins.
3. Inability to obtain peripheral venous access in an emergency.

M. R. K. Chillal (✉)
Critical Care Medicine, Unity Health Network, St. Michaels Hospital, Toronto, Canada

N. Gupta et al. (eds.), *Techniques in Anesthesia, Intensive Care and Emergency Medicine*,
https://doi.org/10.1007/978-981-96-1202-4_11

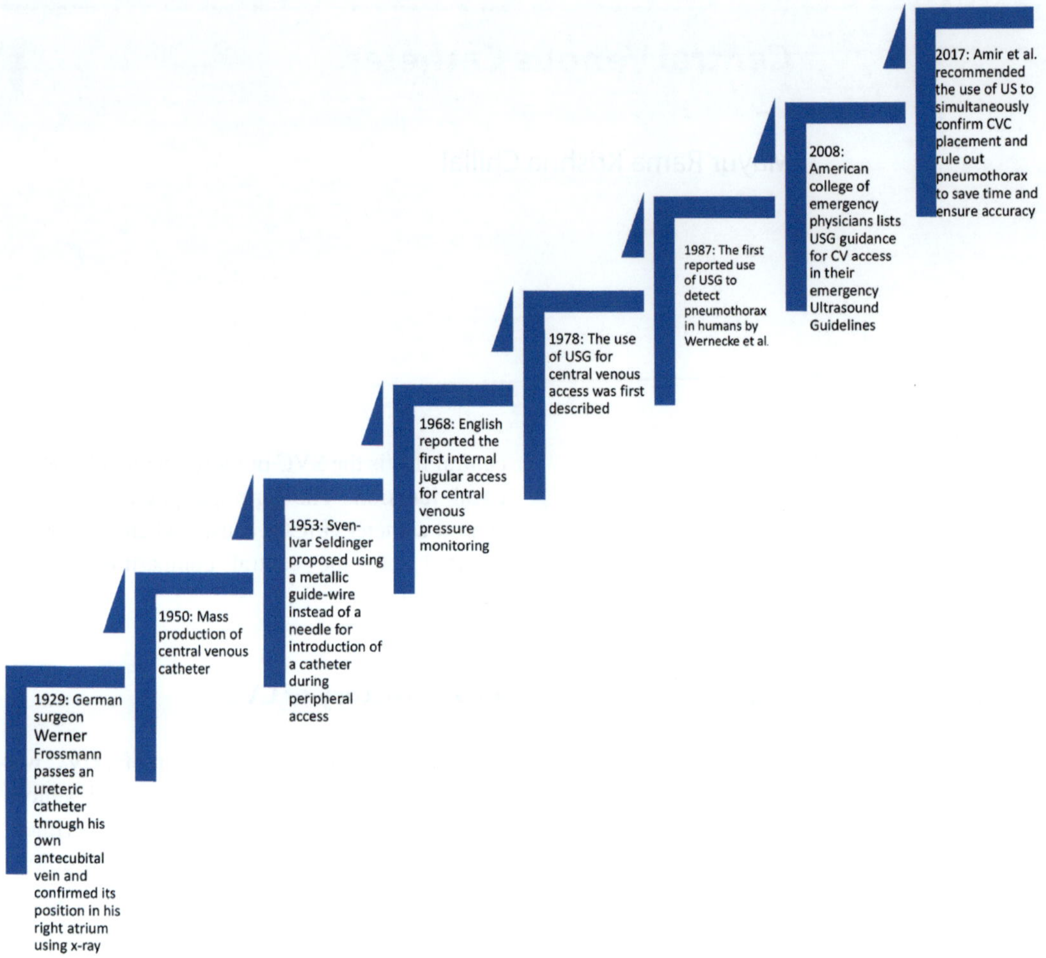

Fig. 11.1 Timeline representing the advances in the evolution of central venous access

4. For extracorporeal therapies, such as plasmapheresis, hemodialysis, and continuous renal replacement therapy.
5. Critical interventions include inferior vena cava filter placement, transvenous pacing, thrombolytic therapy, etc.

Contraindications

Absolute Contraindications

1. Vascular injuries proximal or distal to the site of insertion
2. Active skin and soft tissue infections at the site of insertion

Relative Contraindications

1. Coagulopathy
2. Thrombocytopenia
3. Distorted anatomical landmarks, due to contractures, trauma, etc.
4. Uncooperative awake patient

It may be warranted to consider transfusing fresh frozen plasma and/or platelets before or after the procedure, in certain patients who have an international normalized ratio (INR) of greater than 3.0, or platelets less than 20×10^9/L as there is an increased chance of bleeding. The subclavian (SC) site is usually contraindicated in coagulopathic patients, due to the inability to apply pressure in the event of accidental arterial puncture. Also, the femoral site, especially the right side, should be avoided in a chronic kidney disease patient awaiting a renal transplant.

Equipment

- Personal protective equipment: including gloves, gown, mask
- Drape
- Gauze (4 × 4)
- Chlorohexidine swabs or similar antiseptic agent
- Sterile ultrasound probe cover with sterile ultrasound gel
- Catheter caps for each lumen
- Ultrasound machine with a high-frequency linear transducer probe

Central venous catheter kit, which generally includes:

- Central venous catheter (triple-lumen, dual-lumen, or large bore single-lumen)
- 18-gauge introducer needle, with a syringe
- #11 blade scalpel
- Guidewire
- Venodilator
- Suture material (generally 3–0 silk suture with a straight needle or a needle driver)
- 1% lidocaine, small gauge needle (25 or 27 gauge), syringe

Preparation

The procedure and its potential complications should be explained first to the patient or their relative and written informed consent should be obtained.

An ultrasound scan should be done to evaluate the preferable site, anatomical variations, the compressibility of the vein, and the ease with which the procedure can be performed. The concerned nursing staff must be informed so that the necessary equipment can be ready. Positioning the patient before the procedure is an important key to successful cannulation. For Subclavian and IJV, the patient is placed in a Trendelenburg position to increase the caliber of the vein and better visibility on the USG. The patient is placed in a supine or semi-supine position for the femoral vein. Necessary adjustments with the bed height are done as required. When the primary nurse is present, the patient is prepared, hand hygiene is performed and a sterile gown, gloves, surgical cap, mask, and face shield are donned. The central venous catheter for insertion is prepared by flushing each lumen with saline or heparinized saline. Skin is sterilized with an antiseptic agent and the area is covered with a sterile fenestrated drape. Next, the ultrasound probe is prepared with the help of an assistant who can dispense adequate acoustic gel over the probe. Then the probe is fed into the sterile transducer sheath, over the length of the probe cable. The sheath around the transducer is secured using sterile rubber bands or plastic clips. During the whole procedure, appropriate patient monitoring should be in place, including electrocardiography, blood pressure, pulse oximetry, and, if possible, end-tidal carbon dioxide.

Technique of Insertion

- Once the vein of choice has been decided for cannulation, the proceduralist should stand at the patient's side ipsilateral to the target site. Under USG guidance the vein of insertion is identified before giving 1% lidocaine to anesthetize skin and subcutaneous tissue.
- Align the probe marker with the marker on the screen to be ensure that the image that appears on the USG screen is oriented correctly.
- The introducer needle attached with a 5-cc syringe should be advanced at a 45–90-degree angle under USG guidance through the skin until a flash of blood is seen. Ensure visualization of the needle tip throughout the procedure (Fig. 11.2).
- Once the introducer needle has been confirmed to be inside the vein, it should be stabilized, and the guide wire should be threaded through the needle. The proceduralist should ensure that the wire is advanced easily without any resistance. If there is any resistance then

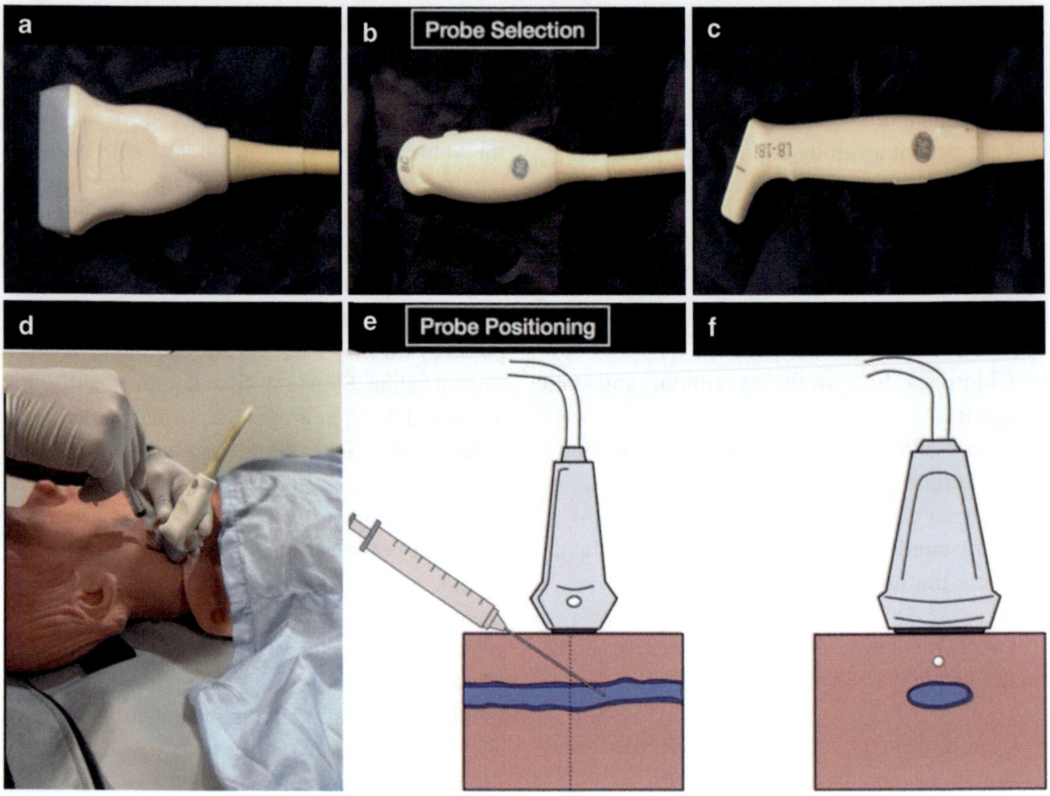

Fig. 11.2 (**a**) High-frequency linear probe. (**b**) Micro-convex ultrasound probe, the lower frequency for subclavian vein assessment. (**c**) Hockey stick high-frequency probe, mainly helpful in obese patients and children. (**d**) probe position for IJV cannulation. (**e**) In-plane or long-axis probe position. (**f**) Out-of-plane or short–axis probe position

the guidewire might not be in the vessel, or there may be an obstruction in the pathway, or it could be advancing in a retrograde direction.

- Once the guide wire has reached around the 15 cm mark, it should be stabilized, and the needle is withdrawn ensuring that the guidewire does not migrate down.
- Confirm guidewire position using USG. Next, thread the dilator onto the guidewire and toward the junction of the skin and the wire. A scalpel can be used to create a nick in the skin, so that dilator can be threaded easily. While threading the dilator, one can use the screwing motion of the hand such that it will help to dilate soft tissue and enable passage of the catheter.
- After adequate dilatation, remove the dilator and thread the CVC should be over the guidewire. Once the CVC has been inserted, the guidewire should be pulled out.
- Aspirate blood from each port with the help of a syringe. All ports should be flushed with saline and attach "Luer locks" to the end of each port.
- CVC should be sutured in place and a bio patch should be placed catheter hub and the skin and a sterile occlusive dressing should be applied over the catheter entry site.
- Adequate measures should be taken for biowaste disposal in a biohazard bin.
- Other than USG guided Confirmation of the CVC it can also be done using a chest X-ray for SCV and IJV.
- Chest X-ray can also be used to rule out any complications such as pneumothorax and also to verify the distal tip of the CVC.

Considerations in the technique of insertion for the individual veins.

11.2.1 IJV

Landmark Technique (Fig. 11.3)

Anterior approach: the needle has to be inserted along the medial edge of the sternocleidomastoid (SCM) muscle, 2–3 finger breadths above the clavicle with an entry angle around 30–45°. The needle should be directed towards the ipsilateral nipple and the carotid artery should be palpated and if needed can be retracted slightly medially.

Central approach: the needle should be inserted at the apex of the triangle formed by the heads of the SCM muscle and the clavicle with an entry angle of around 30°. The needle should be pointed toward the ipsilateral nipple.

Posterior approach: the needle should be inserted at the SCM's posterior (lateral) edge, midway between the mastoid process and the clavicle. During the needle advancement, pressure can be applied to lift the body of the muscle.

USG Guided Technique (Fig. 11.4)

- Anatomically IJV is located laterally (both anterolaterally and posterolaterally) in the neck more than 90% of the time.
- Neck being a rounded structure, scanning it in a true anterior-posterior orientation is not possible. This forces the operator to slide the probe laterally, placing it perpendicular to the skin, and scanning the neck on a lateral to medial axis. This orients the IJV on top of the common carotid artery (CCA). This predisposes CCA cannulation or injury esp. in the short axis.
- Needle insertion point: while using the USG technique needle entry point can be anywhere along the neck, unlike the landmark technique. The head should be placed in a neutral position, as rotating the head increases the incidence of superimposing the IJV over CCA.
- Either a short or long-axis approach can be used based on one's expertise. The needle is inserted very close to the probe (usually <1 cm from the probe), with the angle almost perpendicular to the neck.
- With a short-axis approach the main drawback is visualizing the tip of the needle throughout the insertion period. Hence it becomes important to visualize the intraluminal guidewire proximally towards the heart. Ideally, the guidewire should be demonstrated in the brachiocephalic vein in the long-axis view.

11.2.2 SCV

Landmark Technique (Fig. 11.5)

The tip of the index finger placed on the sternal notch and the thumb at the midpoint of the clavicle, the introducer needle should be inserted inferior to the clavicular midpoint (or 1–2 cm inferior to the junction of the medial and middle third of the clavicle) at a shallow angle to the skin and skirting the underside of the clavicle aiming towards the sternal notch. The introducer needle should be advanced gently until a flash of blood

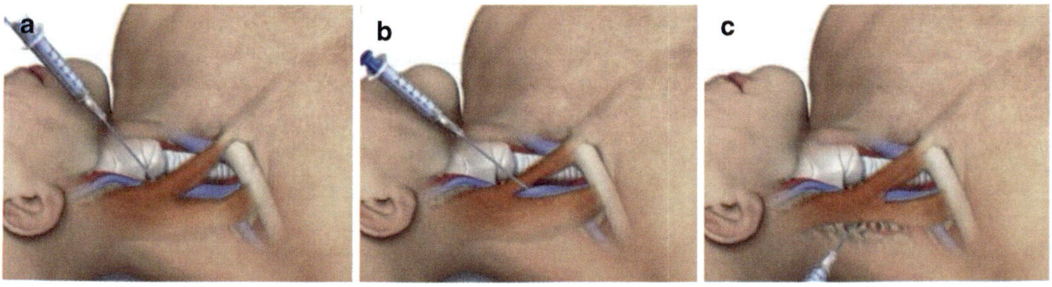

Fig. 11.3 (**a**) Anterior approach. (**b**) Central approach. (**c**) Posterior approach

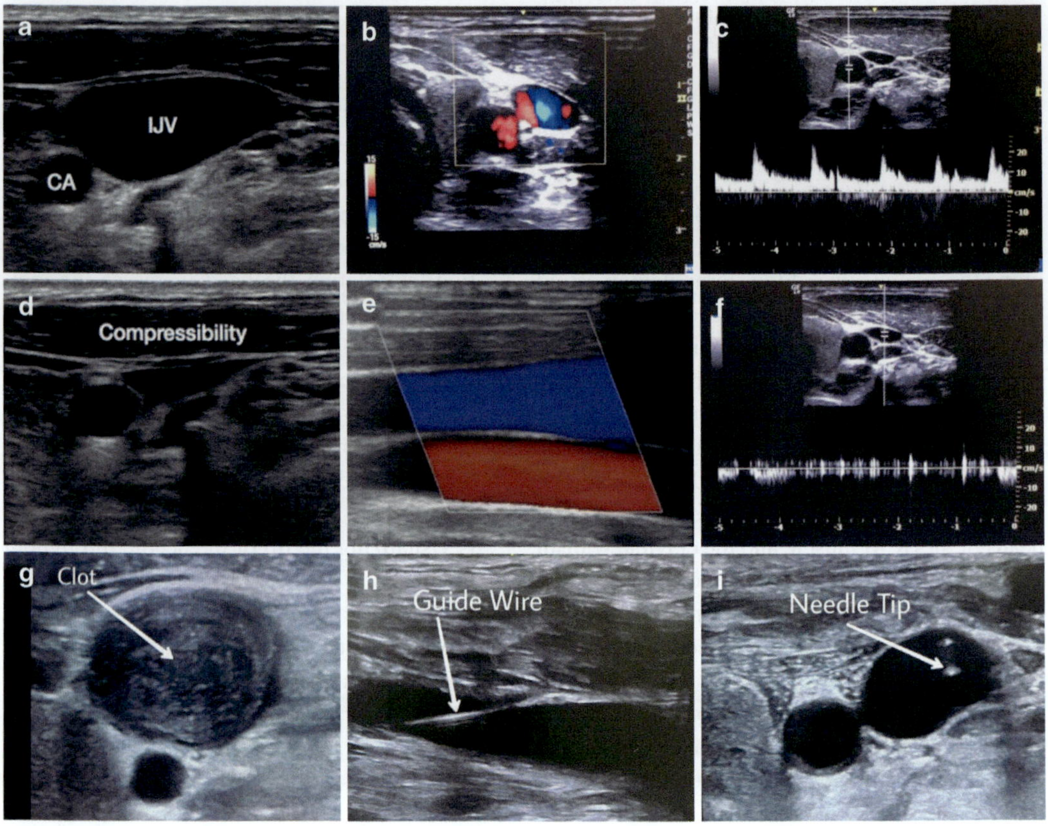

Fig. 11.4 USG images for IJV assessment. (**a**) IJV. (**b**) and (**e**) short and long axis with color flow Doppler. (**c**) and (**f**) Pulse wave Doppler to differentiate between artery and vein. (**d**) IJV compressible compared to the Carotid Artery (CA). (**g**) Clot in IJV causing noncompressibility of the vein. (**h**) Guidewire in the IJV seen in the long-axis view. (**i**) needle tip visualized in the IJV (short-axis view)

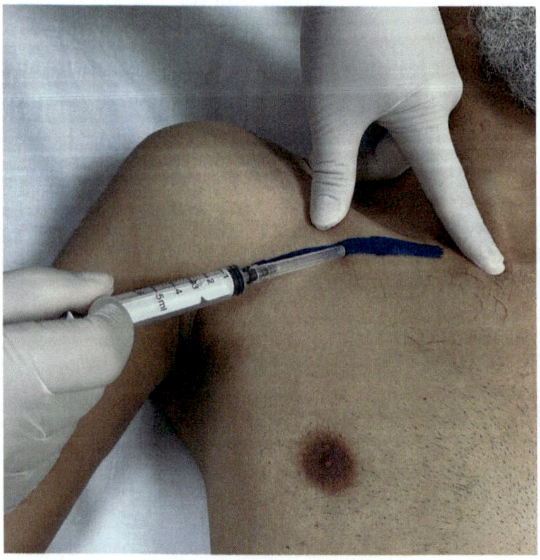

Fig. 11.5 Landmark technique for subclavian cannulation (infraclavicular approach)

is seen, and the syringe should be rotated such that the bevel of the needle faces inferiorly (i.e., away from the IJV and towards the heart). This is followed by the insertion of the guidewire and the rest of the procedure is completed.

USG Guided Technique

Either a short or long-axis approach can be used. The advantage of using a short axis is that it allows visualization of the vessel along with the surrounding structures, such as the artery, nerve, and pleura. Here the probe is placed in the infraclavicular fossa, cephalo-caudally as laterally as possible. The SCV is demonstrated in the short axis, and the probe is slid medially keeping the vein under vision, probe is rotated by 90° to produce a long-axis view. It is important to demonstrate the pleura in this view, the artery can be visualized by tilting the probe slightly cephalad. Also, color and pulse wave Doppler can be used to differentiate between the artery and the vein (Fig. 11.6).

Once the optimal image is obtained, the probe is stabilized, and the needle is inserted in the midpoint of the linear footprint (the in-plane approach). One must make sure that the needle is seen once it is under the skin and advanced under constant visualization. Once inside the vein, the guidewire is inserted, and the rest of the procedure is completed as already described.

11.2.3 Femoral Vein

Landmark Technique

- Palpate the femoral artery inferior to the inguinal ligament with the femoral vein lying medially adjacent to the artery in the femoral canal.
- Puncture the vein at 1–2 cm inferior to the inguinal ligament as shown in the figure and the rest of the procedure remains the same as mentioned already.

The femoral approach has some advantages over the IJV and SCV, that it is distant from the airway and monitoring devices and does not carry the risk of pneumothorax and hemothorax, though it is more prone to infections and thrombosis.

For the ultrasound technique, the probe is placed parallel below the inguinal ligament for out-of-plane and perpendicular for the in-plane technique. Artery and vein can be differentiated with the help of Doppler and anatomy as the vein is medial to the artery in its initial course. Once the vein is identified rest of the procedure is like IJV cannulation (Fig. 11.7).

Complications

Procedural Complications

Arrhythmias—typically ventricular or bundle branch blocks due to guidewire irritation of the atria or ventricles

Arterial puncture

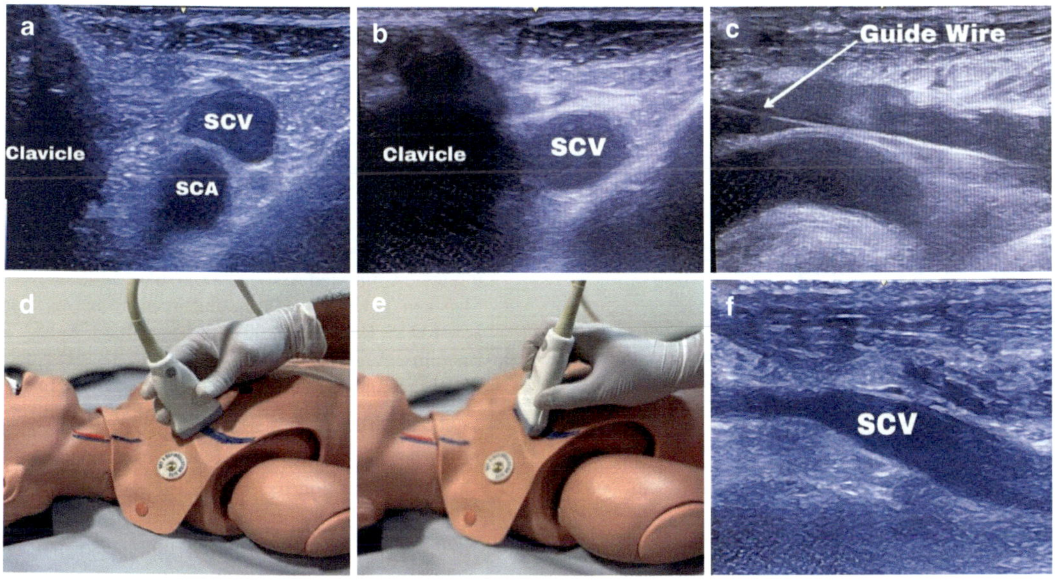

Fig. 11.6. (**a**) and (**d**) showing the USG image of SCV and the position of the USG probe held cephalo caudally respectively. Also, pleura can be appreciated in image **a**. (**b**) As the USG probe is slid medially only SCV can be visualized. (**c**) guidewire seen passing through the SCV. (**e**) and (**f**) Probe rotated 90° to produce long axis view of the SCV

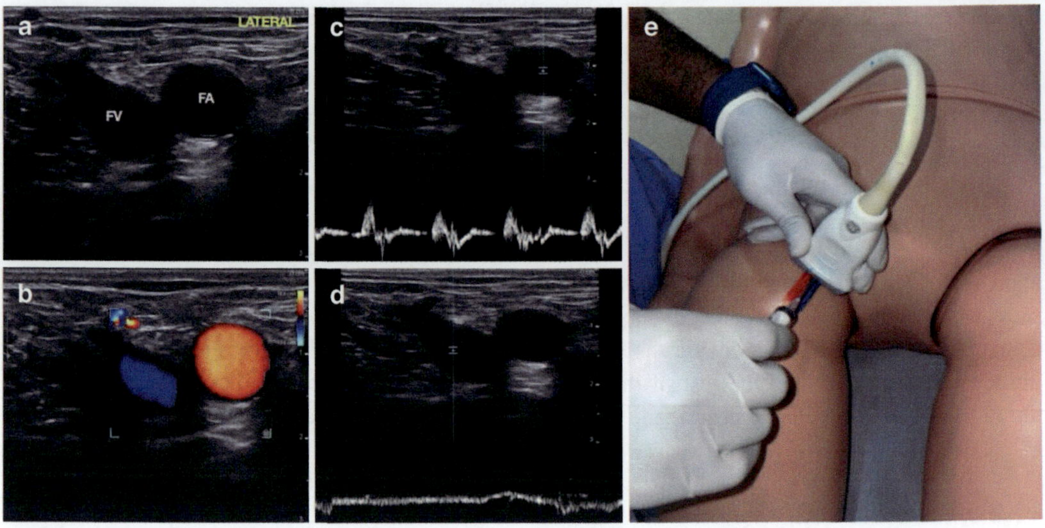

Fig. 11.7 (**a**) Short-axis view of the femoral vein. (**b**) Color Doppler image. (**c**) and (**d**) showing pulse wave Doppler image for differentiation between vein and artery. (**e**) The position of the probe for the short-axis view

Pulmonary puncture with or without resultant pneumothorax Bleeding—hematoma formation, which can obstruct the airway

Tracheal injury

Air emboli during venous puncture or removal of the catheter

Post-procedural complications

Catheter-related bloodstream infections—bacterial or fungal

Central vein stenosis

Thrombosis

Suggested Reading

1. Aslamy Z, Dewald CL, Heffner JE. MRI of central venous anatomy: implications for central venous catheter insertion. Chest. 1998;114(3):820–6.
2. Perin G, Scarpa MG. Defining central venous line position in children: tips for the tip. J Vasc Access. 2015;16(2):77–86.
3. Beheshti MV. A concise history of central venous access. Tech Vasc Interv Radiol. 2011 Dec;14(4):184–5.
4. Seldinger SI. Catheter replacement of the needle in percutaneous arteriography. A new technique. Acta Radiol Suppl (Stockholm). 2008;434:47–52.
5. American Society of Anesthesiologists Task Force on Central Venous Access; Rupp SM, Apfelbaum JL, Blitt C, Caplan RA, Connis RT, Domino KB, Fleisher LA, Grant S, Mark JB, Morray JP, Nickinovich DG, Tung A. Practice guidelines for central venous access: a report by the American Society of Anesthesiologists Task Force on Central Venous Access. Anesthesiology. 2012 Mar;116(3):539–73.
6. Leibowitz A, et al. Ultrasound guidance for central venous access: current evidence and clinical recommendations. J Intensive Care Med. 2019;35(3):303–21.
7. Lu WH, Yao ML, Hsieh KS, Chiu PC, Chen YY, Lin CC, Huang TC, Chen CC. Supraclavicular versus infraclavicular subclavian vein catheterization in infants. J Chin Med Assoc. 2006;69(4):153–6.
8. Maecken T, Grau T. Ultrasound imaging in vascular access. Crit Care Med. 2007;35(5 Suppl):S178–85.
9. Bowdle A, Jelacic S, Togashi K, Ferreira R. Ultrasound identification of the guidewire in the brachiocephalic vein for the prevention of inadvertent arterial catheterization during internal jugular central venous catheter placement. Anesth Analg. 2016;123(4):896–900.

PICC (Peripherally Inserted Central Venous Catheter)

12

Anju Gupta, Nishkarsh Gupta, and Poonam Godhwal

Key Points

- A PICC is a long, thin tube which is inserted through a peripheral vein in the arm and advanced until the tip reaches superior vena cava.
- It is used for a variety reasons including long-term intravenous therapy, chemotherapy, blood transfusions, and parenteral nutrition.
- The complication rates of infection, thrombosis, and bleeding are much lower with PICC as compared to central venous catheters.
- PICCs can retained for several weeks to several months, depending on the patient's needs.
- One should monitor the PICC insertion site closely for signs of infection such as fever, swelling, or redness at the insertion site.

A. Gupta
Anesthesiology, Pain Medicine, Critical Care, All India Institute of Medical Sciences, New Delhi, Delhi, India

N. Gupta (✉) · P. Godhwal
Department Onco-Anesthesiology and Palliative Medicine at DRBRAIRCH, All India Institute of Medical Sciences, New Delhi, Delhi, India

12.1 Introduction

PICC refers to peripherally inserted central venous catheter. It is an advanced skill, desirable to be mastered by the anesthesiologist, to provide prolonged venous access. It is a safe and simple alternate to central venous access. A number of catheter introduction systems are available and the choice of technique depends upon availability, experience of the physician, and the need of the particular patient. We will be discussing about the technique of PICC insertion with a catheter-through-cannula system.

12.1.1 Indications and Contraindications

Indications	Contraindications
1. Difficult venous access. 2. Infusion of irritant or hyperosmolar solutions/drugs. 3. Chemotherapy. 4. Need for prolonged IV access.	1. Inadequate veins. 2. Infection at or near the proposed catheter insertion site. 3. Lymph edema. 4. Anatomical distortion from surgery, injury or trauma. 5. Mastectomy surgery with axillary dissection +/− lymphoedema on affected side.

N. Gupta et al. (eds.), *Techniques in Anesthesia, Intensive Care and Emergency Medicine*,
https://doi.org/10.1007/978-981-96-1202-4_12

12.1.1.1 Relevant Anatomy and Size of PICC Cannula

Relevant clinical anatomy for insertion of a PICC line and a PICC line are shown in the following figure (Fig. 12.1).

12.1.1.2 Size

There are a large range of catheters available and selection should be based on site, reason for insertion and length of use. PICCs are made either polyurethane or silicone and are radi-opaque measuring 30–70 cm in length with an outside diameter of 3–6 French (FR) {22G to 14G}. The catheter may have a single- or double-lumen. The particular device selected should be therapy specific, based on the number of lumens necessary for treatment, recognizing that the potential for infection increases with lumen number.

12.1.1.3 Equipment Required

- Pre-designed consent form with a pen.

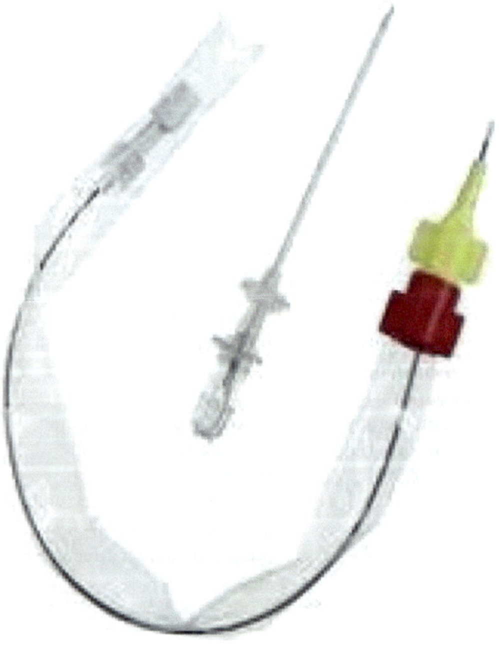

Fig. 12.1 PICC line Cavafix

- Universal precautions (cap, gloves, mask, gown) and surgical drapes.
- PICC line of appropriate size.
- Sterile PICC line insertion set and procedure tray.
- Intra-venous set and intra-venous fluid stand.
- Tourniquet.
- Sterile surgical syringe preloaded with heparin saline.
- Vials for sample collection (optional).
- Label (date and time columns).

12.1.1.4 Pre-procedure Work-Up

- **Equipment:** Inspect the integrity of the equipment, set up the intra-venous fluid stand bedside and preparation of the procedure tray.
- **Patient related:** Take written informed consent (with date) and explain the procedure.
- Confirm the identity of the patient.
- **Physician related:** Check for signed physician's orders to set up PICC line; assess the need to collect blood sample; check for availability of appropriate vials; use aseptic technique) and perform a surgical scrub prior to the procedure.
  - Clean with an antiseptic solution such as 2% chlorhexidine solution with friction for 30–60 s.
  - Allow the site to air-dry for upto 1 min to ensure disinfection.
  - Do not try to palpate the vein again once the region is prepared.
  - Drape the patient using sterile drapes.
- Use properly fitting universal precautions including sterile gown, sterile gloves, cap, mask, eye protection, etc.
- Cephalic or basilic veins or brachial veins may be used. The basilic vein (8 mm) is preferred as it offers the largest diameter of upper extremity vessels and affords a non-tortuous entry into the subclavian vein. The cephalic vein (~6 mm) is smaller and angles 90° to enter the terminal portion of the axillary vein and make the catheter advancement difficult.
- Choose non-dominant hand to make it less incapacitating.

12.1.2 Standard Operating Procedure for Intravenous Line Insertion

- Check for veins and prepare before puncture.
- **Applying the tourniquet** (blood pressure cuff, Foley's catheter, any tubing such as nasogastric tube, assistant's hand) to make them prominent (Fig. 12.2a, b).
- Remove any visible hair (if any) to improve visualization of vein.
- Alternatively squeeze ball may be used to make the veins prominent.
- If the patient's arms are cold, then apply a warm towel/pack may help. The patient's should be in supine position with his hand should be below the level of the heart.
- To prevent the pain of pin-prick, infiltrate 0.5–1 mL of a local anesthetic with a small gauge needle or apply EMLA cream (45–60 min before insertion).
- Use your non-dominant hand to stretch the skin distal to the chosen site of insertion and to stabilize the vein to prevent their slipping under the skin when pricked (especially in elderly).
- Hold the cannula with the dominant hand. With the bevel facing upwards; the skin is penetrated first followed by the vein (Fig. 12.2c–e). Once the needle is inside the vein, you will feel loss of resistance and see a drop of blood in chamber of the cannula (Fig. 12.2d).
- At this point, reduce the angle of the cannula to prevent puncturing the posterior wall; stabilize the cannula at this point.
- In case no blood is seen in the chamber of the cannula, withdrawn the device gradually to just beneath the skin and the reattempt puncture (Fig. 12.2e).
- If a local swelling develops, then withdraw the cannula, release the tourniquet and apply direct pressure for 5 min to prevent hematoma.
- After the vein is punctured.
  - Release the tourniquet.
  - Keeping the outer plastic sheath stable, withdraw the needle from within the sheath and advance the sheath over it (Fig. 12.2e). As soon as the needle is withdrawn out of the sheath, backflow of blood will start from the outer end of the cannula (Fig. 12.2f).
  - Attach the CVC catheter with protective sheath to the cannula by airtight coupling and advance the catheter into the vein through slowly (Fig. 12.2g, h).
  - After the desired position of the catheter is reached, the introducer is peeled off (Fig. 12.2i) and the cannula is withdrawn over PICC (Fig. 12.2j).
  - Remove the inner stylet (Fig. 12.2k) and check for blood return and flush the catheter (Fig. 12.2l).
- A syringe pre-loaded with saline or heparin is use to flush the PICC.
- **Fixing the cannula:** Secure the catheter and the insertion cannula to the skin using an adhesive; a transparent dressing and tape should be preferred. Sutures or securement device can be used to ensure proper fixation.
- Confirm the correct placement of the tip between the carina and the SVC/RA junction using CXR.
- **Apply label** mentioning the date and time of establishing this cannula promptly.
- **Connect the IV fluid** tubing after confirming the patency and position of the cannula.
- Check the physician's orders for the type of fluid to be connected and the rate of administration.

12.1.3 Important Tips (Fig. 12.3)

1. Never set-up intravenous access in absence of specific and complete instructions from the physician in-charge.
2. Never forget to heplock or saline-lock the cannula if not on regular infusion.
3. An X-ray may need to be taken to make sure the PICC tip is in the correct position in a vein in your chest.

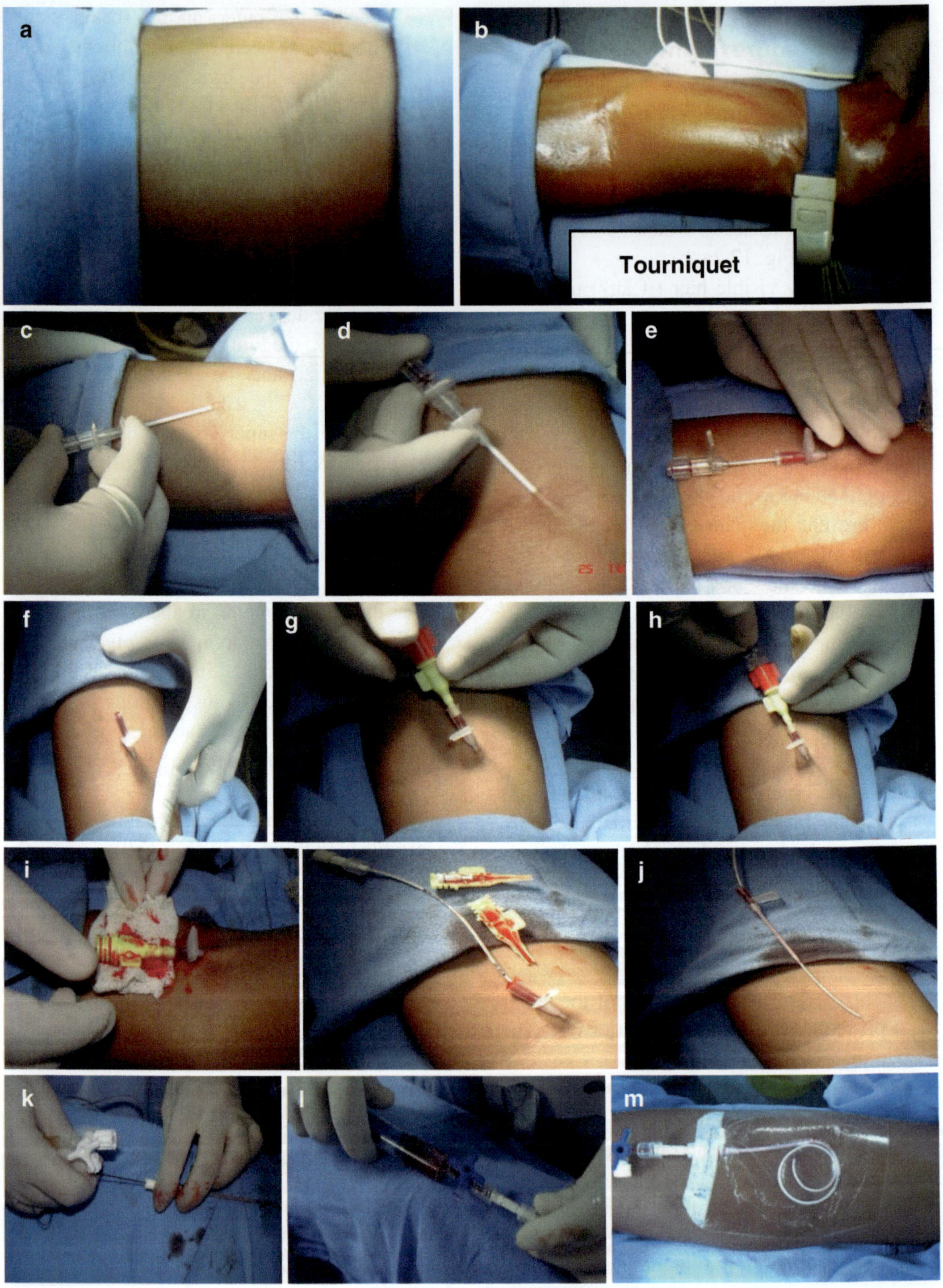

Fig. 12.2 (**a**) Select and make the vein prominent. (**b**) Cleaning and part preparation. Puncture of the overlying skin (**c**) and confirmation of venepuncture by splash of blood (**d**), advancement of the catheter with removal of the needle (**e**), the plastic cannula is left in situ (**f**), introduction of the PICC catheter in sheath (**g**), and advancement of PICC through the cannula (**h**). peel off introducer (**i**); withdraw cannula over PICC (**j**); remove the guide wire (**k**); ensure free flow of blood (**l**) and ensure adequate length is inserted (**m**) lock

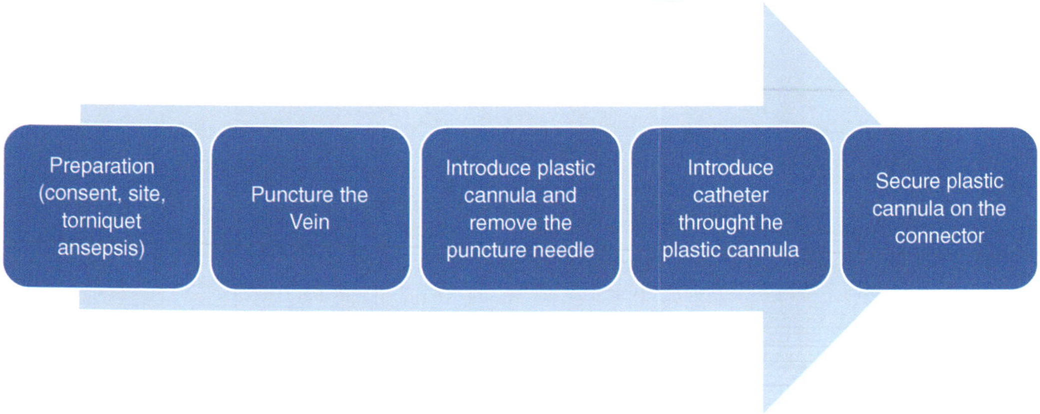

Fig. 12.3 Important steps for PICC insertion

An X-ray may need to be taken to make sure the PICC tip is in the correct position in a vein in your chest.

12.1.4 Post-procedure Care

The dressing of PICC should be changed once a week. Frequent monitoring the site of insertion is important to see signs of local infection like redness, discharge, increased local temperature etc. In case of need dressing can be changed earlier also. However it should be changed under all aseptic precautions.

12.1.5 Complications of PICC

Sometimes, patients who have these catheters experience catheter-related complications (mechanical or infectious), resulting in patient morbidity. In addition, it may lead to bleeding from site of insertion, arrythmias, damage to surrounding structures, thrombus formation, and air embolism.

Suggested Readings

1. Chung DH, Ziegler MM. Central venous catheter access. Nutrition. 1998;14(1):119–23.
2. Linenberger ML. Catheter-related thrombosis: risks, diagnosis, and management. J Natl Compr Canc Netw. 2006;4(9):889–901.
3. Luckianow GM, Smith D, Bullen D, Kaplan LJ. Understanding percutaneous and subcutaneous central venous access devices. JAAPA. 2016;29(1):33–6.
4. Pittiruti M, Hamilton H, Biffi R, MacFie J, Pertkiewicz M, ESPEN. ESPEN guidelines on parenteral nutrition: central venous catheters (access, care, diagnosis and therapy of complications). Clin Nutr. 2009;28(4):365–77.
5. Johansson E, Hammarskjöld F, Lundberg D, Arnlind MH. Advantages and disadvantages of peripherally inserted central venous catheters (PICC) compared to other central venous lines: a systematic review of the literature. Acta Oncol. 2013;52(5):886–92.
6. Duwadi S, Zhao Q, Budal BS. Peripherally inserted central catheters in critically ill patients—complications and its prevention: a review. Int J Nurs Sci. 2018;6(1):99–105. https://doi.org/10.1016/j.ijnss.2018.12.007. Erratum in: Int J Nurs Sci 2020;8(1):IV

13 Swan Ganz Catheter Insertion

Suruchi Hasija and Devishree Das

Key Points

- Swan Ganz catheter is a balloon floatation flow directed catheter inserted into the pulmonary artery.
- Swan Ganz catheter not only estimates pressures of right atrium, right ventricle, pulmonary artery, and pulmonary capillary wedge pressure, but also measures cardiac output, intracardiac shunts, and vascular resistances.
- Cardiac output estimation by Swan Ganz catheter is the gold standard method since 1970; however it is subject to measurement errors introduced by rapid intravenous fluid administration, intracardiac shunts, and tricuspid valve regurgitation.
- Pulmonary artery diastolic or pulmonary artery wedge pressures estimate the left ventricular preload which is subject to many confounding factors, including changes in diastolic ventricular compliance and juxtacardiac pressure.
- Swan Ganz catheter can also be modified to measure continuous cardiac output, continuous mixed venous oxygen saturation, right ventricle ejection fraction, and emergency pacing.
- Swan Ganz catheterization has not been shown to improve patient outcomes because of misinterpretation of catheter-derived data and failure of hemodynamic therapies that are guided by specific hemodynamic indices.

13.1 Introduction

Swan Ganz catheterization or right heart catheterization is insertion of balloon floatation flow directed catheter into the PA in order to measure various hemodynamic variables. This procedure is used for measurement of pressures in the right atrium (RA), right ventricle (RV), PA and pulmonary capillary wedge pressure (PCWP). It also helps in the estimation of cardiac output, intracardiac shunts, and vascular resistances.

13.2 History

Dr. Warner Frossmann in 1929 established right heart catheterization by introducing a catheter into his own heart. However, Dr Andre Cournand and Dickinson Richards developed a catheter which could be inserted into the pulmonary

S. Hasija (✉) · D. Das
Department of Cardiac-Anaesthesia and Intensive care, AIIMS, New Delhi, India

N. Gupta et al. (eds.), *Techniques in Anesthesia, Intensive Care and Emergency Medicine*,
https://doi.org/10.1007/978-981-96-1202-4_13

artery (PA). In 1970 Dr. Jeremy Swan and Dr. William Ganz from Cedars Sinai Medical Center introduced a balloon floatation flow directed catheter that could be used without fluoroscopy at the bedside for assessment of hemodynamics.

13.3 Indications

- *To guide fluid therapy*:
  - Hemodynamic instability
  - Shock
  - Multiple organ failure
  - Acute renal failure
  - Acute respiratory distress syndrome
  - Massive trauma
  - Acute burn
  - Hemorrhagic pancreatitis
- *Surgical procedure*:
  - High risk surgery
  - Pericardiectomy
  - Orthotopic heart transplant
  - LVAD implantation
  - Thoracic aortic aneurysm surgery
  - Sitting craniotomy
  - Liver transplant
  - Portosystemic shunt
  - Severe toxemia of pregnancy
- *Cardiac disease*:
  - Coronary artery disease with left ventricular dysfunction
  - Pulmonary hypertension
  - Pulmonary embolism
  - Heart failure
  - Cardiomyopathy
  - Tamponade
  - Cor pulmonale

13.4 Contraindications

Absolute:

- Infection at insertion site
- Tricuspid stenosis
- Pulmonary stenosis
- Tetralogy of Fallot
- Right sided infective endocarditis
- Right heart masses (tumor/thrombus)

Relative:

- Severe arrythmia
- Left bundle branch block
- Newly placed pacemaker, automatic implantable cardioverter defibrillator, cardiac resynchronization therapy device
- Coagulopathy
- Ebstein anomaly
- Septicemia

13.5 Equipment

The standard pulmonary artery catheter (PAC) (Fig. 13.1) is a multi-lumen catheter of 7–9 Fr circumference and 110 cm length. There are circumferential black lines on the catheter to identify the distance from the tip of the catheter, one thin black line denotes 10 cm whereas a thick black line denotes 50 cm mark. It contains 4 lumens; each lumen is color coded and has a specific function:

1. The blue lumen or central venous pressure (CVP) port: It is the proximal port located in RA 30 cm from the tip used for measurement of CVP.
2. The red port or the balloon port: Air is introduced with a prefixed syringe of 1.5 cc to inflate the balloon near the tip of the catheter in order to measure PCWP.
3. The yellow lumen or PA lumen is the distal lumen located at tip of the catheter. It is used to measure the PA pressure.
4. The red/white connector: It houses a temperature sensitive wire which terminates in a thermistor 4 cm proximal to the tip.

The thermodilution PAC (Fig. 13.2) has an additional white or clear RA infusion port near the proximal CVP port.

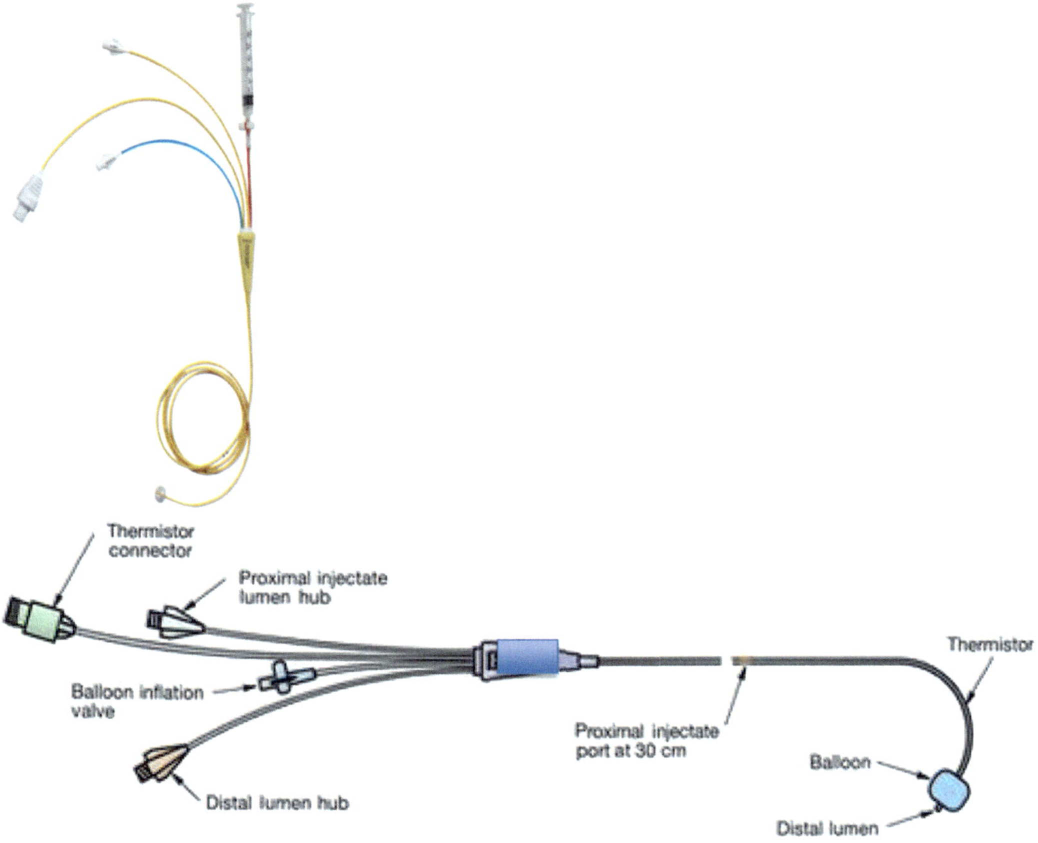

Fig. 13.1 The standard pulmonary artery catheter. (Courtesy Edwards Lifesciences, Irvine, CA, USA)

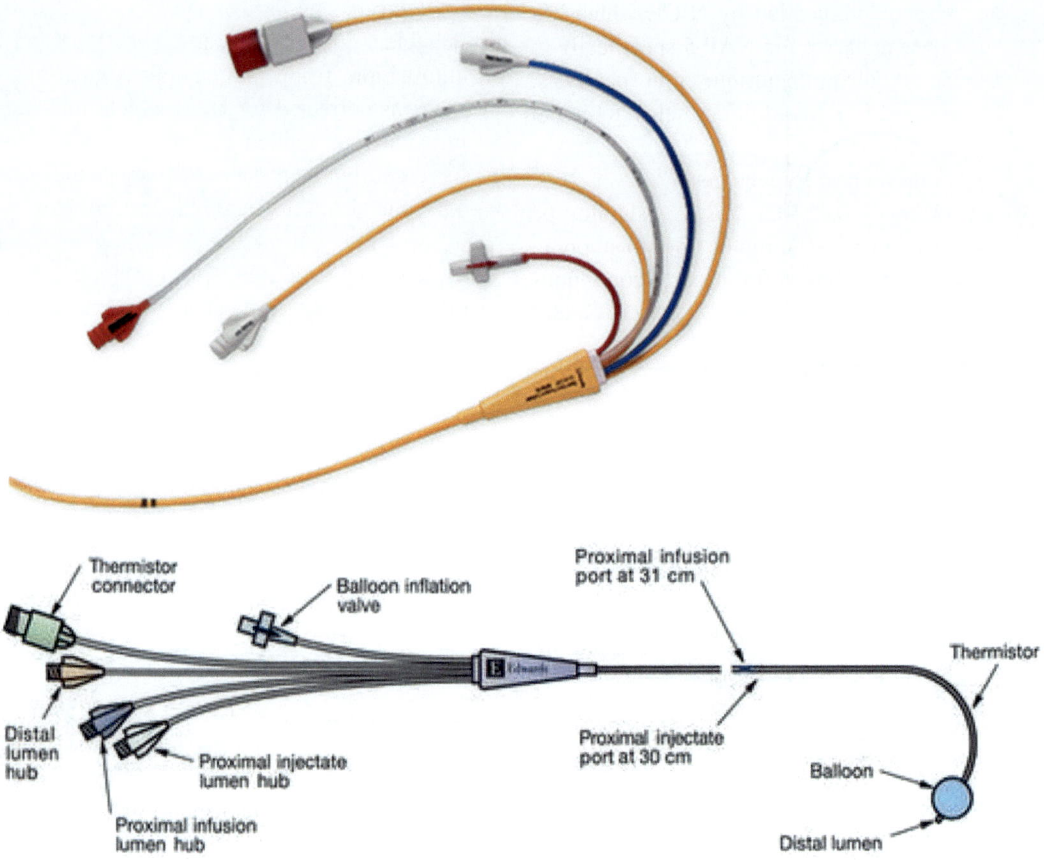

Fig. 13.2 The thermodilution pulmonary artery catheter. (Courtesy Edwards Lifesciences, Irvine, CA, USA)

13.6 Insertion Technique

PAC can be inserted from any central venous site. However, the right internal jugular vein (IJV) is the shortest route to the right sided cardiac chambers. Like central venous cannulation a large introducer sheath is inserted under aseptic conditions. The PAC is connected to pressure transducer and inserted through sterile sheath to a depth of 20 cm into the RA, the balloon at is inflated with air and advanced through the tricuspid valve into the RV, then through the pulmonary valve into the PA and finally into its wedge position (Fig. 13.3). The air-filled balloon tends to float to the non-dependent cardiac chamber. Tilting the patient's head-end downwards will encourage floatation of the PAC into the RV while a rightward and head-up tilt helps to float the PAC into the PA.

Proper catheter placement can be adjudged from the depth at which the desired chamber is reached and the characteristic waveform of each chamber. The RA is typically reached at 20–25 cm, RV at 30–35 cm, PA at 40–45 cm and wedge position at 50–55 cm from the right IJV. The balloon is inflated to obtain the PA wedge pressure tracing while on deflation the PA pressure tracing reappears. Additional 5–10 cm needs to be inserted from the left IJV, and the left and right external jugular venous approaches, an

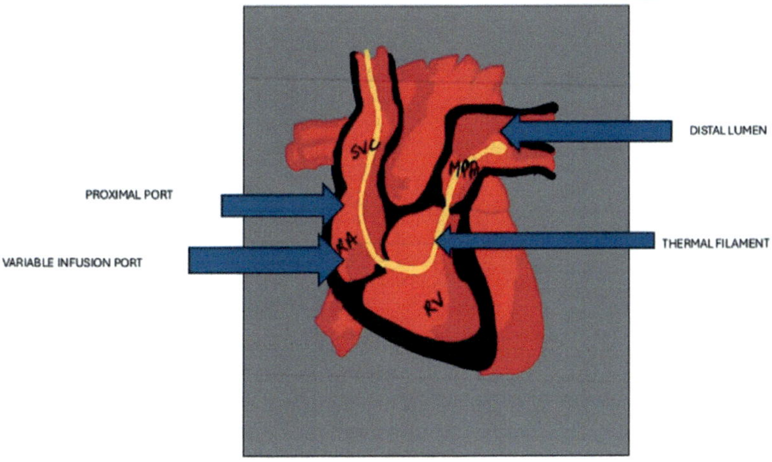

Fig. 13.3 Placement of pulmonary artery catheter through the right internal jugular vein

additional 15 cm is inserted from the femoral vein and an additional 30–35 cm from the antecubital vein.

The position can be confirmed by chest X-ray. The tip ideally lies in the main PA without loops or knots for PAP measurement, and between the medial and middle third of the ipsilateral lung field (West zone 3) during wedging. It should be seen within 2 cm of the cardiac silhouette on standard anteroposterior chest film.

13.7 Complications [9–17]

- *Access related*:
  - Arterial puncture
  - Bleeding
  - Haematoma
  - Pneumothorax
  - Hemothorax
  - Air embolism
  - Guide wire embolization
- *Catheter related*:
  - Catheter shearing
  - Catheter knotting/coiling
  - Incorrect placement
  - Balloon rupture
  - Air embolism
  - Thromboembolism
  - Cardiac valve damage
  - Endocardial injury
  - Ventricular perforation
  - PA rupture
  - Pulmonary infarction
  - Infection
  - Endocarditis
  - PA pseudoaneurysm
  - Thrombocytopenia
  - Misinterpretation of data
- *Arrhythmias*:
  - Atrial tachyarrhythmias
  - Ventricular ectopics
  - Ventricular tachycardia
  - Ventricular fibrillation
  - Right bundle branch block
  - Complete heart block

13.8 Normal Waveform

Characteristic wave forms are recorded as the balloon tipped PAC floats to the appropriate position (Fig. 13.4). In the superior vena cava, the characteristic central venous pressure (CVP) waveform with a, c, v waves and x, y descents are seen. As the balloon is inflated and the PAC is advanced further, the characteristic RV pressure waveform having a rapid systolic upstroke, a low diastolic pressure and a wide pulse pressure is observed. The PAC may stimulate the RV infundibulum causing ventricular ectopics. Further advancement into the PA reveals a step up in diastolic pressure. When the PAC floats to the wedge position, the inflated balloon isolates the distal orifice that monitors PCWP from proximal PAP by creating a static blood column between

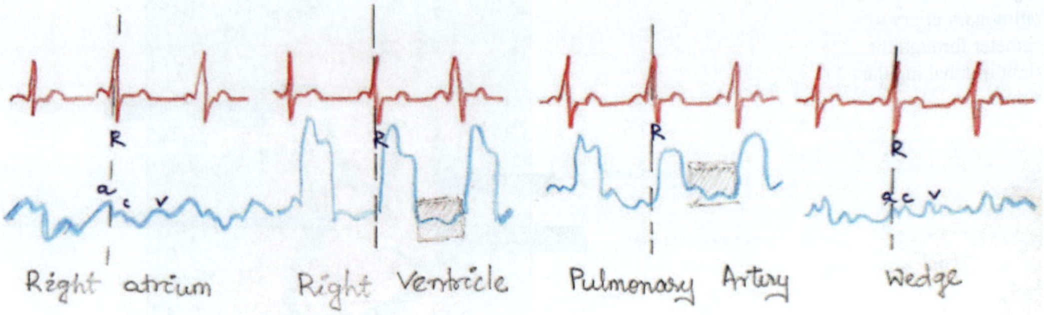

Fig. 13.4 Representative pressure tracings obtained from the pulmonary artery catheter

wedged PAC tip and junction of left atrium (LA) and pulmonary veins. It indirectly measures the LA pressure, left ventricular end-diastolic pressure (LVEDP) and left ventricular end-diastolic volume (LVEDV), providing an indirect estimate of LV preload.

The PCWP resembles CVP waveform with characteristic a, c, v waves and x, y descents. However, it is delayed and damped as the LA pressure wave requires about 160 ms to traverse the pulmonary veins, capillaries, arterioles and finally PA. Also, since atrial depolarization starts in the sinoatrial node in RA and gradually progress to LA.

The v wave is taller in LA pressure waveform than RA suggesting stronger LA contraction. The interval between atrial and ventricular contraction is almost 40 ms longer on right side than on left. Therefore, the a and c waves are separate in the RA trace and composite a-c wave in the LA waveform.

13.9 Abnormal Waveforms

13.9.1 Mitral Stenosis

Mitral stenosis (MS) distorts the diastolic portion of PCWP waveform. It causes increase in the mean PCWP due to a holo-diastolic pressure gradient across the mitral valve. There is a tall end-diastolic a wave and slurred early diastolic y descent. However, in advanced MS with atrial fibrillation a wave may not be present (Fig. 13.5).

A similar waveform is seen in case of mitral inflow obstruction in LA myxoma. The mean PCWP is also raised in LV infarction, aortic stenosis and systemic hypertension, accompanied by a prominent a wave due to increased LV stiffness. But y descent remains steep since there is no obstruction to flow across the mitral valve during diastole.

13.9.2 Mitral Regurgitation

Mitral regurgitation (MR) causes fusion of c-v waves with tall v wave and obliteration of systolic x descent as retrograde ejection of blood into LA obliterates the phase of isovolumetric contraction. The increase in mean PCWP overestimates LVEDP. However, it depicts mean LA pressure and risk of hydrostatic pulmonary edema. The v wave characteristics depend upon LA volume, LA compliance and regurgitant volume. Acute MR cause tall v wave because of smaller, stiffer and less compliant LA compared to long standing MR (Fig. 13.6). Tall v waves are also commonly seen in hypervolemia, congestive heart failure and ventricular septal defect.

13.9.3 Myocardial Infarction

Myocardial infarction (MI) causes ventricular diastolic dysfunction leading to impaired LV relaxation and stiffer less compliant ventricle. As a result of increased LV filling pressure, PCWP

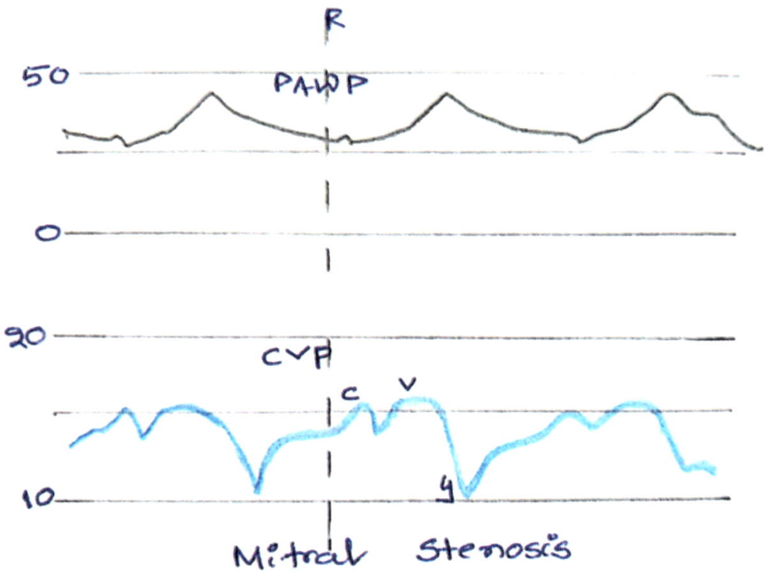

Fig. 13.5 Representative pressure tracings obtained from the pulmonary artery catheter in mitral stenosis

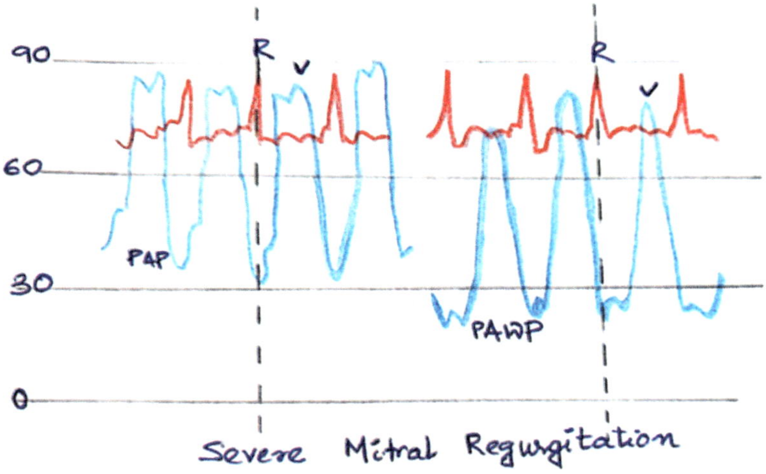

Fig. 13.6 Representative pressure tracings obtained from the pulmonary artery catheter in mitral regurgitation

increases showing prominent a and v waves (Fig. 13.7). Just as RV ischemia causes increase in CVP with prominent v wave due to tricuspid regurgitation described as W or M configuration, similarly LV ischemia increases PCWP.

13.9.4 Pericardial Constriction/ Restrictive Cardiomyopathy

There occurs elevated mean pressure, prominent a and v waves and steep x and y descents due to impaired diastolic compliance of the RV. Similar findings are also seen in restrictive cardiomyopathy, diastolic dysfunction and RV infarction.

In constrictive pericarditis, the rigid calcified pericardium limits chamber filling. Therefore, impaired venous return leads to decrease in end diastolic volume, stroke volume and cardiac output. Equalization of cardiac filling pressure in all four-chambers is seen at end-diastole. The characteristic M or W pattern in the CVP trace may not be apparent on the left side due to damping effect of pulmonary vasculature. Ventricular

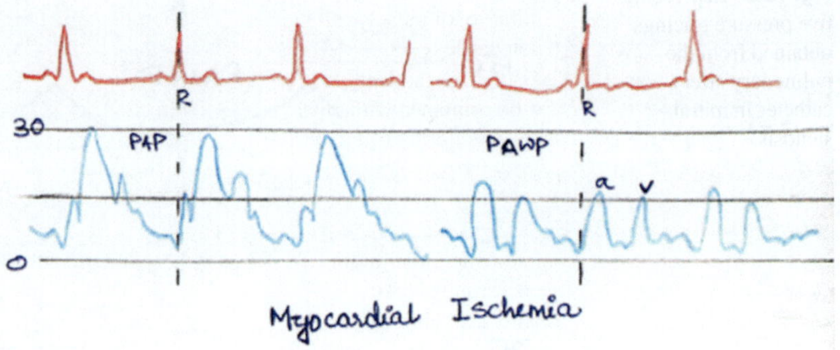

Fig. 13.7 Representative pressure tracings obtained from the pulmonary artery catheter in myocardial ischemia

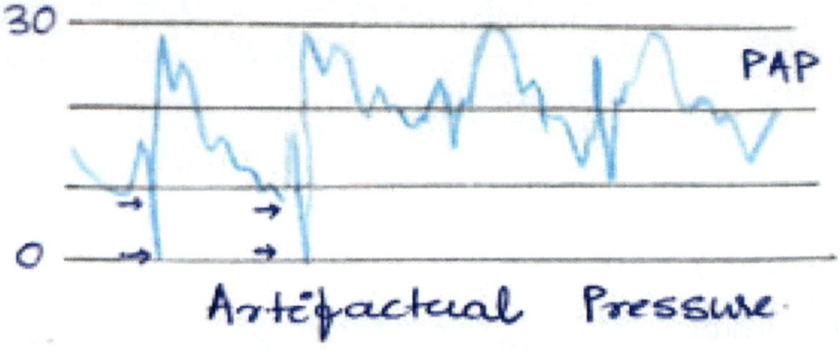

Fig. 13.8 Artifacts in the pulmonary artery catheter waveform

pressure waveform shows characteristic dip and plateau sign or square root pattern due to rapid but short lived early diastolic ventricular filling.

13.9.5 Cardiac Tamponade

In cardiac tamponade compressive pericardial fluid impairs filling of cardiac chambers. As a result, there is marked increase in CVP and decrease in diastolic volume, stroke volume and cardiac output. The CVP waveform become monophasic with dominant systolic x descent and attenuated y descent as early diastolic flow from RA to RV is impaired by surrounding pericardial fluid.

13.9.6 Pulmonary Hypertension

In acute pulmonary hypertension right ventricular end diastolic volume and pressure increases, shifting the ventricular septum leftward. This leads to increase in LVEDP and decrease in LVEDV thereby shifting the LV pressure volume loop to a stiffer steeper curve. The increased gradient across the pulmonary vasculature causes diastolic PA pressure to exceed PAWP.

13.9.7 Positive Pressure Ventilation

During positive pressure ventilation, PAP and PAWP increase in inspiration. In contrast, PAP and PAWP decrease in inspiration during spontaneous ventilation. Therefore, to avoid confounding, cardiac filling pressures are measured at end-expiration.

13.9.8 Artifact

The PAC traverses various cardiac chambers, therefore prone to artifacts because of presence of clot or air bubble, and motion related distortion. During systole, RV contraction and tricuspid valve closure causes excessive catheter motion leading to either low or high pressure occurring simultaneously with CVP c wave (Fig. 13.8).

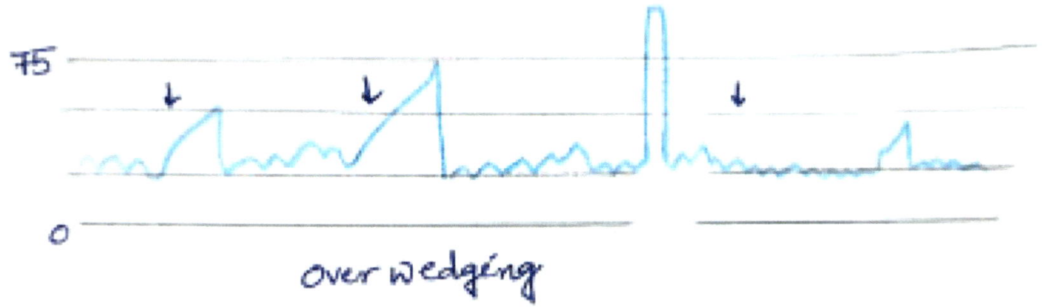

Fig. 13.9 Artifacts in the pulmonary artery catheter waveform

13.9.9 Over Wedging

Over wedging usually occurs due to distal catheter migration causing occlusion of the distal orifice by impinging against the vessel wall. Sometimes the balloon gets inflated eccentrically or unduly resulting in pressure build up obstructing the distal lumen. The PCWP is seen to gradually rise and devoid of pulsatility. Thus, catheter should be slightly withdrawn before wedging (Fig. 13.9).

13.10 Factors Influencing the Relationship Between Left Ventricular Filling Pressure and Preload

One of the important applications of the PAC is their ability to measure PCWP, which is a surrogate of LVEDP and LVEDV. This relationship is dependent on a number of intervening factors, (Fig. 13.10) but may be disturbed by various physiological and pathological conditions.

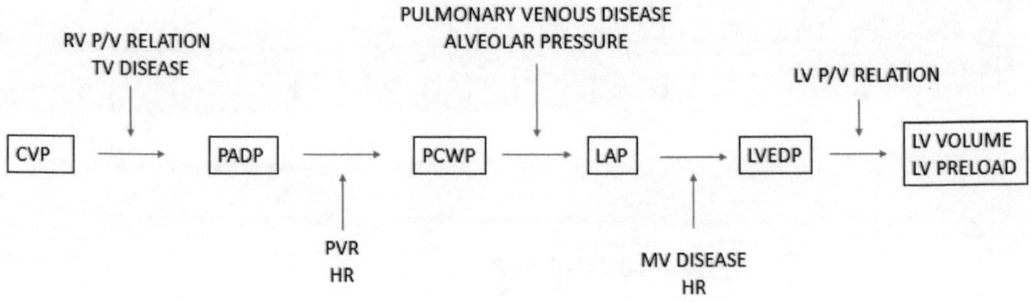

Fig. 13.10 Relationship between PCWP and LVEDP. *CVP* central venous pressure, *PADP* pulmonary artery diastolic pressure, *PCWP* pulmonary capillary wedge pressure, *LAP* left atrial pressure, *LVEDP* left ventricular end diastolic pressure, *LV* left ventricle, *RV* right ventricle, *P/V* pressure-volume, *TV* tricuspid valve, *PVR* pulmonary vascular resistance, *HR* heart rate, *MV* mitral valve

13.11 Discrepancies Between Pulmonary Capillary Wedge Pressure and Left Ventricular End Diastolic Pressure

PCWP < LVEDP:

- Diastolic dysfunction (left ventricle ischemia, hypertrophy)
- Left ventricular failure
- Aortic regurgitation (premature closure of mitral valve)
- Cardiac tamponade
- Constrictive pericarditis

PCWP > LVEDP:

- Positive pressure ventilation
- High level of positive end-expiratory pressure
- Raised intrathoracic pressure
- Catheter tip outside West lung zone III placement
- Raised pulmonary vascular resistance
- Tachycardia
- Left atrial myxoma
- Mitral stenosis or regurgitation
- Pulmonary disease:
  - Chronic obstructive pulmonary disease
  - Acute respiratory distress syndrome
  - Embolism

13.12 Measured Chamber Pressures

Location	Range (mm Hg)	Mean (mm of Hg)
Right atrium	1–10	5
Right ventricle	15–30/0–8	25/5
Pulmonary artery	15–30/5–15/10–20	23/9/15
Pulmonary capillary wedge pressure	5–15	10
Left atrial pressure	4–12	8
Left ventricular pressure	90–140/4–12	130/8

13.13 Cardiac Output Estimation

Cardiac output estimation by PAC is the gold standard method since 1970. The most common principles used by PAC for determination of cardiac output are Fick principle and indicator (thermal) dilution technique.

13.13.1 Fick Principle

It states that uptake or release of a substance (oxygen) by an organ is the arteriovenous concentration difference of the substance and blood flow to the organ. Therefore, cardiac output is oxygen consumption divided by difference in arteriovenous oxygen content.

$$\begin{aligned} CO &= O_2\ \text{consumption} / \text{arterial}\ O_2\ \text{content}\quad \text{mixed venous}\ O_2\ \text{content} \\ &= VO_2 / CaO_2 - CvO_2 \\ &= 200 / 0.15 - 0.10 = 4000\,\text{ml} / \text{min} \end{aligned}$$

Where, CO is cardiac output.

13.13.2 Indicator Dilution Technique

This method is based on the fact that, for a known amount of indicator injected into circulation at one point, the same amount would be detected at the downstream point. The final amount of indicator detected is equal to the product of cardiac output and change in indicator concentration over time. Thus, cardiac output is calculated using the **Stewart-Hamilton equation:**

$$CO = I \times 60 \div \int Cdt$$

Where, CO is cardiac output, I is amount of indicator and $\int Cdt$ is integral of the indicator concentration over time.

Cold saline (thermodilution) or lithium ions are used as indicators. However, thermodilution is the preferred technique nowadays. Other dyes are rarely used in current practice.

13.13.3 Thermodilution Technique

A know volume of iced or room temperature fluid is injected to the RA as a bolus (2.5, 5, 10 ml) through proximal port of PAC and the change in PA blood temperature is recorded by the thermistor at the tip. After injection, the **thermodilution curve** is plotted which is change in temperature over time. Cardiac output is inversely proportional to area under the curve. In adults, 10 ml whereas in children 0.15 ml/kg injectate volume is recommended. Usually three measurements are performed and averaged to provide reliable result. Accurate measurement depends upon the presence of regurgitant lesions, intracardiac shunts, timing of respiratory cycle, rapid and smooth injection, correct calibration factors, thermistor malfunction and electrocautery interference during measurements.

The rate of blood flow is inversely proportional to the change in temperature over time as per **modified Stewart-Hamilton equation**:

$$CO = \frac{V\left(T_B - T_I\right) \times K_1 \times K_2}{\int_0^{\infty} \Delta T_B\left(t\right) dt}$$

Where, CO is cardiac output (L/min), V is volume of injectate (ml), T_B is initial blood temperature (°C), T_I is initial injectate temperature (°C), K_1 is density factor, K_2 is computation constant, and ${}_0\int^{\infty} \Delta T_B(t)dt$ is integral of blood temperature change over time.

13.14 Derived Hemodynamic Parameters

Parameter	Formula	Normal value
Cardiac index (CI)	CI = CO/BSA	2.6–4.4 L/min/m^2
Stroke volume (SV)	SV=CO × 1000/HR	50–110 ml/beat
Stroke index (SI)	SI=SV/BSA	30–65 ml/beat/m^2
Left ventricular stroke work index (LVSWI)	LVSWI = 1.36 × (MAP-PCWP) × SI/100	45–60 g.m/m^2
Right ventricular stroke work index (RVSWI)	RVSWI = 1.36 × (MPAP-CVP) × SI/100	5–10 g.m/m^2
Systemic vascular resistance (SVR)	SVR = (MAP-CVP) × 80/CO	900–1400 dynes.s.cm^{-5}

Parameter	Formula	Normal value
Systemic vascular resistance index (SVRI)	SVRI = (MAP-CVP) × 80/CI	1500–2400 dynes.s.cm^{-5}/m^2
Pulmonary vascular resistance (PVR)	PVR = (MPAP-PCWP) × 80/CO	150–250 dynes.s.cm^{-5}
Pulmonary vascular resistance index (PVRI)	PVRI = (MPAP-PCWP) × 80/CI	250–400 dynes.s.cm^{-5}/m^2

CO cardiac output, *BSA* body surface area, *HR* heart rate, *MAP* mean arterial pressure, *PCWP* pulmonary capillary wedge pressure, *MPAP* mean pulmonary artery pressure, *CVP* central venous pressure

13.15 Oxygen Delivery Parameters

Parameter	Formula	Normal value
Arterial oxygen content (CaO_2)	$CaO_2 = (1.39 \times Hb \times SaO_2) + (0.0031 \times PaO_2)$	18–20 ml/dL
Mixed venous oxygen content (CvO_2)	$CvO_2 = (1.39 \times Hb \times SvO_2) + (0.0031 \times PvO_2)$	13–16 ml/dL
Arteriovenous oxygen content difference ($avDO_2$)	$avDO_2 = CaO_2 - CvO_2$	4–5.5 ml/dL
Pulmonary capillary oxygen content (CcO_2)	$CcO_2 = (1.39 \times Hb \times ScO_2) + (0.0031 \times PcO_2)$	19–21 ml/dL
Pulmonary shunt fraction (Qs/Qt)	$Qs/Qt = 100 \times (CcO_2 - CaO_2)/(CcO_2 - CvO_2)$	2–8%
Oxygen delivery (DO_2)	$DO_2 = 10 \times CO \times CaO_2$	800–1100 ml/min
Oxygen consumption (VO_2)	$VO_2 = 10 \times CO \times (CaO_2 - CvO_2)$	150–300 ml/min

Hb haemoglobin, SaO_2 arterial oxygen saturation, PaO_2 arterial oxygen tension, SvO_2 venous oxygen saturation, PvO_2 venous oxygen tension, ScO_2 pulmonary capillary oxygen saturation, PcO_2 pulmonary capillary oxygen tension, *CO* cardiac output

13.16 Special Purpose Pulmonary Artery Catheters

13.16.1 Continuous Cardiac Output

Modification of thermodilution technique allows continuous measurement of cardiac output by a specialized catheter (Fig. 13.11). It contains a thermal filament which ejects small pulses of heat into the blood column proximal to pulmonary valve and a thermistor which measures change in blood temperature in PA. The cardiac output and other hemodynamic parameters are measured by computer-based algorithm (stochastic analysis) and displayed on a special monitor.

13.16.2 Continuous Mixed Venous Oximetry

The mixed venous oxygen saturation (SvO_2) provides a global estimate of oxygen delivery versus oxygen requirement of various tissues, i.e., oxygen supply–demand ratio. The SvO_2 is derived from modified Fick equation:

$$SvO_2 = SaO_2 - \frac{\dot{V}O_2}{CO \cdot 1.34 \cdot Hb}$$

The fiberoptic bundles embedded in the PAC enables continuous monitoring of SvO_2 using reflectance spectrophotometry. SvO_2 is calculated from the difference in absorption spectrum of various wavelengths of light by saturated and desaturated Hb (Fig. 13.12).

13.16.3 Thermodilution Right Ventricular Ejection Fraction

The RV ejection fraction is measured by a special type of PAC equipped with a rapid response thermistor and intracardiac ECG electrodes. The proximal lumen facilitates mixing of cold bolus above tricuspid valve. It analyses exponential

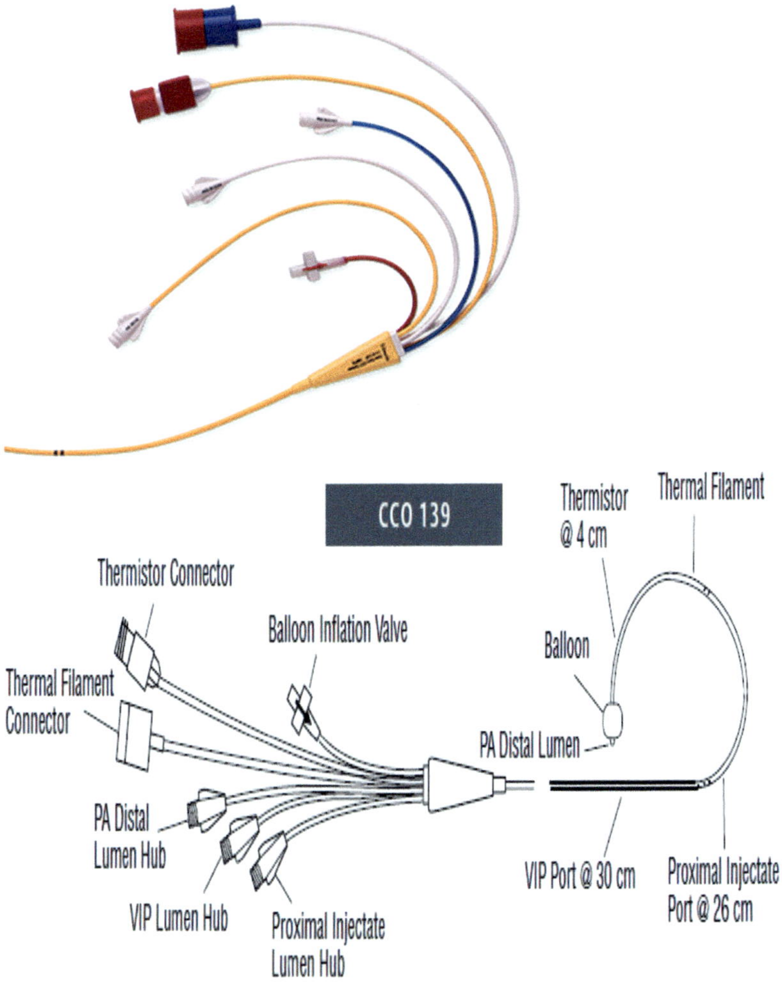

Fig. 13.11 The continuous cardiac output pulmonary artery catheter. (Courtesy Edwards Lifesciences, Irvine, CA, USA)

decay of PA temperature over several cardiac cycles to calculate RV ejection fraction. It is useful for assessment of RV end diastolic volume or preload in RV dysfunction.

13.16.4 Pacing

Currently electrode PACs and pacing wire PACs are available for symptomatic bradycardia, sinus node dysfunction, second-degree (Mobitz II) block, complete heart block and left bundle branch block.

Electrode catheters are multipurpose PACs which contains three atrial and two ventricular electrodes for atrial, ventricular or AV sequential pacing whereas pacing wire catheters have lumen for insertion of a ventricular wire (Paceport catheter) or both atrial and ventricular wires (A-V Paceport) for temporary transvenous pacing (Fig. 13.13).

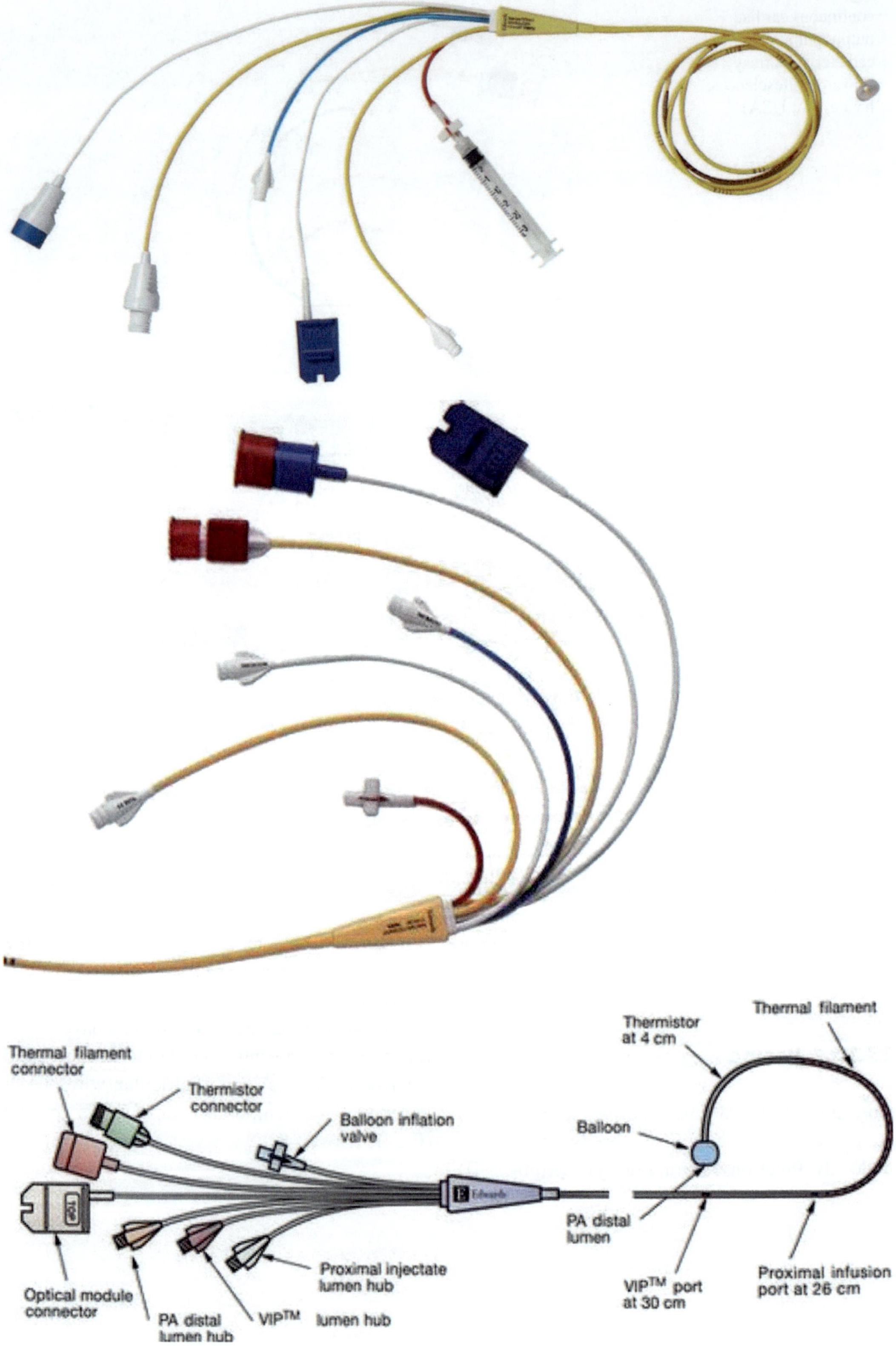

Fig. 13.12 Pulmonary artery catheter with capability of measuring SvO_2. (Courtesy Edwards Lifesciences, Irvine, CA, USA)

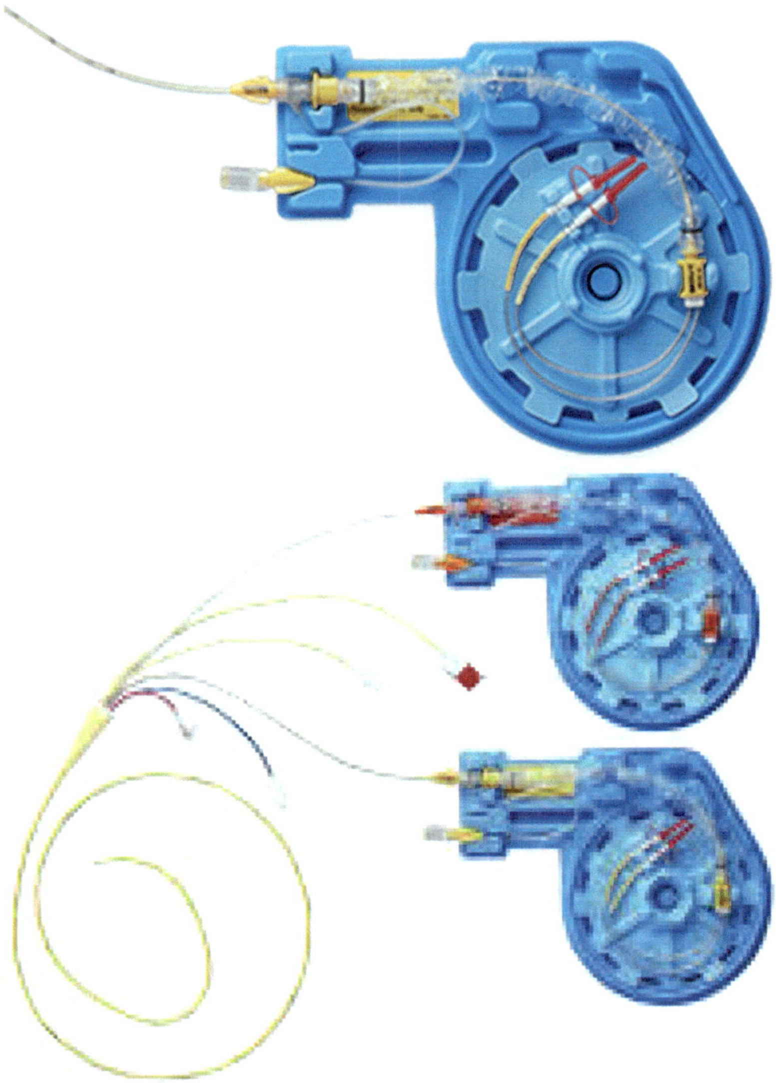

Fig. 13.13 Pulmonary artery catheter with temporary pacing capability

Suggested Reading

1. Frossmann W. Die Sondierung des Rechten Herzens. Klin Wochenschr. 1929;8:2085–7.
2. Cournand A. Cardiac catheterization; development of the technique, its contributions to experimental medicine, and its initial application in man. Acta Med Scand Suppl. 1975;579:3–32.
3. Swan HJ, Ganz W, Forrester J, Marcus H, Diamond G, Chonette D. Catheterization of the heart in man with the use of a flow-directed balloon-tipped catheter. N Engl J Med. 1970;283:447–51.
4. Chatterjee K, Swan HJC, Ganz W, Gray R, Loebel H, Forrester JS, Chonette D. Use of a balloon-tipped flotation electrode catheter for cardiac monitoring. Am J Cardiol. 1975;36:56–61.
5. Forrester JS, Ganz W, Diamond G, McHugh T, Chonette DW, Swan HJ. Thermodilution cardiac output determination with a single flow-directed catheter for cardiac monitoring. Am Heart J. 1972;83:306–11.
6. Keusch DJ, Winters S, Thys DM. The patient's position influences the incidence of dysrhythmias during pulmonary artery catheterization. Anesthesiology. 1989;70:582–4.
7. Mark JB. Pulmonary artery pressure. In: Mark JB, editor. Atlas of cardiovascular monitoring. New York: Churchill Livingstone; 1998. p. 27–37.
8. Bennett D, Boldt J, Brochard L, et al. Expert panel: the use of the pulmonary artery catheter. Intensive Care Med. 1991;17:I–VIII.
9. Evans DC, Doraiswamy VA, Prosciak MP, et al. Complications associated with pulmonary artery catheters: a comprehensive clinical review. Scand J Surg. 2009;98:199–208.

10. Morris D, Mulvihill D, Lew WYW. Risk of developing complete heart block during bedside pulmonary artery catheterization in patients with left bundle-branch block. Arch Intern Med. 1987;147:2005–10.
11. Troianos CA, Stypula RW. Transesophageal echocardiographic diagnosis of pulmonary artery catheter entrapment and coiling. Anesthesiology. 1993;79:602–4.
12. Huang GS, Wang HJ, Chen CH, et al. Pulmonary artery rupture after attempted removal of a pulmonary artery catheter. Anesth Analg. 2002;95:299–301.
13. Arnaout S, Diab K, Al-Kutoubi A, Jamaleddine G. Rupture of the chordae of the tricuspid valve after knotting of the pulmonary artery catheter. Chest. 2001;120:1742–4.
14. Sherman SV, Wall MH, Kennedy DJ, Brooker RF, Butterworth J. Do pulmonary artery catheters cause or increase tricuspid or pulmonic valvular regurgitation? Anesth Analg. 2001;92:1117–22.
15. Rowley KM, Clubb KS, Smith GJW, Cabin HS. Right-sided infective endocarditis as a consequence of flow-directed pulmonary artery catheterization. N Engl J Med. 1984;311:1152–6.
16. Barash PG, Nardi D, Hammond G, et al. Catheter-induced pulmonary artery perforation. J Thorac Cardiovasc Surg. 1981;82:5–12.
17. Hoar PF, Wilson RM, Mangano DT, et al. Heparin bonding reduces thrombogenicity of pulmonary-artery catheters. N Engl J Med. 1981;305:993–5.
18. Mark JB. Pulmonary artery wedge pressure. In: Mark JB, editor. Atlas of cardiovascular monitoring. New York: Churchill Livingstone; 1998. p. 39–48.
19. Levy MM. Pulmonary capillary pressure. Clinical implications. Crit Care Clin. 1996;12:819–39.
20. Mark JB. Patterns of valvular heart disease. In: Mark JB, editor. Atlas of cardiovascular monitoring. New York: Churchill Livingstone; 1998. p. 287–312.
21. Sanchez R, Wee M. Perioperative myocardial ischemia: early diagnosis using the pulmonary artery catheter. J Cardiothorac Vasc Anesth. 1991;5:604–7.
22. Trager MA, Feinberg BI, Kaplan JA. Right ventricular ischemia diagnosed by an esophageal electrocardiogram and right atrial pressure tracing. J Cardiothorac Anesth. 1987;1:123–5.
23. Kushwaha SS, Fallon JT, Fuster V. Restrictive cardiomyopathy. N Engl J Med. 1997;336:267–76.
24. Hirschmann JV. Pericardial constriction. Am Heart J. 1978;96:110–22.
25. Kern MJ, Aguirre F. Interpretation of cardiac pathophysiology from pressure waveform analysis: pericardial compressive hemodynamics, Part III. Cathet Cardiovasc Diagn. 1992;26:152–8.
26. Cengiz M, Crapo RO, Gardner RM. The effect of ventilation on the accuracy of pulmonary artery and wedge pressure measurements. Crit Care Med. 1983;11:502–7.
27. Mark JB. Predicting left ventricular end-diastolic pressure. In: Mark JB, editor. Atlas of cardiovascular monitoring. New York: Churchill Livingstone; 1998. p. 59–79.
28. Kaplan JA, Augoustides JGT, Manecke GR Jr, Maus T, Reich DL. Kaplan's cardiac anesthesia: for cardiac and noncardiac surgery. 7th ed. Philadelphia: Elsevier; 2017.
29. Guyton AC. The Fick principle. In: Guyton AC, Jones CE, Coleman TG, editors. Circulatory physiology: cardiac output and its regulation. 2nd ed. Philadelphia: WB Saunders Company; 1973. p. 21.
30. Kurita T, Morita K, Kato S, et al. Comparison of the accuracy of the lithium dilution technique with the thermodilution technique for measurement of cardiac output. Br J Anaesth. 1997;79:770–5.
31. Forrester JS, Ganz W, Diamond G, McHugh T, Chonette DW, Swan HJ. Thermodilution cardiac output determination with a single flow-directed catheter. Am Heart J. 1972;83:306–11.
32. Nishikawa T, Dohi S. Errors in the measurement of cardiac output by thermodilution. Can J Anaesth. 1993;40:142–53.
33. Jakobsen CJ, Melsen NC, Andresen EB. Continuous cardiac output measurements in the perioperative period. Acta Anaesthesiol Scand. 1995;39:485–8.
34. Pond CG, Blessios G, Bowlin J, McCawley C, Lappas DG. Perioperative evaluation of a new mixed venous oxygen saturation catheter in cardiac surgical patients. J Cardiothorac Vasc Anesth. 1992;6:280–2.
35. Urban P, Scheidegger D, Gabathuler J, Rutishauser W. Thermodilution determination of right ventricular volume and ejection fraction: a comparison with biplane angiography. Crit Care Med. 1987;15:652–5.
36. Risk SC, Brandon D, D'Ambra MN, Koski EG, Hoffman WJ, Philbin DM. Indications for the use of pacing pulmonary artery catheters in cardiac surgery. J Cardiothorac Vasc Anesth. 1992;6:275–9.

14 Intra-arterial Blood Pressure Monitoring

Vinayak PS

Key Points

- Intra-arterial blood pressure monitoring (IABP) is typically used in critical care settings for close monitoring blood pressure of patients.
- Strict aseptic precautions should be used for insertion of IABP insertion.
- The IABP system should be calibrated and zeroed to ensure accurate measurements.
- The patients should be monitored for possible complications of IABP insertion including bleeding, infection, artery damage, and nerve injury.

14.1 Accurate, Continuous, Invasive

Intra-arterial blood pressure (IABP) measurement is considered to be the gold standard in blood pressure measurement. It is used for "beat – to- beat" monitoring of blood pressure for any reason (surgical or non-surgical) and/or need for frequent blood sampling. Recent indications also include measurement of cardiac output. IABP is used extensively in anesthesia, ICU, and emergency department.

Indications for IBP monitoring

1. Perioperative management of major surgical procedures, long duration procedures, and procedures associated with significant anticipated blood loss.
2. Patients with comorbidity predisposing them to perioperative hemodynamic instability and risk of cardiovascular complications.
3. High risk patients undergoing non- surgical procedures requiring anesthesia.
4. Contraindications to noninvasive blood pressure monitoring, relative or absolute.
5. Hemodynamic instability or need for monitoring in ICU or emergency department.
6. Post-resuscitation monitoring following cardiac arrest.
7. Need for repeated blood sampling or ABG monitoring in ICU.
8. Transfer of high-risk patients.
9. Monitoring of cardiac output.

Vinayak PS (✉)
Manipal Hospital, Bangalore, India

N. Gupta et al. (eds.), *Techniques in Anesthesia, Intensive Care and Emergency Medicine*,
https://doi.org/10.1007/978-981-96-1202-4_14

14.2 Equipment Description

14.2.1 For Intra-arterial Access

1. Cannula: A 20G arterial cannula should be used in adults and a 22G arterial cannula can be used in children (Fig. 14.1).

> Venous cannulas with a side port should not be used for arterial cannulation as there is a chance of inadvertent injection of medication or air through it.

2. **Transducer, pressure bag, and tubing setup.**
   (i) The transducer is a device that changes one form of energy to another form, an arterial line pressure transducer converts the pressure inside the artery to an electrical energy that can be displayed as a number (Fig. 14.2).
   (ii) The transducer is connected to the arterial catheter by saline filled tubing. The tubing should be stiff, non- compliant and ideally no longer than 120 cm to prevent damping. The other end of the transducer is connected to a pressurized saline bag via another saline filled tubing (Fig. 14.3).
   (iii) An infusion or flushing system: the other end other end of the transducer is connected to pressurized saline bag which counteracts the systemic arterial pressure. Although the author adds 1000 IU of heparin to the bag to prevent catheter thrombosis, but studies have shown that non- heparinized saline has no higher risk of catheter thrombosis (Fig. 14.4).

The bag is pressurized to 300 mmHg, it serves two purposes one is to flush the catheter and the other is some systems allow a continuous infusion at 3–4 ml/h to prevent catheter thrombosis.

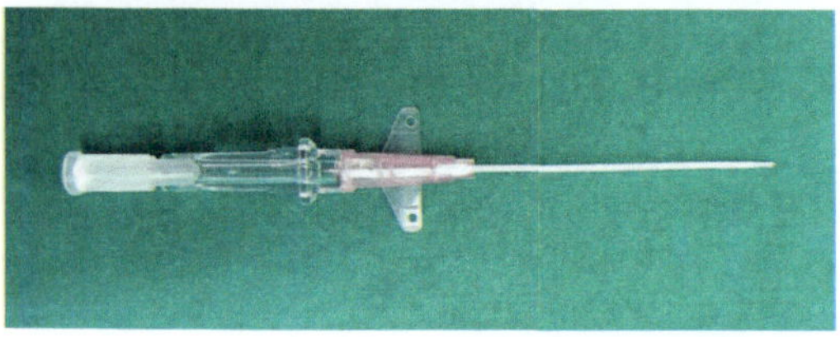

Fig. 14.1 One 20 G arterial cannula

> **Pro Tip** Use a collapsible fluid bag rather than a regular fluid bottle as there will be fluid leaks associated with the later.

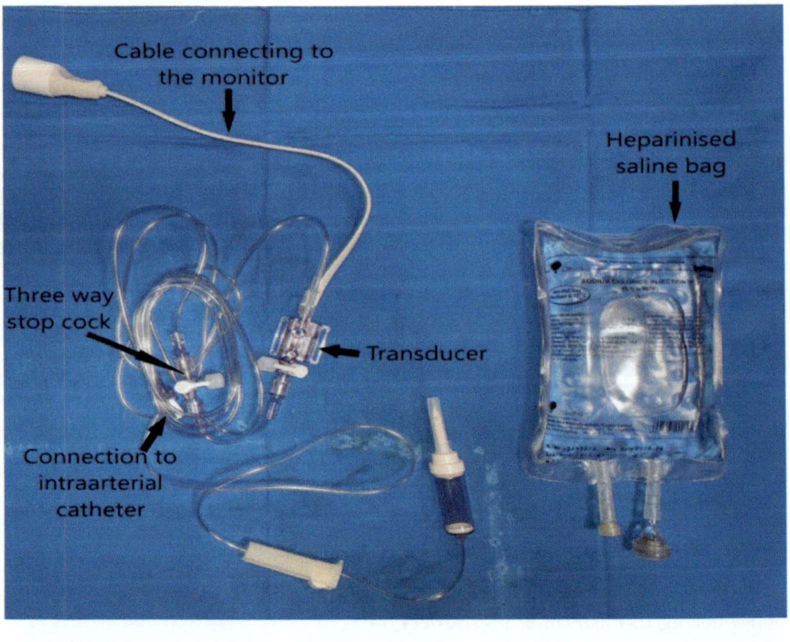

Fig. 14.2 Transducer, pressure bag and tubing setup

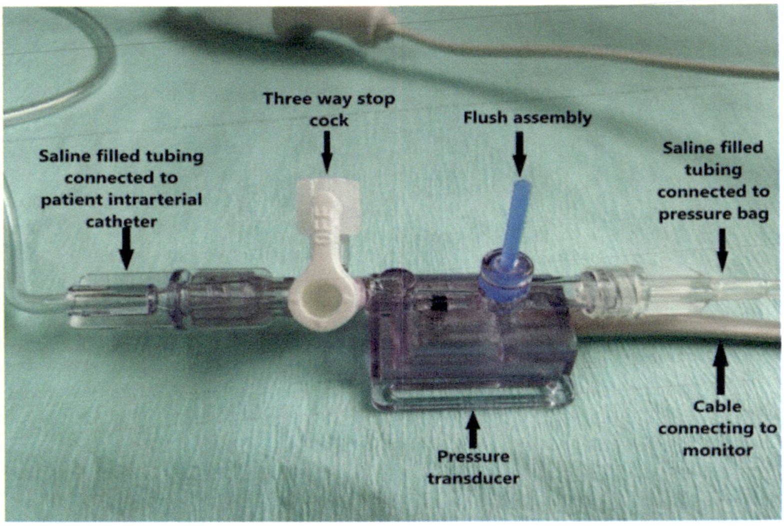

Fig. 14.3 The transducer has a flush assembly to rapidly flush the system, a three way stop cock for zeroing to the atmosphere and a cable which connects to the monitor

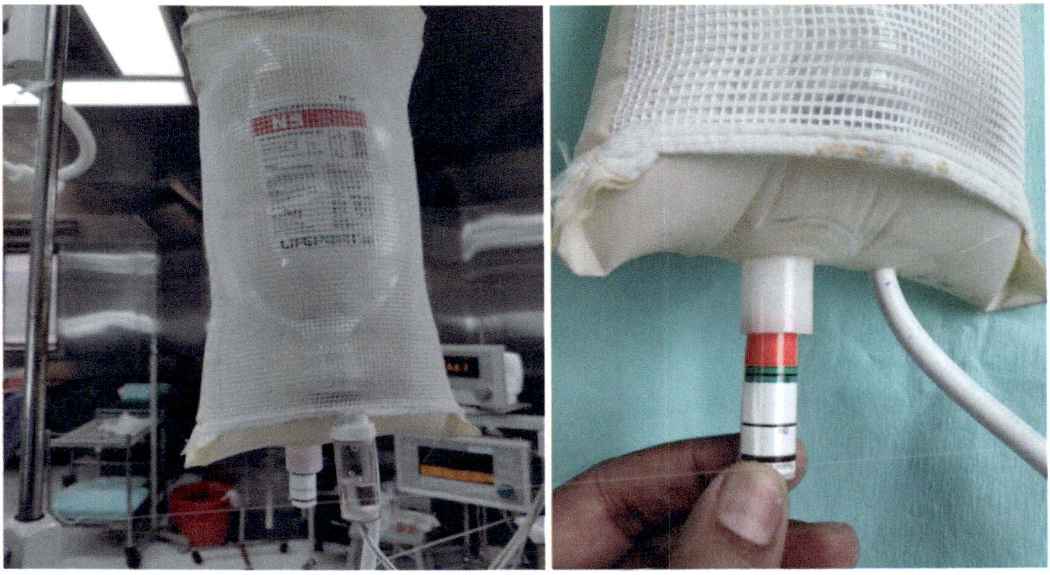

Fig. 14.4 Pressure bag assembly

(iv) Three way stop cocks: there are two three way stop cocks in the system one is part of the transducer assembly which can be used for zeroing of the transducer. The other stop cock is closer to the patient end, it is used to draw blood and to deair the system.

3. **Monitor and cable:** The configuration of the adaptor of the cable connecting to the monitor is not standardized i.e. it is different for each transducer manufacturer. Always make sure that the cable is compatible with the transducer and monitor (Fig. 14.5).

14.2.2 Transducer Setup

1. Assemble the pressure monitoring set, the equipment should be assembled for use prior to line insertion and confirm that the connections are secure.

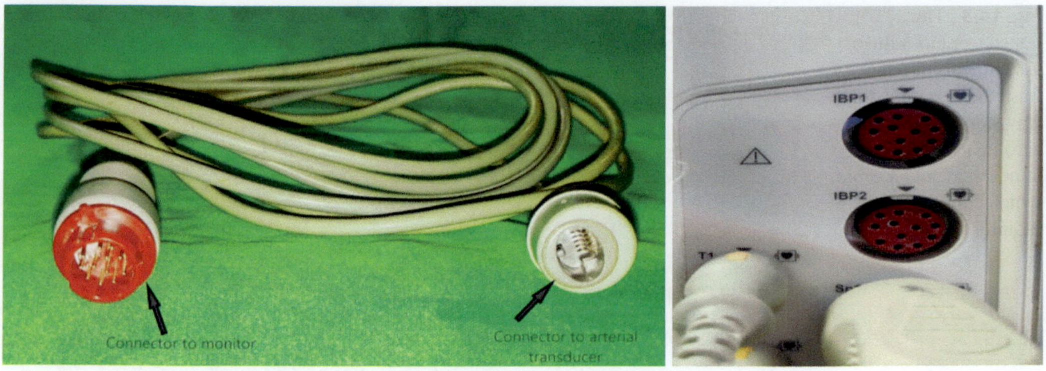

Fig. 14.5 Cables for IAP measurement other equipment required

2. Add heparin 1000 IU to the saline bag. Ensure that the flush system is free of air bubbles, and that all parts are primed with fluid.
3. Ensure the pressure bag is inflated to 300 mmHg.

14.2.3 Preparation

- Personal protective equipment: sterile gloves, cap, mask, and goggles.
- Antiseptic prep solution.
- Sterile fenestrated drape.
- Sterile dressing/Transparent occlusive dressing.
- Pressure bag.
- Arterial pressure transducer kit.
- Arterial catheter 20 G/22 G.
- 0.9% sodium chloride 500 mL
- Lignocaine 2% 5 mL for local infiltration.
- 5 ml syringe with heparinized saline for flushing
- Monitor with pressure cable.
- Line labels.

14.2.4 Procedure

Steps: 1. Selection of artery
2. Allen's or Modified Allen's Test
3. Assembly of Equipment, Cannula and Heparinized Saline
4. Asepsis
5. Insertion of Arterial Cannula, Flushing and Fixation
6. Connecting to the Transducer System and Monitoring

Explain the patient regarding the procedure and written consent should be taken.

14.2.5 Selection of Artery

Radial artery of the non- dominant hand is the ideal site for cannulation due to its accessibility. It is recommended to perform the Allen's test (or modified Allen's test) to detect adequacy of collateral supply to the hand via the ulnar artery before cannulation.

Other sites which are less commonly used are the femoral artery, ulnar artery, dorsalis pedis, posterior tibial and the axillary artery. The distal limb should be monitored regularly for signs of ischemia and care should be taken to avoid emboli.

> The brachial artery should be avoided as there is no collateral blood supply.

Position the patient (if the radial artery is to be used, an intravenous fluid bottle/rolled towel may be used to hyperextend the wrist to allow easier visualization of landmarks) (Fig. 14.6).

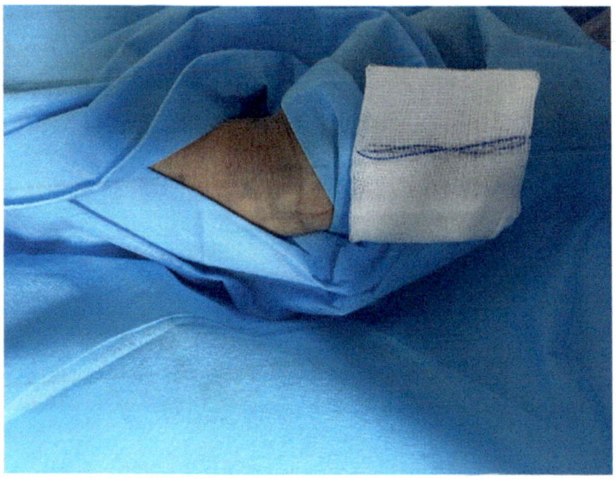

Fig. 14.6 Positioning for radial artery catherization

14.2.6 Insertion of a Radial Arterial Line

Allen's test: Perform Allen's test to detect adequacy of collateral supply to the hand via the ulnar artery. The test can only be performed in an awake and cooperative patient; also, it is not fail-safe putting the patient for higher risk of distal ischemia.

Aseptic precautions and local anesthesia: the site should be cleaned with antiseptic prep solution prior to cannulation. In conscious patients, the skin should be infiltrated with 1% plain lignocaine.

Position: The arm should be abducted and the wrist should be hyper-extended over a rolled towel or saline bag to aid cannulation. This can be done by an assistant or use tape to secure the patients hand fingers extended over a bag of fluid.

Cannula insertion: All arterial catheters should be inserted using aseptic technique. Personal protective equipment should be worn during the insertion and removal of an arterial line and for whenever the arterial line is accessed. Strict aseptic technique should be followed during insertion and management The usual insertion technique is to palpate the artery with the fingers of one hand and locate the artery with the cannula at an angle of about 30°. Once a "flashback" has been obtained the cannula is brought level with the skin and then advanced 2–3 mm further which will ensure that the entire tip of the cannula, rather than just the needle, is within the arterial lumen. Then the cannula can be advanced over the needle.

Flush with heparinized saline or connect the transducer tubing. Apply transparent occlusive dressing. While still scrubbed, the operator must connect the transducer to the arterial line to confirm arterial placement. Ensure sampling port is in "ON" position, the transducer is attached to the pressure cable and monitor.

Once there is an identifiable arterial trace line, zero the arterial line. Label the line appropriately, including "ARTERIAL" close to the arterial blood sampling port. Document the insertion in the case notes, include the site, date and time.

Nowadays, ultrasound can be used to guide arterial line placement. Ultrasound-guided arterial catheterization is an effective technique for placing an arterial catheter. It can reduce the risk of complications and improve patient outcomes. An ultrasound probe (linear high frequency preferably small footprint) should be used to localization of artery (Fig. 14.7). Thereafter the probe can be rotated to view the long axis view for insertion of arterial cannula under real time ultrasound guidance.

14.2.7 Zeroing and Leveling

Zeroing is a process which confirms that atmospheric pressure results in a zero reading by the measurement system. The device is zeroed when the air-fluid interface is opened to atmospheric pressure. Re-zeroing must be done regularly as both the transducer and the atmospheric pressure will gradually drift away from the calibration point.

Procedure: Once the transducer tubing is connected to the arterial line.

Observe the arterial line trace on the monitor. Open the three-way stopcock (off to the patient and exposing the transducer to the atmosphere) and the tracing should disappear on the monitor.

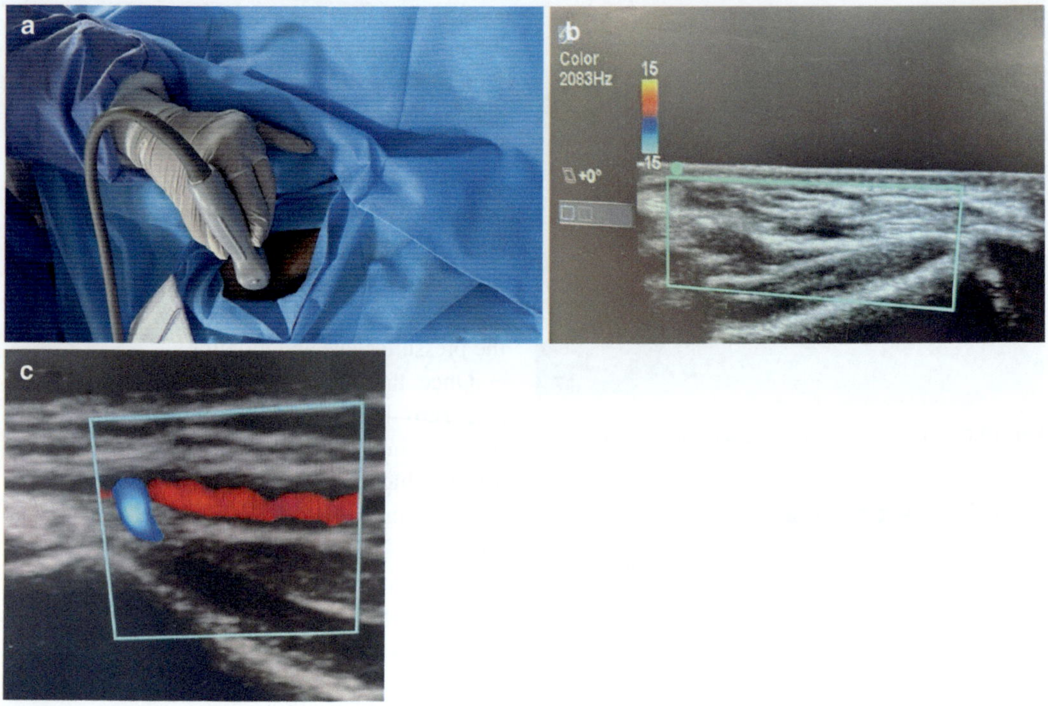

Fig. 14.7 USG linear probe placed on draped hand for radial artery puncture (**a**); short axis (**b**) and long axis view (**c**) of the radial artery under USG guidance

Press art line zero on the monitor, the monitor should confirm that the arterial line is zeroed and should display the arterial BP as zero. Turn the 3-way stopcock back and ensure that the arterial blood pressure waveform and value are displayed. Close the three-way stopcock with a cap and label it.

Leveling can be defined as "a position of interest at which the reference standard (zero) is set." The transducer is leveled at the intersection of the fourth intercostal space and the mid thoracic anterior-posterior diameter.

This is an external landmark used to identify the level of the root of aorta/atria which corresponds to the phlebostatic axis in the supine patient.

In intracranial surgeries, the transducer is leveled at the external auditory meatus to reflect the pressure at the circle of Willis.

Clinical pearl

A 10 cm error in leveling causes an error of 7.4 mmHg in the pressure reading. If the transducer is moved below the zeroed level shows falsely high reading and if it is moved above the reading is falsely low.

To avoid leveling errors due to movement of the table the author tapes the transducer to the patient's midarm or to a stand attached to the table.

Damping In an oscillating system, anything that reduces the energy will reduce the amplitude of the oscillation this is known as damping.

A small air bubble can lower the natural resonant frequency resulting in a spuriously elevated systolic blood pressure. A large air bubble will lead to excessive signal damping and cause underestimation of the systolic blood pressure. The causes for damping are

- Three-way stopcocks: resistance or turbulence in the system should be avoided.
- Bubbles/clots.
- Vasospasm.
- Narrow, long or compliant tubing.
- Kinking of the arterial cannula or tubing.

14.2.8 Complications

Temporary vascular occlusion/thrombosis
Rare: nerve damage and severe ischemia
Distal ischemia
Hematoma formation
Catheter-related infection and sepsis

Suggested Readings

1. Kim JM, Arakawa K, Bliss J. Arterial cannulation: factors in the development of occlusion. Anesth Analg. 1975;54:836–41.
2. Nuttall G, Burckhardt J, Hadley A, Kane S, Kor D, Marienau MS, et al. Surgical and patient risk factors for severe arterial line complications in adults. Anesthesiology. 2016;124:590–7.
3. Gleich SJ, Wong AV, Handlogten KS, Thum DE, Nemergut ME. Major short-term complications of arterial cannulation for monitoring in children. Anesthesiology. 2021;134:26–34.
4. Tiru B, Bloomstone JA, McGee WT. Radial artery cannulation: a review article. J Anesth Clin Res. 2012;3:209.
5. Lamperti M, Biasucci DG, Disma N, Pittiruti M, Breschan C, Vailati D, et al. European Society of Anaesthesiology guidelines on peri-operative use of ultrasound-guided for vascular access (PERSEUS vascular access). Eur J Anaesthesiol. 2020;37:344–76.
6. Melhuish TM, White LD. Optimal wrist positioning for radial arterial cannulation in adults: a systematic review and meta-analysis. Am J Emerg Med. 2016;34:2372–8.
7. Belda FJ, Aguilar G, Teboul JL, Pestaña D, Redondo FJ, Malbrain M, et al. PICS Investigators Group. Complications related to less-invasive haemodynamic monitoring. Br J Anaesth. 2011;106:482–6.
8. Scheer B, Perel A, Pfeiffer UJ. Clinical review: complications and risk factors of peripheral arterial catheters used for haemodynamic monitoring in anaesthesia and intensive care medicine. Crit Care. 2002;6:199–204.

Arterial Blood Gas Sampling and Pitfalls

15

Bhavna Kayarat, Nishkarsh Gupta, and Anju Gupta

Key Points

- ABG sampling is an important skill for management of critical patients in ICU.
- The measurement of pH, pO2, and pCO2 in the ABG sample is a vital procedure.
- Intensivists need to be proficient in the procedure, interpretation, and pitfalls of the procedure.
- One must be familiar with the anatomy of the arteries one needs to puncture for sampling.

15.1 Introduction

Arterial blood sampling remains an extremely important procedure for the critical care physician. In 1711, Stephan Hales performed the first blood vessel cannulation by inserting brass pipes in the arterial and venous vasculature of a horse. Since then, the practice of arterial blood sampling and cannulation has evolved and remains a vital procedure, performed daily in the critically ill population. Measurements of arterial pH and partial pressures of oxygen and carbon dioxide provide precise information regarding a patient s acid–base balance and gas exchange. Although a majority of the critically ill patients have an arterial catheter in situ, all medical trainees and intensivists need to be proficient with the procedure, interpretation, and pitfalls of arterial blood puncture. In this chapter, we discuss the anatomy of the vasculature; indications, the procedure, common complications; and pitfalls associated with the interpretation of arterial blood gas sampling.

15.2 Indications

The common indications for arterial blood sampling include

- Management of patients with severe acid/base disturbances.
- Patients with respiratory distress/potential respiratory derangements.
- In primary evaluation of any critically ill patient to assess electrolytes and hemoglobin.
- To assess arterial lactate levels.
- To assess carboxyhemoglobin in CO poisoning.

B. Kayarat · A. Gupta
Anesthesiology, Pain Medicine, Critical Care, All India Institute of Medical Sciences, New Delhi, Delhi, India

N. Gupta (✉)
Department Onco-Anesthesiology and Palliative Medicine at DRBRAIRCH, All India Institute of Medical Sciences, New Delhi, Delhi, India

N. Gupta et al. (eds.), *Techniques in Anesthesia, Intensive Care and Emergency Medicine*,
https://doi.org/10.1007/978-981-96-1202-4_15

- To assess response to therapy in critically ill patients.
- Situations associated with fallacies of pulse oximetry monitoring.

15.3 Contraindication

The contraindications for arterial blood puncture include

- Infection over the sampling site.
- Severe peripheral vascular disease in the selected artery to be sampled.
- Known deficiency of collateral circulation to the artery to be sampled.
- Severe coagulopathy.
- Presence of arterial venous fistula at the site of sampling artery.
- Patients with history of Raynaud's phenomenon.

15.4 Relevant Anatomy

An understanding of normal arterial anatomy and common anatomic variants is of utmost importance. The radial artery, although smaller than the ulnar artery, is more commonly preferred for arterial puncture. The rationale being that is more superficial and is often stabilized more easily. The use of the brachial artery is another safe and reliable alternative site. At times, the femoral artery is also used for arterial puncture. Another notable landmark is the flexor carpi radialis tendon that runs immediately medial to the radial artery. The recommended point of needle insertion is at the proximal flexor crease of the wrist and directly above the radial artery pulse.

The radial artery is a branch of the brachial artery. It courses over the flexor digitorum and flexor pollicis muscles and lies just lateral to the flexor carpi radialis in the forearm. A notable landmark is that the radial artery can be palpated just medial and proximal to the radial styloid process on the ventrolateral wrist. A 45–60° dorsiflexion of the wrist can aid in palpating the arterial pulse. As the artery enters the floor of the palm, it ends in the deep volar arterial arch and communicates with the ulnar artery. A second site of collateral flow for the radial artery occurs via the dorsal arch running in the dorsum of the hand. In the hand, the ulnar artery runs over the transverse carpal ligament and forms the superficial volar arch, which forms the third minor anastomosis with a the radial artery. These three anastomoses thus contribute to good collateral flow to the hand. It is to be noted that one of these anastomoses could be absent in up to 20% of individuals.

The brachial artery is a continuation of the axillary artery. It then bifurcates just below the elbow to the ulnar and radial arteries. The brachial artery courses along the medial side of the antecubital fossa just lateral to the median nerve. An important landmark is that it is lateral to the medial epicondyle of the humerus and medial to the biceps brachii muscle and therefore easily identified when the elbow is fully extended. In order to locate the artery, start by palpating the medial epicondyle of the humerus. The brachial artery is best palpated in the antecubital fossa at the level of the proximal flexor crease.

The femoral artery courses under the inguinal ligament near the junction of the medial and the middle third of a line drawn between the tubercle of the pubic symphisis and the anterior superior iliac spine. The femoral artery is larger than other arteries and is deeper than the radial or brachial arteries, necessitating the usage of a longer cannula. Extension and slight abduction of the hip improves access to the femoral triangle enabling easier palpation.

15.4.1 Evaluation of Collateral Circulation of the Hand

Before the procedure, to evaluate collateral circulation of the head, the modified Allen's test is performed. Poor collateral perfusion is noted in 10–12% of the population. If the perfusion to ulnar artery is poor and a cannula or the puncturing occludes the radial artery, blood flow to the hand may be impaired.

The test is performed by asking the patient to clench his hand. The ulnar and radial arteries are together occluded with digital pressure. The hand is subsequently unclenched and pressure over the ulnar artery is released. If there is adequate collateral circulation, the palm should flush in less than 6 s. In practice, the usefulness of this test is questionable in patients with altered sensorium and patients on sedation and paralysis. The Allen test is subjective, often improperly performed, and has poor sensitivity and specificity to predict complications. Although an abnormal Allen test may not preclude radial artery puncture or cannulation, it may indicate a greater need for caution and the possibility of complications including thrombosis, hand ischemia, and necrosis.

An alternative method of assessing the collateral circulation in an unconscious or an uncooperative patient is the usage of a pulse oximeter with a pulse waveform display. The pulse oximeter sensor is placed on the patient's thumb and waveform is observed. The radial artery is occluded and the waveform is then observed. In a radial-dominant or an ulnar-dominant system with adequate collateral circulation, the waveform is likely to remain unchanged while the radial artery is occluded. The Doppler ultrasound is yet another alternate method to ascertain collateral hand perfusion.

15.4.2 Site Selection

Several factors are to be considered while selecting the site for arterial puncture. The ideal artery has to have extensive collateral circulation that will maintain the viability of distal tissues in the event of thrombosis. Sites involved by infection, any disruption of the epidermis, vessel ischemia, or thrombosis need to be avoided. The most commonly used sites for arterial puncture in adults are the radial, femoral, and brachial arteries. Each site has unique complications, and they should be taken into account by the proceduralist.

The radial artery is often chosen first. The radial artery is small and easily stabilized because it passes over a bony groove located at the wrist. The brachial artery is larger than the radial artery, but the risk of median nerve injury due to its proximity to the brachial artery remains. Hemostasis after an arterial puncture is enhanced by the vessels proximity to bone. The femoral artery is generally preferred when there is altered perfusion to the upper limbs or limited access as in the case of cardiopulmonary arrest. Complications related to femoral artery puncture include hemorrhage and hematoma because bleeding could be difficult to control; inadvertent puncture of the femoral vein because of the close proximity of the vein to the artery; infection because aseptic technique in the groin area is difficult to maintain; and limb ischemia if the femoral artery is damaged.

15.5 Sonoanatomy

Ultrasonography has useful application related to arterial catheterization. Although ultrasound guidance to decrease complication rates of central venous catheter insertion has become relatively commonplace, fewer clinicians are familiar with the use of ultrasound to guide arterial puncture and catheterization.

Arterial puncture can be especially challenging for patients with obesity, edema, small vessel caliber, and shock states that obscure pulsatility. Additionally, repeated attempts after initial failure often result in arterial spasm, leading to further failed attempts with increased risk of complications. Multiple studies and meta-analyses have proven the benefits of real-time ultrasound-guided arterial catheterization by demonstrating increased success rates and overall reductions of rates of complications.

15.6 Procedure

15.6.1 Preparation (Fig. 15.1)

- Asepsis:
- Equipment needed for arterial blood sampling:
  1. Blood gas syringe (pre-heparinized, if available).
  2. 1 mL tuberculin syringe (for local infiltration)
  3. Needle size 23 G–25 G (longer needles may be needed for brachial and femoral artery puncture).

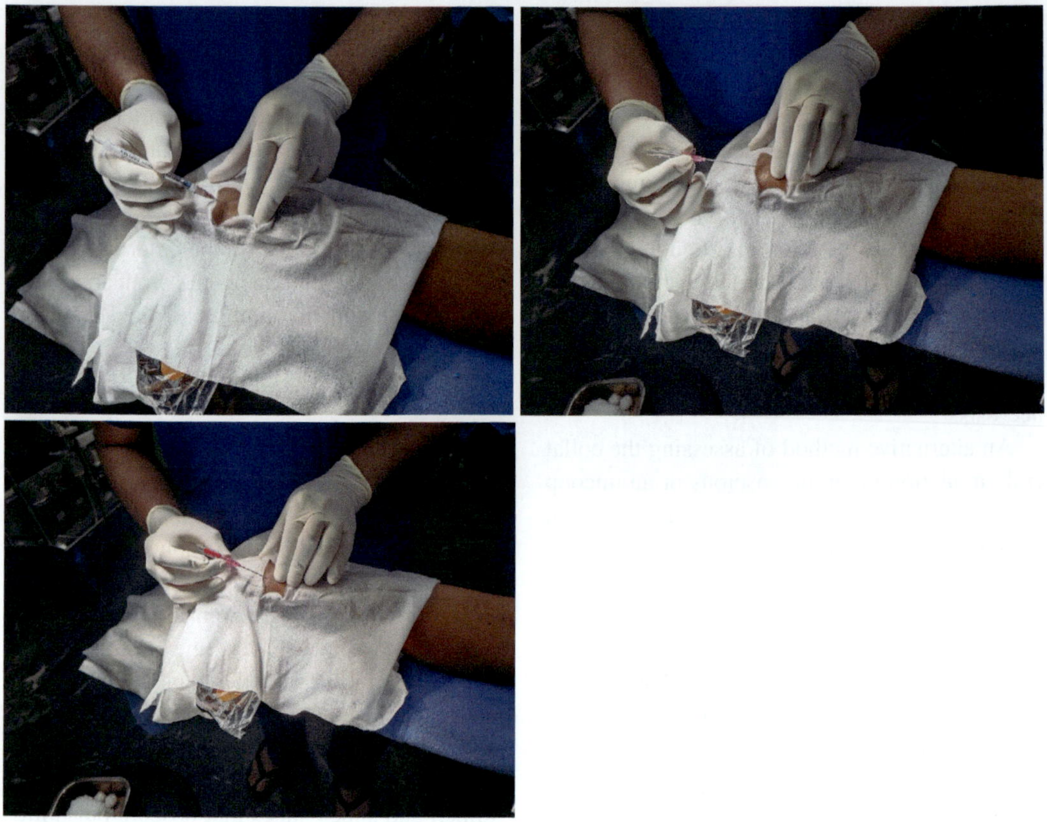

Fig. 15.1 Positioning and procedure for ABG sampling

4. Liquid heparin flush: 0.05 mL of 1000 IU/mL concentration of heparin for per mL of blood drawn (e.g., 0.1 mL of 1000 IU/mL of heparin for 2 mL of blood sample).
5. Rolled towel to aid in positioning of wrist (for radial artery puncture).

15.6.2 Procedure

- Explain procedure to the patient.
- Assess for factors that can interfere with the blood gas measurements, including patient anxiety, suctioning, use of nebulizer treatment, change in oxygen therapy/ventilator settings, and body temperature.
- Reconfirm the patient s past history (e.g., use of radial artery for coronary artery bypass surgery, presence of arterio venous fistulas or shunts).
- If the patient is on oxygen or mechanical ventilation, ensure that the current settings are ongoing for at least 20–30 min before obtaining the sample.
- Site selection and position (radial/brachial/femoral):
- Prefer nondominant hand for radial artery punctures. The hand is positioned in 30–60° of dorsiflexion with the aid of a rolled towel, avoiding hyperabduction of thumb.
- This aids in bringing the radial artery to a more superficial position.
- For femoral puncture, the patient is positioned in supine, straight-leg position.
- Feel for strongest point of maximal arterial impulse. Ultrasound can also be used to localise the artery.
- Part preparation with 2% chlorhexidine with 70% alcohol. Allow antiseptic to dry.

- Around 0.5 mL of lidocaine is infiltrated through a 25 G or smaller needle. Aspirate prior to injection to ensure that the vessel has not been punctured.
- Hold the heparinized syringe-needle assembly.
- Slowly insert the needle and after skin puncture. Once the artery is hit, the blood is seen in needle hub and then gently apply a slight negative pressure and the syringe fills in quickly.
- Another technique to insert needle all the way till it hits the bone, and then to slowly retract it till syringe starts filling.

To confirm that the sample is arterial, look for the pulsation when blood enters hub of the needle. The syringe will also autofill with blood without any withdrawal effort. Under normal conditions, arterial blood is bright red in color, but the color could be altered when oxygenation is hampered.

- Sample handling: After sampling, the needle is quickly retracted, and sealed to prevent contact with air. Remove any air/air bubble from the syringe.
  - Post-sampling compression: Immediately after needle is withdrawn, digital pressure is applied for 3–5 min.

15.6.2.1 Arterial Blood Gas Sampling from an Arterial Line

Prior to taking blood sample from the arterial line, ensure patency of arterial line, i.e., the pressure in pressure bag is raised up to 300 mm Hg, the tubing from the arterial cannula site to the three-way tap is clear and the arterial line flushes easily.

- Insert a 5 mL syringe into the three-way tap, subsequently turn the tap OFF to the flush solution and slowly withdraw 5 mL of blood. Subsequently discard both syringe and blood.
- Turn the three-way tap OFF half way between transducer line and syringe.
- Insert a heparinized 2 ml syringe into three-way tap. Turn the tap OFF to flush solution, gently apply a negative pressure and blood will slowly fill into the syringe.
- Turn three-way tap OFF to patient and remove the syringe. Thereafter flush the line and ensure that the arterial line and threeway stopcock are clear of blood.
- Replace the needle or stopper on the blood gas syringe. Remove air/air bubble, if any from the syringe.

15.7 Complications

The most common technical difficulties associated with arterial puncture are the failure to obtain a blood sample because of vasospasm and the collection of venous blood instead of arterial blood. If vasospasm is suspected, the procedure can be stopped and reattempted at a different site. Compartment syndrome, radial arterial aneurysm and limb ischemia, and hematoma though described in literature are relatively rare.

Nerve injury from direct puncture of the nerve has also been reported. Neuropathy as a result of a hematoma formation and subsequent nerve compression has been described as well. This can be prevented by applying direct compression to the vessel for 3–4 min after the arterial puncture. Although small hematomas are common, major bleeding is unusual and generally observed as concealed retroperitoneum after femoral artery puncture or cannulation.

15.8 Sources of Error in Interpretation of an Arterial Blood Gas

The most common problems that are encountered include nonarterial or mixed arterial venous samples, presence of air bubbles, inadequate or excessive anticoagulant in the sample, and delayed analysis of a noncooled sample.

(i) Air bubbles in the sample: Any air bubble in the sample must be removed as soon as possible. An air bubble whose relative volume is up to 1% of the blood in the syringe is a potential source of error. The presence of air bubbles in the syringe could result in a significant increase of PaO2 and a decrease in PaCO2.

(ii) Sample with excessive anticoagulant: Excess liquid heparin causes a dilution of the sample, i.e., dilutes the plasma, but not the contents of the blood cells which can interfere with the values of pCO2 and electrolytes. The dilution effect will also depend on the hematocrit value. Plasma electrolytes, pCo2 and glucose levels decrease proportionately with the dilution, whereas pH and pO2 values are relatively unaffected by dilution.

Heparin binds to positive ions such as Ca2+, K+, and Na+. Electrolytes bound to heparin cannot be measured by ion-selective electrodes, hence leading to false low values. The use of electrolyte-balanced heparin significantly reduces this effect and the resulting inaccuracy.

(iii) Inappropriate type of syringe used: Gas-tight syringe rather than evacuated tubes are to be used ideally.

(iv) Leucocyte larceny: If the sample measured contains an excessive number of leukocytes, they tend to consume the oxygen leading to a spurious hypoxemia, commonly referred to as "leukocyte larceny." Studies have observed a blood samples a PaO2 drop of up to 72 mmHg with high WBC counts.

(v) Delayed analysis of sample: The samples are to be analyzed within 30 min. For samples with high paO2, e.g., shunt or with high leukocyte or platelet count they need to be analyzed within 5 min.

With delay in sampling; pH decreases; HCO3- decreases; SBE decreases; lactate increases and glucose decreases. PaO2 decreases and PaCO2 increases as a consequence of RBC metabolism.

(vi) Hemolyzed sample: Hemolyzed by inappropriately small needle; hemolyzed by syringe vacuum can interfere with the measurements.

Suggested Reading

1. Ruengsakulrach P, Brooks M, Hare DL, Gordon I, Buxton BF. Preoperative assessment of hand circulation by means of Doppler ultrasonography and the modified Allen test. J Thorac Cardiovasc Surg. 2001;121:526–31.
2. Gurjar M. Manual of ICU procedures. 1st ed. Jaypee Brothers Medical Publishers (P) Ltd; 2016. English ISBN: 978-93-5152-422-9.717
3. Barone JE, Madlinger RV. Should an Allen test be performed before radial artery cannulation? J Trauma. 2006;61:468–70.
4. Agrifoglio M, Dainese L, Pasotti S, et al. Preoperative assessment of the radial artery for coronary artery bypass grafting: is the clinical Allen test adequate? Ann Thorac Surg. 2005;79:570–2.
5. Halpern AA, Mochizuki R, Long CE III. Compartment syndrome of the forearm following radial-artery puncture in a patient treated with anti-coagulants. J Bone Joint Surg Am. 1978;60:1136–7.
6. Pillow K, Herrick IA. Pulse oximetry compared with Doppler ultrasound for assessment of collateral blood flow to the hand. Anaesthesia. 1991;46:338–90.
7. AARC Clinical Practice Guidelines. Sampling for arterial blood gas analysis. Respir Care. 1992;37(8):913–7.
8. National Committee for Clinical Laboratory Standards. Procedures for the collection of diagnostic blood specimens by skin puncture. 3rd ed. Pennsylvania: NCCLS; 1992.
9. Okeson GC, Wulbrecht PH. The safety of brachial artery puncture for arterial blood sampling. Chest. 1998;114(3):748–51. [PubMed: 9743161]
10. Nevasier RJ, Adams JP, May GI. Complications of arterial puncture in anticoagulated patients. J Bone Joint Surg Am. 1976;35:1118–23.

16 Total Intravenous Anesthesia (TIVA)

Rohini Dattatri, Poonam Godhwal, and Nishkarsh Gupta

Key Points

- It is an increasingly popular choice for maintenance of anesthesia using sedative hypnotic anesthetic (typically Propofol) and an analgesic component (typically an opioid).
- Benefits are seen in outcomes like quality of recovery, adequate analgesia, less impact on neurocognitive function, and survival advantages in cancer patients.
- Propofol is typically chosen as has rapid onset and recovery with added advantage of its antiemetic, anticonvulsant, antipruritic, and bronchodilator's properties.
- Remifentanyl is the most suitable opioid for TIVA technique mainly during variable noxious stimulus during procedure.
- Both remifentanyl and Propofol have similar pharmacokinetic profile of rapid elimination and shorter half life.
- Target controlled infusion (TCI) systems are designed using pharmacokinetic and pharmacodynamic properties of drugs, patient's covariate based on computer assisted IV infusion pumps to maintain target concentration at an effect site.
- Three compartment model is typically used and computer constantly calculates agent required to achieve target effect site concentration, than recalculates how much drug is in the tissues. For this, TCI pump initially gives a bolus followed by administration of infusion to maintain the target concentration.
- Some disadvantages include inter subject variability in pharmacodynamics and pharmacokinetic properties.

16.1 Introduction

Total intravenous anesthesia (TIVA) is a technique of maintenance of general anesthesia without the use of inhalational anesthetics. A combination of hypnotics with or without analgesics is used to achieve the desired clinical end-point. A clear understanding of the pharmacokinetics of TIVA/TCI (target-controlled infusion) is necessary as improper usage can lead to

R. Dattatri
Department of Anesthesiology, AIIMS, Bibinagar, Telangana, India

P. Godhwal · N. Gupta (✉)
Department Onco-Anesthesiology and Palliative Medicine at DRBRAIRCH, All India Institute of Medical Sciences, New Delhi, Delhi, India

N. Gupta et al. (eds.), *Techniques in Anesthesia, Intensive Care and Emergency Medicine*,
https://doi.org/10.1007/978-981-96-1202-4_16

accidental awareness during anesthesia as reported in the Fifth National Audit Project (NAP) on accidental awareness during general anesthesia (NAP5) report. TIVA has definite advantages in certain scenarios where the use of inhalational anesthetics might not be possible such as non-operating room anesthesia (NORA), during transfer of the patients, airway surgeries, high risk of postoperative nausea and vomiting (PONV), patients with malignant hyperthermia. During TIVA, anesthesia can be induced and maintained by either manual dosing where the provider determines the bolus dose and infusion rate, or by using a TCI pump where the anesthetist enters the desired "target" concentration to be achieved in the patient's plasma or brain. This chapter provides an overview of practical aspects related to TIVA.

16.2 Indications for TIVA

Few indications for TIVA have been given in Table 16.1.

Table 16.1 Indications of TIVA

SI	Indications
1.	History of PONV
2.	Tubeless ENT and thoracic surgery
3.	Anticipated difficult intubation/extubation
4.	Neurosurgery
5.	Intra-operative neurophysiological monitoring
6.	Myasthenia gravis/ neuromuscular disorders to avoid neuromuscular blockers
7.	Day care surgery
8.	Risk of malignant hyperthermia
9.	Long QT syndrome
10.	Non- operating room anesthesia
11.	Transfer of anesthetised patients
12.	Choice of the patient

16.3 Practice of TIVA

Society for Intravenous Anesthesia (SIVA) and Association of Anesthetists have produced guidelines for the safe conduct of TIVA. The recommendations include –

- Need for competency and training in TIVA for all anesthetists.
- Use of TCI during propofol-based anesthesia maintenance is recommended.
- The clinical situations, co-administered drugs, and patient characteristics should be considered when choosing target concentrations. Setting a low initial target concentration with repeated small incremental increases is helpful in older, frail, and sick patients.
- To reduce drug errors, Remifentanil should be diluted to a single standard concentration and a single concentration of propofol should be stocked preferably.
- The infusion set should have a Luer-lock connector, an anti-syphon valve on the drug delivery line, and an anti-reflux valve on the fluid administration line. The dead space should be minimized by ensuring that the fluid lines join as close to the patient. It is preferable to use TIVA- specific administration sets.
- Programme the infusion pumps only after the syringe containing the drug to be infused has been placed in the pump.
- If possible, ensure the visibility of the intravenous cannula or central venous catheter through which the infusion is being delivered during anesthesia delivery.
- It is recommended to use a processed EEG (pEEG) monitor when a neuromuscular blocking drug is used with TIVA.
- The provider should be familiar with processed electroencephalogram (EEG) monitoring.
- The same standards of practice and monitoring should apply for the administration of TIVA during NORA as for anesthesia in the operating room.

16.4 Pharmacological Agents Used During TIVA

Any combination of iv hypnotics and opioids as well as opioid-free techniques can be used during TIVA. The use of drugs with faster onset and offset times is useful for balancing adequate hypnosis/analgesia with rapid recovery. Propofol and remifentanil with minimal context-sensitive half-time are preferred drugs. The synergy of this drug combination is effective in obtunding responses to noxious stimuli.

16.5 Pharmacokinetic Principles and Models for TIVA

Three-compartment model is used to predict the pharmacokinetic behaviour of most anesthetic drugs. The exponential decline in the plasma concentration of a drug administered iv can be explained by the distribution of the drug between the **central compartment (V1, principally plasma**) and **two compartments** which equilibrate rapidly (**V2, well-perfused tissue like muscle**) and slowly (**V3, mainly fatty tissue**) (Fig. 16.1). The drug is administered into the central compartment (V1) which is the initial volume of distribution. The second (V2) and third (V3) compartments are mathematical constructs that explain the rapid and slow re-distribution of drugs from V1 into highly perfused (V2) and less well perfused (V3) tissues. The proportion of drug moving between compartments is given by **rate constants**. k_{12} indicates movement from V1 to V2 and k_{21}, the movement from V2 to V1. The proportion of the drug in V1 that is metabolized or eliminated in any unit of time is given by the **metabolic rate constant (k_{10}).** The transfer of the drug from the central compartment to the effect site (brain) is given by the **rate constant k_{e0}.** It represents the speed of equilibration between the plasma and the brain, a higher k_{e0} equates to a more rapid equilibrium. A bolus dose or infusion or both is administered to volunteers or patients and timed blood samples are obtained to assay drug concentrations and determine volumes and rate constants. Mathematical modeling software is used to estimate the pharmacokinetic variables in individual subjects and to determine the influence of potential covariates such as body weight and age on these variables.

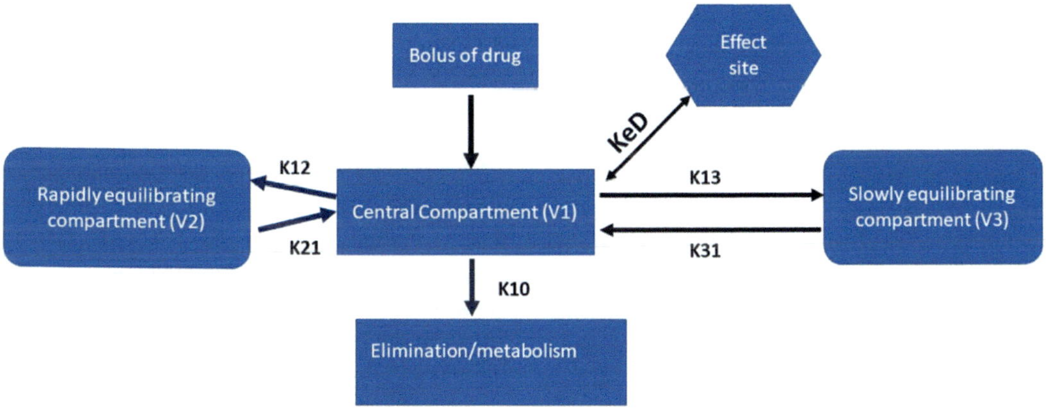

Fig. 16.1 Three-compartment model showing the various compartments and the associated rate constants. V1–3 represents the compartment volumes. K12 is the rate constant between V1 and V2, K21 between V2 and V1, etc. K10 is the rate constant for drug elimination from the central compartment. ke0 is the rate constant for equilibration between plasma and effect-site concentrations

16.6 What Is TCI?

A TCI pump helps to maintain clinically appropriate concentrations of drug in the brain in an accurate manner in equilibrium with the plasma concentration of the drug with the help of a microprocessor programmed with pharmacokinetic models for relevant drugs. The key components of a TCI pump include- a user interface, a microprocessor programmed with pharmacokinetic software, an infusion pump that can deliver up to 1200 ml/hr., and visual and audible safety systems and alarms. The drug and pharmacokinetic model to be used by the TCI pump is to be selected by the user along with entering the patient characteristics (covariates) such as body weight and age, and the target plasma or "brain" (effect-site) concentration, which allows the pump to determine the initial bolus and subsequent infusion rates.

16.7 Principles of TCI

The TCI pump uses complex mathematical equations to determine the distribution of a drug between compartments and allow rapid adjustments in targets to achieve the desired clinical effect. This is mainly based on BET (**Bolus, Elimination, Transfer**) principle. As the initial bolus dose of 600–1200 ml/hr. fills the central compartment V1, the rate of subsequent infusion is adjusted by the pump so as to compensate for the rapid and slow transfer of the drug to V2 and V3, the target concentration as well as the elimination of the drug from V1 as described by the rate constant K_{10} (rate constant for drug elimination from the central compartment in a pharmacokinetic model). This estimation is done every 10 seconds. Once a steady state concentration is reached between all three compartments, the rate of infusion slows to match elimination only. The bolus and subsequent infusion rate are calculated to maintain the target plasma concentration (Cpt).

In case the target concentration is unchanged, the infusion rate will be slowly decreased while a new bolus will be administered and the infusion rate increased if the target concentration is increased by the user. If the target concentration is decreased, the infusion is paused until the plasma concentration has reached the new target, taking into consideration the drug metabolism and flux of drug between compartments, after which time the infusion will restart at a lower rate. In the absence of an appropriate bolus with just a constant propofol infusion at 10 mg kg − 1 h − 1, it would require 40–90 min (depending on the pharmacokinetic model) to achieve a clinically useful plasma concentration of 4 μg ml − 1 in an 85 kg adult male. This might lead to an inadequate clinical effect.

16.8 Effect-Site Targeting

In this TCI mode, the user inputs a target effect-site (brain) concentration. Whenever the effect-site target concentration is increased, a bolus of the drug is administered, increasing the plasma concentration higher than the target effect-site concentration to an optimal level for a brief time so as to hasten the increase in effect-site concentration after which the infusion is stopped temporarily until the plasma concentration decreases to the level of target effect-site concentration. So, the plasma concentration is manipulated to achieve the effect site concentration rapidly. In contrast, when a target plasma concentration is used, a similar effect can be achieved on the induction by setting a higher initial plasma target which is reduced after the patient has lost consciousness. **V1, V2, and k_{eo}** in the pharmacokinetic model determine the **size of the bolus and the "overshoot" in plasma concentration** in effect-site targeting. The estimated rate of decline in plasma concentration also influences the magnitude of the overshoot in plasma concentration. If the rate of decline in plasma concentration estimated is slower, then the system will administer a lesser plasma overshoot than when faster decline so as to avoid an eventual effect-site concentration overshoot. If **k_{eo}** is smaller, a greater overshoot in the peak plasma concentration is needed so as to produce a larger concentration gradient between the plasma and the effect site and thereby hasten plasma-effect-site equilibration. The magnitude of the optimal plasma concentration overshoot-the peak plasma concentration that is generated should be sufficient to cause a rapid increase in effect-site concentration but without an over-shoot of it above the target concentration. If the effect-site target concentration is decreased, the TCI pump pauses the infusion until the estimated effect-site concentration has reduced to the new target.

16.9 TCI Models

Marsh and Schneider models are the two most commonly used propofol models. **Marsh model** is the simplest model. In this model, the **compartment volumes** are **variable** parameters scaled to **body weight** only while the **rate constants are fixed**. The age of the patient is not taken into consideration for calculating the bolus dose although it is entered to ensure that the patient's age is >16 years and used in the appropriate age group. As a result, a similar bolus dose is administered to all patients of a given body mass for any chosen Cpt leading to hemodynamic instability in elderly patients. Another major difference between Marsh and Schneider model is the volume of V1 (Marsh **19.4 liter** vs Schnider **4.27 liter** for an 85 kg individual), and therefore a bolus administered as mg kg − 1 shows a fourfold difference in calculated peak plasma concentrations. Hence, in frail patients, it is better to start the infusion at a lower Cpt with an incremental increase to obtain the desired effect.k_{e0} was not used in the original model as in the Diprifusor (AstraZeneca Limited, Macclesfield, UK) devices and can be used only for plasma targeting. However, most of the currently used newer "TCI" pumps offer effect-site targeting with the Marsh model using a more rapid ke0 (e.g., 1.2 /min) with an estimated TTPE of 1.6 minutes (Modified Marsh model) that helps to avoid excessively large loading doses. In morbidly obese patients, the induction dose is based on total body weight (TBW) leading to an increased dose being administered, and during maintenance lean body weight (LBW) is used. **Time to peak effect (TTPE)** which is the time delay between the bolus dose administered and the peak clinical effect can be used to estimate ke0 for a given pharmacokinetic model and patient group.

Schneider model considers **V1, V3** compartment volumes, rate constants **k_{13} and k_{31}** as **fixed parameters** while **V2** compartment volume along with rate constants **k_{12} and k_{21}** are **variable parameters.** Age, gender, total body weight, and height are used as covariates. Total weight, height, and lean body mass influence the metabolic rate constant k10. This model incorporates a Ke0 of 0.26/min with an estimated time-to -peak effect (TTPE) of 1.69/min. There is less hemodynamic instability as bolus doses and infusions are age adjusted. As the volume of V1 is fixed and small, a lower propofol dose suffices to achieve the Cpt. At times, this bolus dose is inappropriately small leading to inadequate clinical effect. Hence, it is preferable to use Schneider model with effect-site targeting as larger bolus doses are used. But still, the dose would be smaller as compared to the Marsh model. The cumulative dose of the drug administered by the two models using two modes of operation follows a similar pattern. The highest dose to lowest dose administered is in the following order—Marsh model (effect site), Marsh model (plasma site), Schneider (effect site), Schneider (plasma site). The comparison of the two models in plasma site and effect site is shown in Tables 16.2 and 16.3.

Table 16.2 Comparison of the propofol dose administered in Marsh and Schneider models to a 40-yr-old male, 178 cm tall, and 85 kg in weight when a 4 µg ml−1 target concentration is set in plasma concentration

Model	Plasma targeting Cpt		Cumulative dose	
	Initial bolus (mg)	Time to equilibrium (min)	At equilibrium (mg)	After 30 minutes of infusion (mg)
Marsh	86	16	360	570
Schneider	18	9.8	142	414

Table 16.3 Comparison of the propofol dose administered in Marsh and Schneider models to a 40-yr-old male, 178 cm tall, and 85 kg in weight when a 4 μg ml−1 target concentration is set in effect site concentration

Model	Effect site targeting Cet		Cumulative dose	
	Initial bolus (mg)	Time to equilibrium (min)	At equilibrium (mg)	After 30 minutes of infusion (mg)
Marsh	119	1.6	119	574
Schneider	73	1.6	73	444

Minto model is a validated model for remifentanil, and it can be used for plasma or effect-site targeted TCI in patients aged ≥12 yr., and weighing ≥30 kg. It incorporates age, weight, height, and sex as covariates. Paedfusor and Kataria models have been used in pediatric patients.

16.10 How to Choose an Appropriate Target Concentration for a Patient?

The target concentration chosen should be based on the patient characteristics, co-drugs used as well as the degree of the surgical stimulus. It should be sufficient to produce loss of consciousness, and prevent movement in response to noxious stimuli but not produce marked hypotension or delay the recovery. Older, frail patients, ASA 3–5 require lower brain anesthetic concentration compared to younger healthy adults. Propofol/remifentanil combination exhibits good synergy and allows to achieve the desired clinical effect (Table 16.4). The clinical calibration of an individual patient's response can be done by noting the effect site concentration at which there is loss of response to speech; absence of hemodynamic response or limb movement with vigorous jaw thrusting and absence of tachycardia or even bradycardia with laryngoscopy and intubation. This may be used as a guide to approximate the concentration required during the maintenance of anesthesia. The neuromuscular blocker should be administered only after the lack of response to jaw thrusting has been achieved. **Tivatrainer** pharmacokinetic software (www.eurosiva.eu) may be used to predict the necessary effect-site concentrations in real time during drug administration. It graphically plots the 50 and 95% probabilities of the absence of response to a noxious event when propofol and remifentanil TCIs are used simultaneously. Using processed EEG will help to avoid excessive hypnosis. The steps to operate TCI have been shown in Figs. 16.2, 16.3, and 16.4.

If slower induction of anesthesia is desirable, a lower initial target concentration of propofol (1 ug/ml) with repeated increments of 0.5–1 ug/ml can be used.

Table 16.4 Suggested minimum effect-site concentrations for propofol and remifentanil in adult patients

	Spontaneous breathing Age < 50 years	Spontaneous breathing Age > 50 years	IPPV Age < 50 years	IPPV Age > 50 years
Propofol(ug/ml)	4–6	2–4	3–4	2–3
Remifentanil (ng/ml)	1–3	1–2	5–8	3–6

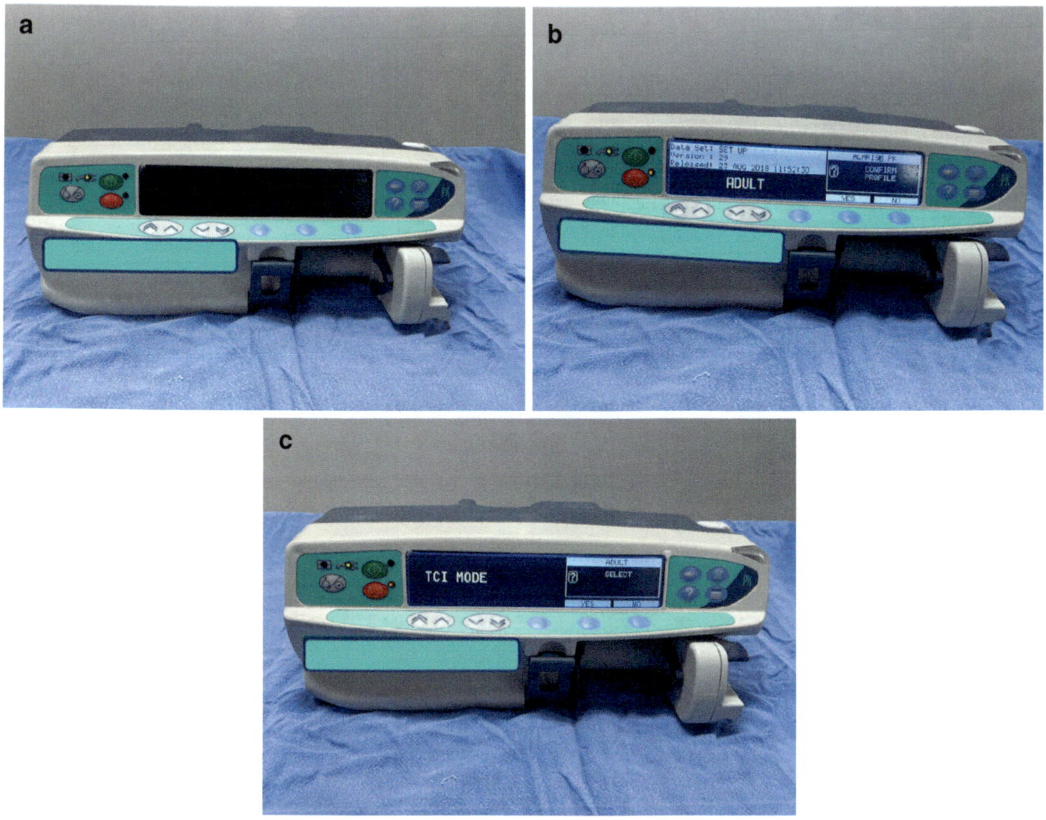

Fig. 16.2 (**a**) Place the TCI pump near the patient end. (**b**) Switch on the TCI pump. (**c**) Choose option adult followed by TCI mode

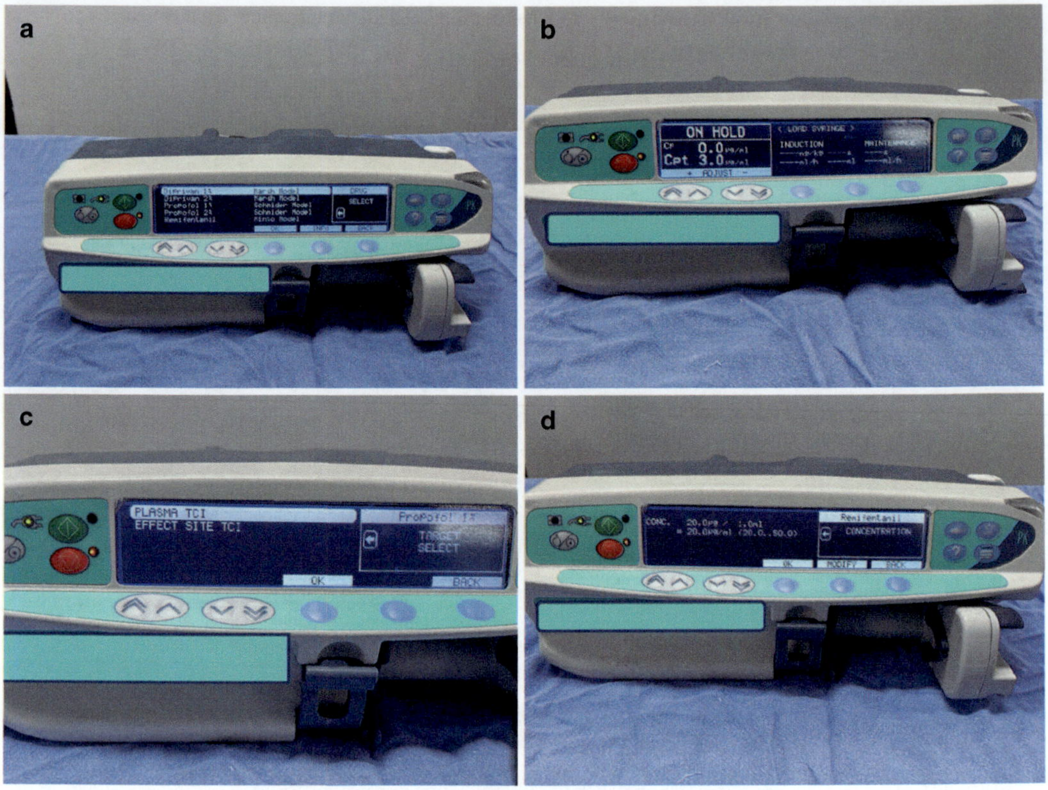

Fig. 16.3 (**a**) multiple modes will be displayed after TCI mode is selected (**b**) with diprivan 1% or 2% marsh model, next option is target plasma concentration CP that we can adjust according to Cpt (target plasma concentration) (**c**) Propofol 1% or 2% Schnider model: shows plasma TCI and effect site TCI (**d**) Remifentanyl Minto model showing target site concentration

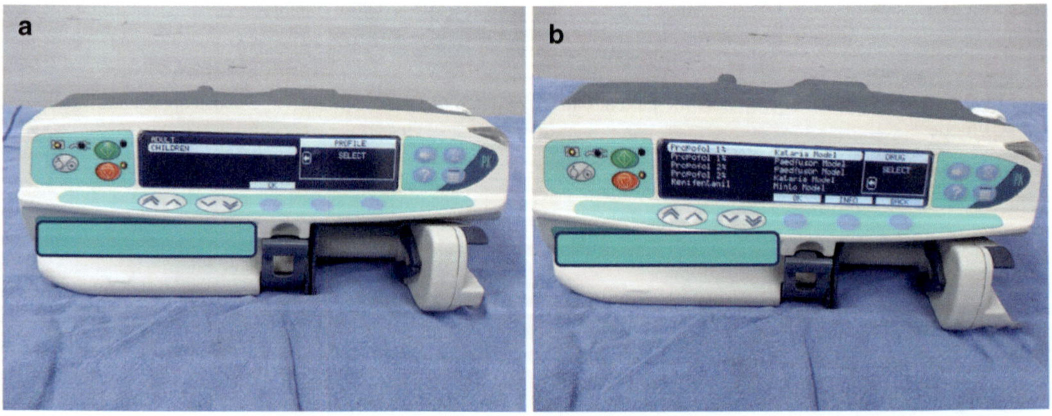

Fig. 16.4 (**a**) patient profile as children (**b**) Different models available are: Propofol 1% or 2% Katerina & paedfusor models; Minto model for remifentanyl

16.11 Terminating the Infusions

TCI targets may be reduced by the end of surgery if loco-regional techniques are used in addition to general anesthesia. Inappropriate reduction in the presence of noxious stimulus such as during wound closure should be avoided. If smooth extubation is desirable, remifentanil infusion can be continued at a target of 1–2 ng ml − 1 to smooth. Recovery may be delayed with the use of the Marsh model in obese patients and the administration of high doses of morphine. There is a risk of post-extubation apnea remains a risk until remifentanil is completely cleared from the effect site.

16.12 Potential Problems with TIVA

1. **Awareness**

   Awareness during anesthesia has been cited as the potential reason for TIVA being not so popular technique. Though the randomised controlled trials are few and these have failed to demonstrate an increased incidence with the use of TIVA [13–15]. Few studies have shown similar rates of responsiveness in subjects receiving TIVA as well as volatile anesthetics titrated to bispectral index. NAP5 has reported technical errors and poor knowledge on application as major factors for awareness during TIVA highlighting the need for education and training which can prevent this problem in 75% of cases. Use of processed EEG device when administering TIVA has been recommended by NICE which has been re- emphasized in NAP 5 specifically in patients requiring neuromuscular paralysis. Processed EEG in addition helps to avoid excessive hypnosis.

   Analgesia and hyperalgesia

   Morphine 0.15–0.3 mg/kg should be administered 30–40 minutes prior to stopping remifentanil infusion to ensure continuous analgesia post-extubation. A recent meta-analysis has addressed the phenomenon of acute opioid tolerance with the use of a high dose of intra-operative opioids which leads to a small and significant increase in acute post-operative pain. This can be dealt with by the use of adjunctive non-opioid analgesics and locoregional techniques and by using opioids as rescue drugs.

2. **Propofol-related infusion syndrome (PRIS)**

   Propofol-related infusion syndrome (PRIS) is a complication with the use of propofol infusion for a long duration, especially in critical care settings. It presents as acute metabolic acidosis and cardiac dysfunction together with rhabdomyolysis, hypertriglyceridemia, or renal failure. However, there are no published case reports of PRIS occurring in association with TIVA. TIVA in pediatric practice is safe even though it is more likely to occur in this age group when used in propofol sedation in critical care settings.

   Morbid obesity

   Providing TIVA in morbidly obese patients is challenging. Current TCI models are not validated for use in morbidly obese although it is being used in these patients. In the Marsh model, the input weight is limited to 150 kg though it can be increased with their proprietary software. The problem here is the use of actual body weight to calculate bolus dose leading to undesirable cardiovascular side effects at induction. In contrast, the Schnider and Minto models use the "James equation" to derive lean body mass (LBM) generating a paradoxically diminishing value of LBM as BMI exceeds 42 in men and 35 in women. In Schneider model, the rate constant for drug elimination from the central compartment (K10) is corrected for LBM which limits the infusion rate applied as actual body weight increases, but increase in BMI above the critical value leads to insufficient correction of infusion rate with a high rate of drug administration producing exaggerated haemodynamic effects. The converse occurs in Minto model where the central and rapidly equilibrating compartment volumes and the K10 rate constant increase proportionately with LBM. When the BMI exceeds the critical value, the bolus dose and infusion rate are progressively reduced along with inadequate analgesic effect. Continuous clinical assessment and use of processed EEG monitoring is recommended in these patients.

16.13 Conclusion

TIVA has definite advantages in certain scenarios and competency in TIVA allows for the safe administration. A good understanding of pharmacokinetics of TCI reduces the accidental awareness during the use of this technique. At present, there is no "best" TCI model for propofol and anesthesiologist should use the model which matches the patient characteristics of their usual patient population. Close monitoring of the patient is essential.

Suggested Reading

1. Nimmo AF, Cook TM. Total intravenous anesthesia. 5th National Audit Project (NAP5). Accidental Awareness during General Anaesthesia in the United Kingdom and Ireland Report and Findings—Chapter 18. The Royal College of Anaesthetists and the Association of Anaesthetists of Great Britain and Ireland, 2014.
2. Nimmo AF, Absalom AR, Bagshaw O, Biswas A, Cook TM, Costello A, Grimes S, Mulvey D, Shinde S, Whitehouse T, Wiles MD. Guidelines for the safe practice of total intravenous anesthesia (TIVA): Joint Guidelines from the Association of Anaesthetists and the Society for Intravenous Anaesthesia. Anaesthesia. 2019;74(2):211–24. https://doi.org/10.1111/anae.14428. Epub 2018 Oct 31. PMID: 30378102.
3. Vuyk J, Lim T, Engbers FH, et al. The pharmacodynamic interaction of propofol and alfentanil during lower abdominal surgery in women. Anesthesiology. 1995;83:8–20.
4. Al-Rifai Z, Mulvey D. Principles of total intravenous anaesthesia: basic pharmacokinetics and model descriptions. BJA Edu. 2016;16(3):92–7. https://doi.org/10.1093/bjaceaccp/mkv021.
5. Engbers FH, Sutcliffe N, Kenny G, Schraag S. Pharmacokinetic models for propofol: defining and illuminating the devil in the detail. BJA. 2010;104(2):261–4. https://doi.org/10.1093/bja/aep385.
6. Marsh B, White M, Morton N, Kenny GN. Pharmacokinetic model driven infusion of propofol in children. Br J Anaesth. 1991;67:41–8. 2.
7. Schnider TW, Minto CF, Gambus PL, et al. The influence of method of administration and covariates on the pharmacokinetics of propofol in adult volunteers. Anesthesiology. 1998;88:1170–82. 3.
8. Schnider TW, Minto CF, Shafer SL, et al. The influence of age on propofol pharmacodynamics. Anesthesiology. 1999;90:1502–16.
9. Minto CF, Schnider TW, Gregg KM, Henthorn TK, Shafer SL. Using the time of maximum effect-site concentration to combine pharmacokinetics and pharmacodynamics. Anesthesiology. 2003;99:324–33.
10. Minto CF, Schnider TW, Egan TD, et al. Influence of age and gender on the pharmacokinetics and pharmacodynamics of remifentanil. I. Model development. Anesthesiology. 1997;86:10–23. 7.
11. Minto CF, Schnider TW, Shafer SL. Pharmacokinetics and pharmacodynamics of remifentanil. II. Model application. Anesthesiology. 1997;86:24–33.
12. Al-Rifai Z, Mulvey D. Principles of total intravenous anaesthesia: practical aspects of using total intravenous anaesthesia. BJA Edu. 2016;16(8):276–80. https://doi.org/10.1093/bjaed/mkv074.
13. Sandin R, Nordstrom O. Awareness during total intravenous anaesthesia. Br J Anaesth. 1993;71:782–7. 8.
14. Nordstrom O, Englstrom AM, Persson S, Sandin R. Incidence of awareness in total i.v. anaesthesia based on propofol, alfentanil and neuromuscular blockade. Acta Anaesthesiol Scand. 1997;41:978–84. 9.
15. Sandin RH, Enlund G, Samuelsson P, et al. Awareness during anaesthesia: a prospective study. Lancet. 2000;355:707–1.
16. Whyte SD, Booker P. Monitoring depth of anaesthesia by EEG. Contin Educ Anaesth Crit Care Pain. 2003;3:106–10.
17. Fletcher D, Martinez V. Opioid-induced hyperalgesia in patients after surgery: a systematic review and a meta-analysis. Br J Anaesth. 2014;112:991–1004.
18. Lauder GR. Total intravenous anesthesia will supercede inhalational anesthesia in pediatric anesthetic practice. Paediatr Anaesth. 2015;25:52–64.

Intracranial Pressure Monitoring 17

Bharath Srinivasaiah and Sriganesh Kamath

17.1 Introduction

Intracranial pressure (ICP) is the pressure exerted within the cranium by the intracranial contents. The normal range of ICP is 7–15 mmHg for adults in the supine position, 3–7 mmHg for young children, and 1.5–6 mmHg for infants. The ICP can vary under normal physiological processes like brain activity, posture, respiration, cardiac function, and adrenergic tone.

ICP monitoring is essential in the armamentarium of clinicians caring for neurological patients. Many studies have shown that ICP monitoring leads to better clinical outcomes. However, the current ICP monitoring techniques cannot reliably define the limits of the brain's compensatory reserve to manage the raised ICP, which can allow for proactive ICP management. Hence, current efforts at live-streaming ICP waveforms and integration with multimodality monitoring could encourage better clinical utility of ICP monitoring.

B. Srinivasaiah · S. Kamath (✉)
Department of Neuroanaesthesia and Neurocritical Care, National Institute of Mental Health and Neurosciences (NIMHANS),
Bengaluru, Karnataka, India

17.2 Pathophysiology of Raised ICP

The physiological processes behind ICP changes can be understood by the Monro-Kellie doctrine. The intracranial volume is comprised of three components—brain volume, blood volume (arterial and venous), and cerebrospinal fluid (CSF) (Fig. 17.1). As the intracranial space is constant, a rise in the volume of any component can lead to raised ICP. Further, the ICP can be raised due to a fourth component, like mass, hematoma, cerebral edema, etc. There is some variability in ICP

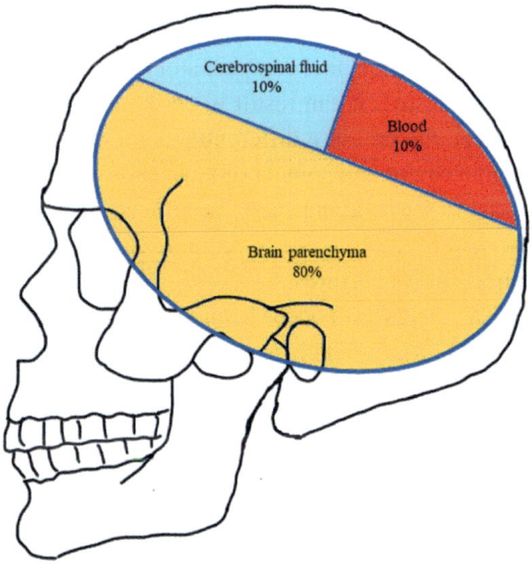

Fig. 17.1 Monro-Kellie doctrine

N. Gupta et al. (eds.), *Techniques in Anesthesia, Intensive Care and Emergency Medicine*,
https://doi.org/10.1007/978-981-96-1202-4_17

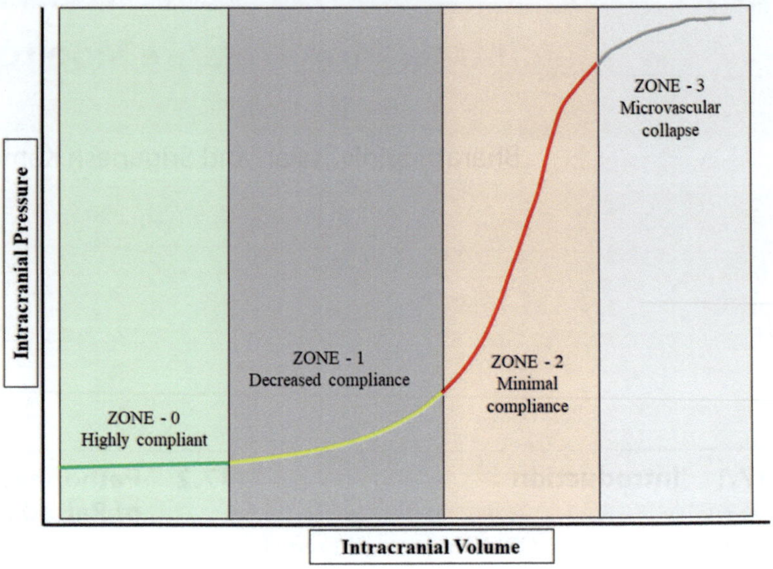

Fig. 17.2 Intracranial pressure—volume curve

under physiological conditions. However, the ICP is largely maintained stable by modification in the brain venous blood pool and reduction in the CSF volume. This compensatory reserve is finite; when depleted, a small increase in volume will result in a catastrophic rise in the ICP (Fig. 17.2).

An increase in ICP results in brain injury predominantly through cerebral ischemia and herniation. The elevation in ICP is compensated by an increase in mean arterial pressure (MAP) to maintain cerebral perfusion pressure (CPP). However, when the compensatory mechanisms are exhausted, it can result in cerebral ischemia. Further, the pressure differential across the intracranial cavity and spinal cord can cause the brain tissue to move along the path of least resistance (herniation), resulting in compression of vital intracranial structures.

Raised ICP can occur from various neurological pathologies, such as traumatic brain injury (TBI), brain tumors, aneurysmal subarachnoid hemorrhage (aSAH), arterial and venous stroke, hemorrhage from vascular anomalies (arteriovenous malformations), status epilepticus, neuroinfections, and hydrocephalus. The common contributors to the worsening of elevated ICP in the neurointensive care unit(ICU) include inappropriate (hypotonic and large quantity) fluid choices, positioning (supine, prone, vs. reverse Trendelenburg), mechanical ventilation with high airway pressures, hypoxia and hypercarbia, extremes of blood pressure such as hypo- and hypertension, chest physiotherapy, oro-tracheal suctioning, other painful ICU procedures and stimuli, seizures, fever, and agitation. In contrast, interventions such as removal of CSF and osmotherapy with mannitol or hypertonic saline contribute to reduction of raised ICP in the neuro ICU.

17.3 Indications of ICP Monitoring

Some of the common indications of ICP monitoring include TBI with Glasgow Coma Scale (GCS) < 9 and abnormal computed tomography (CT) scan; severe TBI with normal CT scan when any two of the three factors are present—age > 40 years, motor posturing, and systolic blood pressure < 90 mmHg; acute brain pathology where clinical assessment is difficult; decision for, and part of surgery (decompressive craniectomy decision for diffuse axonal injury, ICP changes during cranial remodeling for craniosynostosis); and as a guide for assessing the need and effect of interventions such as osmotherapy and hyperventilation.

17.4 Techniques of ICP Monitoring

Both invasive and non-invasive techniques are used to monitor the ICP and guide therapy for managing raised ICP. Given the shape of the intracranial pressure-volume curve (Fig. 17.2) and the relative position of the intracranial compliance, clinical management can be proactive rather than reactive. The advantages and disadvantages of both techniques are depicted in Table 17.1.

17.4.1 Invasive Techniques

Invasive ICP monitoring techniques include fluid-based transducer systems and implantable micro-transducers (Fig. 17.3).

Ventricular Catheter It is the most common technique of ICP measurement and is considered gold standard for ICP monitoring. It facilitates accurate ICP monitoring and allows therapeutic CSF drainage to reduce the raised ICP. An external ventricular drain (EVD) catheter is placed in the lateral ventricle through a burr hole under strict aseptic precautions. The catheter is connected to a saline-filled tubing that transmits the pressure within the ventricle to a strain-gauge transducer connected to the tubing. The transducer connected to a monitor will display the measured ICP and the waveforms. The insertion of EVD is often difficult in patients with small or compressed ventricles due to the raised ICP. Further, there is a 5.7% risk of bleeding at insertion and a 5% risk of infection after five days of insertion of EVD. Another fluid-based system used for ICP monitoring is the epidural or subdural bolt/screw. Through a burr-hole, the tip of the device is inserted into the epidural space (epidural bolt) or through the duramater into the subarachnoid space (subdural bolt). These devices cannot drain the CSF but carry the risk of local infection.

Parenchymalcatheter The sensor tip is placed within the brain parenchyma close to the area of interest, but it can also be placed in the ventricle,

Table 17.1 Advantages and disadvantages of various ICP monitoring techniques

ICP monitoring technique	Advantages	Disadvantages
Invasive:		
Ventricular catheter	Low cost Serves both diagnostic and therapeutic purposes Zeroing frequently is possible Familiarity of nurses with its maintenance	Most invasive Bleeding risk Infection risk Difficulty to place in slit ventricle scenario Short duration of monitoring
Parenchymal catheter	Easy to place the probe Can be combined with other neuro-monitoring techniques	Bleeding Infection Seizure Technical failure High cost
Non-invasive:		
Optic nerve sheath diameter	Point of care monitoring Short learning curve	Inter and intra observer variability Difficult in facial trauma or eye diseases
Trans-cranial Doppler	Readily available at bedside Continuous monitoring possible Provides additional information about cerebral autoregulation and intracranial compliance	Inter and intra observer variability Inability to monitor with thick skull Requires expertise Equipment cost

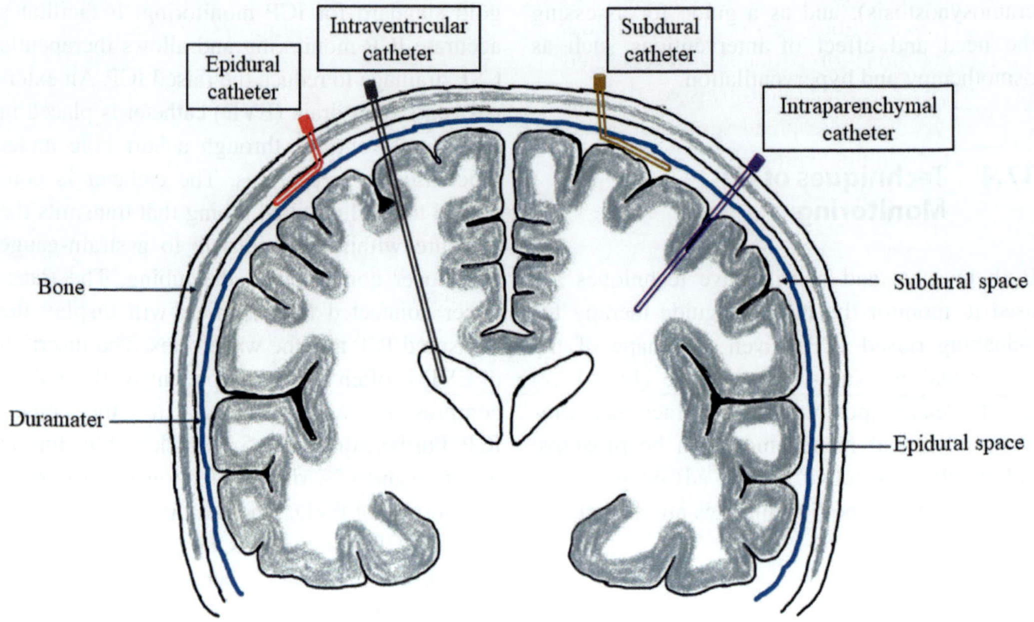

Fig. 17.3 Invasive ICP monitoring techniques

subdural or epidural space. There are three main types of commercially available parenchymal catheters based on the principle of measurement.

1. Strain gauge (e.g., Codman Microsensor)
2. Fiberoptic device (e.g., Camino ICP monitor)
3. Pneumatic sensor (e.g., Spiegelberg ICP monitor)

The strain gauge sensor contains a diaphragm that bends with changes in ICP. The change in electrical resistance is used to calculate the ICP. The fiberoptic device has a displaceable mirror at the tip, which moves with changes in the ICP. The intensity of light reflected back along the fiberoptic cable varies, which helps to calculate the ICP. The pneumatic sensors contain a balloon at the tip of the probe. The surrounding pressure on the balloon is sensed to measure the ICP. Parenchymal sensors have a lower rate of infection and bleeding risk compared to ventricular ICP monitoring catheters. However, they are expensive and cannot be recalibrated or zeroed. Therefore, these sensors are usually placed when the EVD placement is unsuccessful or CSF drainage is not deemed necessary.

17.4.1.1 ICP Waveform and Analysis

The ICP is derived from the time average of the ICP waveform (Fig. 17.4). The ICP waveform is visualized using an intraventricular catheter connected to a monitor or using software (ICM$^+$). The ICP waveforms are described as follows:

1. Pulse waveform—this is equal to the heart rate (Fig. 17.4A). It can be subdivided into three components—P1 (percussion wave), P2 (tidal wave), and P3 (dicrotic wave), representing arterial pulsation, intracranial compliance, and closure of the aortic valve, respectively. A prominent P2 (> P1) amplitude reflects a decrease in intracranial compliance.
2. Respiratory waveform—0.1 to 0.3 Hz, represents the changes in ICP with respiration (Fig. 17.4B).
3. Slow vasogenic waves—Lundberg A and B (Fig. 17.4C). The presence of Lundberg A wave, a sharp increase in ICP sustained over

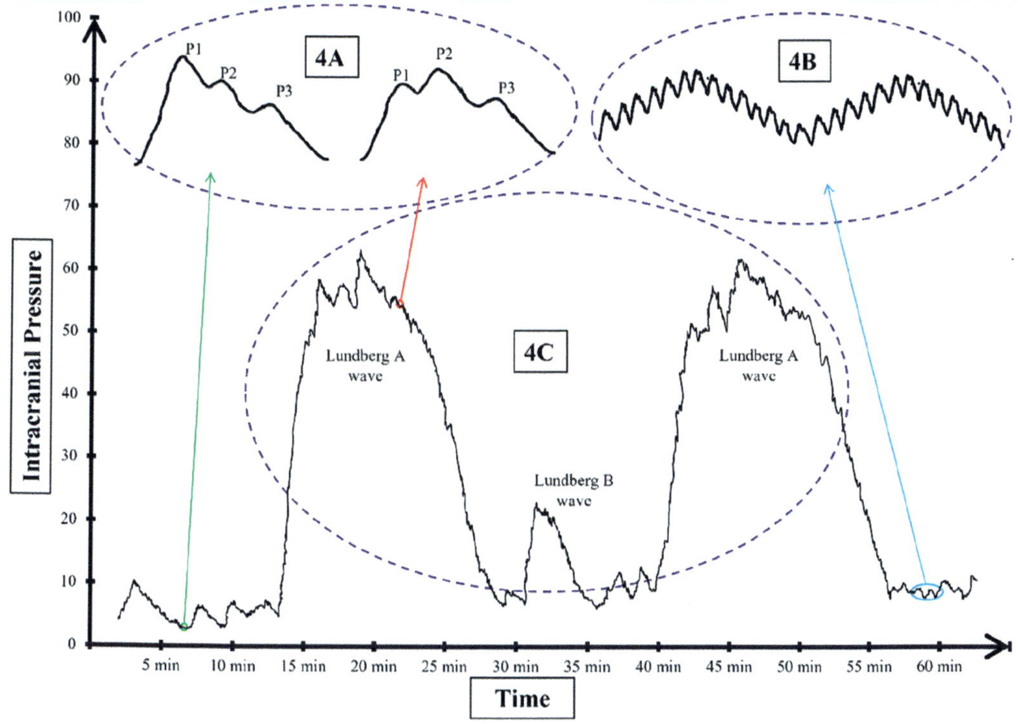

Fig. 17.4 ICP waveforms

5–20 minutes, indicates decreased intracranial compliance. Lundberg B wave, a cyclical elevation in ICP at the rate of 0.33–3 cycles/minute with a cluster duration of 5–30 minutes, is considered a nonspecific indicator of decreased compliance.

The pulse amplitude (AMP) can be isolated from the ICP waveform with spectral analysis. Higher AMP is associated with lower intracranial compliance. The RAP (R-correlation, A-amplitude, and P-pressure) coefficient is a correlation coefficient between AMP and mean ICP, and is a measure of compensatory reserve. The linear part of the curve (Fig. 17.2, Zone 1) is where RAP = 0 is suggestive of a good reserve. The steep part of the curve (Fig. 17.2, Zone 2) is where RAP = +1 is suggestive of a low reserve. The higher part of the curve (Fig. 17.2, Zone 3), where RAP is negative, is suggestive of a decompensated state with collapse of cerebral microvasculature. The RAP-weighted ICP-guided management has been shown to improve TBI outcomes. The RAP algorithms developed based on machine learning can help predict ICP elevation 30 minutes prior based on ICP and AMP data of the preceding 4 hours. This can help institute measures early and reduce the occurrence of adverse outcomes.

17.4.1.2 ICP and Cerebral Autoregulation

An intact cerebral autoregulation is essential to maintain constant cerebral perfusion with changes in ICP. The pressure reactivity index (PRx) is a time-averaged correlation coefficient of ICP and MAP. A positive PRx indicates impaired autoregulation, whereas a negative PRx indicates normal autoregulation. Individual patient-specific optimal ICP and CPP thresholds can be estimated from autoregulation-weighted ICP and CPP. This approach is considered a better predictor of patient outcomes than conventional fixed ICP thresholds of 20–25 mmHg.

17.4.2 Non-invasive Techniques

Non-invasive ICP monitoring techniques provide an indirect measurement of ICP. Non-invasive monitoring may be desirable when invasive techniques are not promptly available or when there is a relatively low suspicion of raised ICP. This can decrease the complications associated with invasive ICP monitoring. The advantages and disadvantages of both techniques are described in Table 17.1.

Optic Nerve Sheath Diameter (ONSD) The optic nerve is surrounded by the dural optic nerve sheath. The CSF within the optic nerve sheath is in a continuum with the intracranial subarachnoid space. The optic nerve sheath diameter (ONSD) changes with the changes in the CSF pressure within the optic nerve sheath. An increased ICP is transmitted from the intracranial cavity to the optic nerve sheath leading to an increase in ONSD. This increased ONSD can be detected by trans-ocular ultrasonography examination at a 3 mm distance behind the posterior pole of the globe (Fig. 17.5). A good correlation has been shown between invasive ICP and non-invasive ONSD values. A cutoff of 5 mm of ONSD on ultrasonography is considered appropriate for diagnosing raised ICP, though some studies report a higher cutoff of >5.6 mm. Thus, ONSD can be an important bedside quick and simple screening tool to identify patients who require invasive ICP monitoring. The benefits of common interventions in the neuro ICU, such as positive end-expiratory pressure to improve oxygenation and hyperventilation to reduce ICP, can be assessed using ONSD measurements in patients with raised ICP.

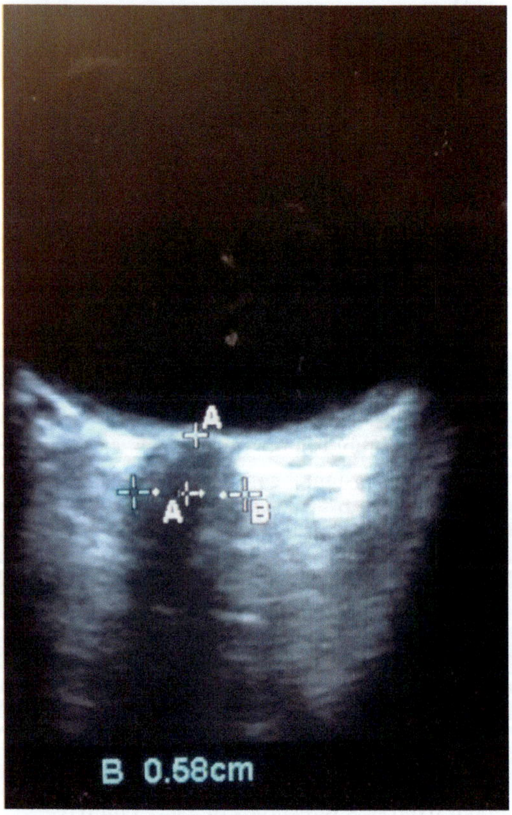

Fig. 17.5 Optic nerve sheath diameter

Transcranial Doppler (TCD) TCD monitoring is used to measure cerebral blood flow (velocity) in patients with different brain pathologies in operating rooms and ICU. The TCD-derived parameters of systolic, diastolic, and mean flow velocities (SFV, DFV, MFV) in cerebral arteries and derived pulsatility index (PI) are useful indirect estimations of ICP. Studies have shown a good correlation between PI and invasive ICP measurements. The ICP values can be obtained from PI using the formula of ICP = 10.927 * PI—1.284. The TCD waveform spectrogram changes with changes in ICP. Figure 17.6a shows a normal TCD FV when the ICP is normal. When the ICP increases, initially there is a decrease in DFV and an increase in PI (Fig. 17.6b). Subsequently, with further increase in ICP, DFV becomes zero resulting in only systolic spikes (Fig. 17.6c). A further increase in ICP beyond MAP will result in reversed blood flow (Fig. 17.6d). Lastly, when ICP breaches the threshold of systolic blood pressure, no FV waveforms are visible (absent flow) on the TCD monitor (Fig. 17.6e).

There are several other less commonly used non-invasive techniques for surrogate assessment of ICP. Some of these are described below.

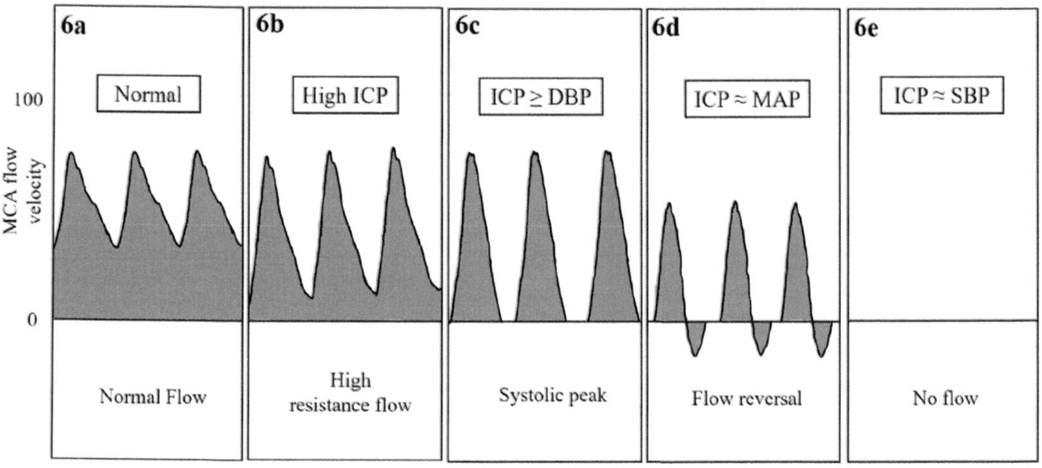

Fig. 17.6 Transcranial doppler changes with intracranial pressure (ICP) changes. 6a: normal ICP, 6b high ICP, 6c: ICp more than DBP, 6d: ICP similar to mean arterial pressure9 MAP), 6e: ICP similar to systolic blood pressure (SBP)

- Radiological imaging (CT, magnetic resonance imaging): The presence of midline shift, cerebral edema (loss of gray-white matter differentiation), and compression of basal cisterns are indicative of raised ICP.
- Electroencephalogram (EEG): Specific EEG patterns are described in patients with raised ICP. These are closely related to changes in cerebral blood flow consequent to raised ICP.
- Pupillometry: An oval pupil observed prior to the manifestation of fixed nonreactive pupils is suggestive of raised ICP. Impaired pupillary light reflexes, such as decreased neurologic pupil index and constriction velocity, are suggestive of raised ICP.
- Brain oxygenation assessment using Near Infrared Spectroscopy (NIRS): Increased ICP results in brain ischemia and cerebral hypoxia, which can be detected by measuring regional cerebral oxygen saturation. Changes in NIRS-derived parameters may help in the non-invasive detection of vasogenic ICP waves.
- Tympanic membrane displacement (TMD): Changes in ICP are reflected in the perilymphatic fluid pressure. Assessment of TMD provides a useful non-invasive method for assessment of raised ICP.

17.5 Management During ICP Monitoring

The important points to remember during ICP monitoring include the following:

1. Have clear thresholds and treatment plan (22–25 mmHg ICP)
2. Limit the duration of monitoring to <5 days to reduce infection
3. Maintain the transducer at the level of the internal auditory canal
4. Calibration at regular intervals
5. Maintain maximum infection prevention measures and check coagulation
6. Seizure prophylaxis

17.6 Raised ICP Management Strategies

The commonly followed protocol for the management of raised ICP is given below

1. General prophylactic measures (sedation, analgesia, ventilation, reverse Trendelenburg position, neutral neck position, etc.).
2. Resection of mass lesion/ CSF drainage when indicated.

3. Hyperosmolar therapy with mannitol or hypertonic saline.
4. Hyperventilation to not <25 mmHg.
5. Barbiturate coma for refractory raised ICP.
6. Decompressive craniectomy.

17.7 Conclusions

Monitoring the ICP is an important part of caring for patients with acute brain injury. Various invasive and non-invasive techniques are available for monitoring ICP. ICP monitoring-based management has been shown to improve patient outcomes.

Suggested Reading

1. Rangel-Castillo L, Gopinath S, Robertson CS. Management of Intracranial Hypertension. Neurol Clin. 2008;26:521.
2. Harary M, Dolmans RGF, Gormley WB. Intracranial pressure monitoring—review and avenues for development. Sensors (Basel). 2018;18:465.
3. Härtl R, Stieg PE. Intracranial pressure is still number 1 despite BEST:TRIP study. World Neurosurg. 2013;79:599–600.
4. Robba C, Graziano F, Rebora P, Elli F, Giussani C, Oddo M, et al. Intracranial pressure monitoring in patients with acute brain injury in the intensive care unit (SYNAPSE-ICU): an international, prospective observational cohort study. Lancet Neurol. 2021;20:548–58.
5. Munakomi S, Das JM. Intracranial pressure monitoring [Internet]. StatPearls. In: StatPearls [Internet]. Treasure Island, FL: StatPearls Publishing; 2022. Available from: https://www.ncbi.nlm.nih.gov/books/NBK542298/.
6. Jagannatha AT, Sriganesh K, Devi BI, Rao GSU. An equiosmolar study on early intracranial physiology and long term outcome in severe traumatic brain injury comparing mannitol and hypertonic saline. J Clin Neurosci. 2016;27:68–73.
7. Binz DD, Toussaint LG, Friedman JA. Hemorrhagic complications of ventriculostomy placement: a meta-analysis. Neurocrit Care. 2009;10:253–6.
8. Czosnyka M, Pickard JD. Monitoring and interpretation of intracranial pressure. J Neurol Neurosurg Psychiatry. 2004;75:813–21.
9. Raboel PH, Bartek J, Andresen M, Bellander BM, Romner B. Intracranial pressure monitoring: invasive versus non-invasive methods-a review. Crit Care Res Pract. 2012;2012:950393.
10. Zhang X, Medow JE, Iskandar BJ, Wang F, Shokoueinejad M, Koueik J, et al. Invasive and non-invasive means of measuring intracranial pressure: a review. Physiol Meas. 2017;38:R143–82.
11. Hall A, O'Kane R. The best marker for guiding the clinical management of patients with raised intracranial pressure—the RAP index or the mean pulse amplitude? Acta Neurochir. 2016;158:1997.
12. Calviello L, Donnelly J, Cardim D, Robba C, Zeiler FA, Smielewski P, et al. Compensatory-reserve-weighted intracranial pressure and its association with outcome after traumatic brain injury. Neurocrit Care. 2018;28:212–20.
13. Güiza F, Depreitere B, Piper I, Van Den Berghe G, Meyfroidt G. Novel methods to predict increased intracranial pressure during intensive care and long-term neurologic outcome after traumatic brain injury: development and validation in a multicenter dataset. Crit Care Med. 2013;41:554–64.
14. Lazaridis C, DeSantis SM, Smielewski P, Menon DK, Hutchinson P, Pickard JD, et al. Patient-specific thresholds of intracranial pressure in severe traumatic brain injury. J Neurosurg. 2014;120:890–900.
15. Needham E, McFadyen C, Newcombe V, Synnot AJ, Czosnyka M, Menon D. Cerebral perfusion pressure targets individualized to pressure-reactivity index in moderate to severe traumatic brain injury: a systematic. Review. 2017;34:963–70.
16. Wang J, Li K, Li H, Ji C, Wu Z, Chen H, et al. Ultrasonographic optic nerve sheath diameter correlation with ICP and accuracy as a tool for non-invasive surrogate ICP measurement in patients with decompressive craniotomy. J Neurosurg. 2019;133:514–20.
17. Koziarz A, Sne N, Kegel F, Nath S, Badhiwala JH, Nassiri F, et al. Bedside optic nerve ultrasonography for diagnosing increased intracranial pressure: a systematic review and meta-analysis. Ann Intern Med. 2019;171:896–905.
18. Jeon JP, Lee SU, Kim SE, Kang SH, Yang JS, Choi HJ, et al. Correlation of optic nerve sheath diameter with directly measured intracranial pressure in Korean adults using bedside ultrasonography. PLoS One. 2017;12:e0183170.
19. Balakrishnan S, Naik S, Chakrabarti D, Konar S, Sriganesh K. Effect of respiratory physiological changes on optic nerve sheath diameter and cerebral oxygen saturation in patients with acute traumatic brain injury. J Neurosurg Anesthesiol. 2022;34:E52–6.
20. Robba C, Taccone FS. How I use transcranial Doppler. Crit Care. 2019;23:420.
21. Bellner J, Romner B, Reinstrup P, Kristiansson KA, Ryding E, Brandt L. Transcranial Doppler sonography pulsatility index (PI) reflects intracranial pressure (ICP). Surg Neurol. 2004;62:45–51.
22. Kayhanian S, Young AMH, Piper RJ, Donnelly J, Scoffings D, Garnett MR, et al. Radiological correlates of raised intracranial pressure in children: a review. Front Pediatr. 2018;6:32.

23. Connolly M, Vespa P, Pouratian N, Gonzalez NR, Hu X. Characterization of the relationship between intracranial pressure and electroencephalographic monitoring in burst suppressed patients. Neurocrit Care. 2015;22:212.
24. Al-Obaidi SZ, Atem FD, Stutzman SE, Olson DM. Impact of increased intracranial pressure on pupillometry: a replication study. Crit Care Explor. 2019;1:e0054.
25. Weerakkody RA, Czosnyka M, Zweifel C, Castellani G, Smielewski P, Brady K, et al. Near infrared spectroscopy as possible non-invasive monitor of slow vasogenic ICP waves. Acta Neurochir Suppl. 2012;114:181–5.
26. Dhar R, Sandler RH, Manwaring K, Kostick N, Mansy HA. Non-invasive detection of elevated ICP using spontaneous tympanic membrane pulsation. Sci Reports 2021 111 [Internet]. Nature Publishing Group; 2021 [cited 2022 Nov 30];11:1–13. Available from: https://www.nature.com/articles/s41598-021-01079-8.

18 Transesophageal Echocardiography

Priya R. Menon and P. S. Nagaraja

Key Points

- TEE is a diagnostic ultrasound modality which involves inserting a flexible tube with an attached ultrasound probe into the patient's esophagus.
- It is typically performed under sedation and may require a local anesthetic to anesthetize the throat. It may be useful when standard echocardiogram is unable to provide sufficient information.
- It provides high-quality, detailed images of the heart and its blood vessels, and help to diagnose a variety of heart conditions like valvular heart disease, blood clots, etc.
- The risks associated with TEE include bleeding, infection, and injury to the esophagus.

P. R. Menon (✉)
Department of Critical Care, Abu Dhabi, UAE

P. S. Nagaraja
Sri Jayadeva Institute of Cardiovascular Sciences and Research, Bangalore, India

18.1 Introduction

Transesophageal echocardiography (TEE) was introduced in 1980s and has earned popularity and advancement as it provides an opportunity to overcome many of the transthoracic echocardiography limitations of chest wall acoustic windows. Frazin et al. used M mode echocardiography for the first time in 1976. The transducer with biplane was introduced in 1984, and multiplane transducers in 1992. Intraoperative use of TEE offers real time dynamic monitoring tool of cardiac anatomy and physiology. It opens up a cardiac window with great spatial resolution. The clinical utility of TEE as a diagnostic and guide for therapeutic management in cardiac surgery is widely reported. The sequential assessment of TEE views will be discussed in this chapter.

18.2 Indications

Cardiac surgery and thoracic aortic procedures:

1. Adult open heart, Coronary artery bypass surgeries and thoracic aortic surgeries to: confirm and refine the preoperative diagnosis. Detect new or unanticipated pathology. Guide for anesthetic and surgical management. Assess the surgical intervention.

N. Gupta et al. (eds.), *Techniques in Anesthesia, Intensive Care and Emergency Medicine*,
https://doi.org/10.1007/978-981-96-1202-4_18

2. In pediatric patients it is indicated based on the benefits and the risks (bleeding, bronchial obstruction)involved.
3. Catheterisation guided intracardiac interventions: it is used in transcatheter intracardiac procedures.

Noncardiac Surgery
1. TEE may be used in noncardiac surgeries if the patient has known or suspected cardiovascular pathology, which may result in severe hemodynamic, pulmonary or neurological compromise.
2. TEE may be used when unexpected life threatening circulatory instability persists despite optimal corrective therapy.

Critical Care
1. TEE may be used in critically ill patients when the diagnostic information obtained by TTE or other modalities are inconclusive.

Indications of TEE based on the guidelines:

Appropriate
1. Non coronary cardiac intervention
2. Acute aortic pathology
3. Valvular structure and function with suitability of intervention
4. Diagnose infective endocarditis
5. In atrial fibrillation, to assess the need for anticoagulation, cardioversion and/ radiofrequency ablation
6. TTE is inconclusive
7. Follow up of prior TEE (resolution of thrombus post anticoagulation)
8. Evaluation of cardiovascular emboli with unidentified non cardiac source

Uncertain
1. Evaluation for cardiovascular source of emboli when previously identified noncardiac source

Inappropriate
1. Diagnose infective endocarditis with low pretest probability.
2. Atrial fibrillation/flutter patient evaluation, when decision has been made to anticoagulate and not to cardiovert.
3. Assessment of pulmonary veins in asymptomatic status post pulmonary vein isolation.
4. Surveillance of prior TEE when no change in therapy is anticipated.
5. Routine use of TEE when TTE is inconclusive.

18.3 Contraindications

Absolute
1. Oesophageal pathology: diverticulum, stricture, trauma, tumour, Mallory Weiss tear
2. Active or recent upper GI bleed
3. Esophagectomy, esophagogastrectomy
4. Perforated viscous
5. Patient refusal

Relative
1. Esophagitis
2. Barrett's esophagus
3. Esophageal varices
4. Bleeding diasthesis
5. Previous GI surgery
6. History of dysphagia
7. History of radiation to the neck or chest
8. Symptomatic hiatal hernia
9. Restricted cervical mobility

Probe: The TEE probes are of various sizes to cater all age groups, infant, pediatric, and adult probes with extended operating frequency ranging from 3 to 7 MHz. Modern TEE probe distal tip is flexible to allow range of motion, anteriorly antero-flexion, posteriorly retro-flexion, laterally to the right and to the left. It also has a multiplanar angle rotation of 180 degrees. The TEE probe has the probe shaft, handle, cable and the pin connector. The probe shaft is flexible containing coaxial cables carrying signals to and from the transducer. There are depth markers on the shaft to guide the clinician to various views. The handle of the adult TEE probe possess two round dials, the bigger dial performs anteflexion and retroflexion when rotated clockwise and anti-clockwise respectively, whereas the smaller dial is used to flex in either right or left direction. The multiplane angle (mpa) controller buttons are also housed in the handle. The connector attaches the handle to the echo machine through the cable.

18.4 Comprehensive TEE Examination

The American society of echocardiography recommends twenty standard views and eight modified views. It's important to do the TEE imaging sequentially to obtain the standard views so that, it allows the clinician to compare the images pre and post intervention. It further ensures nothing is missed out during imaging. However, it may not be possible to obtain the similar images at a particular depth or multiplanar angle due to the difference in anatomy or body habitus. There are four different depths at which the imaging planes are obtained. Upper esophageal, mid esophageal, transgastric, and deep transgastric views are obtained approximately at 25 cm, 35 cm, 40 cm, and 50 cm depth of the probe from the teeth respectively. The 20 comprehensive views will be discussed in this chapter.

18.5 Mid Esophageal (ME) Views

1. Mid esophageal four chamber (ME4C) view: The probe is inserted to a depth of 35 cm to obtain mid esophageal views. When the multiplanar angle is at 0 to 10^0 the imaging plane is anterior to the oesophagus and posterior to the left atrium. The right sided structures are displayed on the left side of the imaging sector and the left sided structures onto the right of the sector. The ME4C view displays the four chambers of the heart (Fig. 18.1).

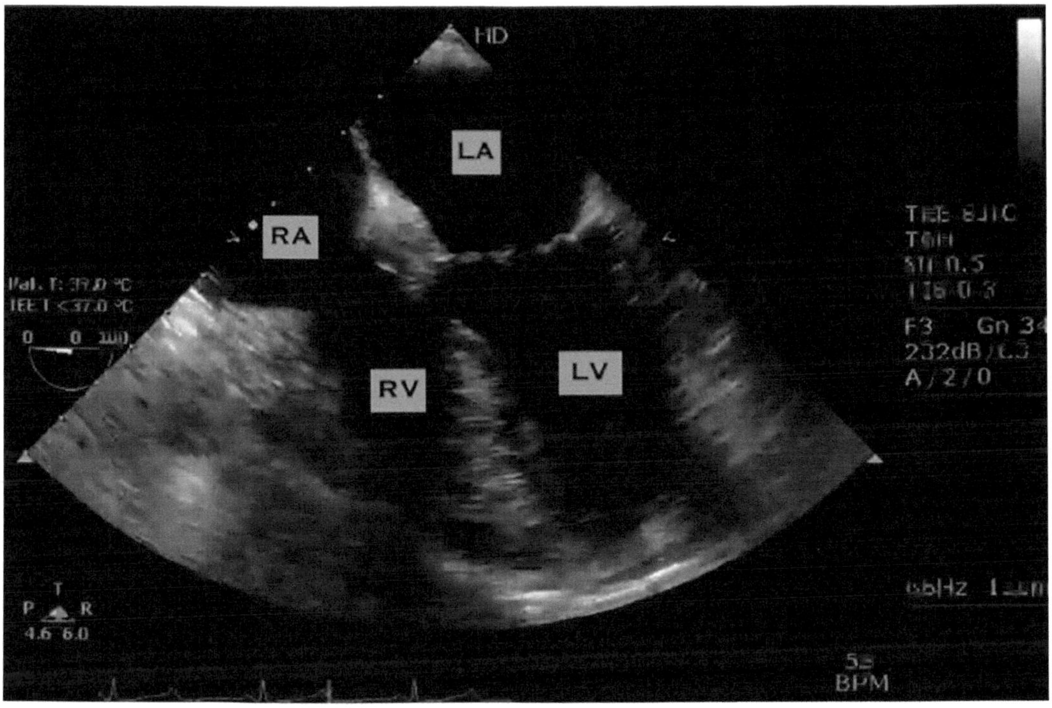

Fig. 18.1 Mid esophageal views

Acquisition guide	Imaging structures		Information obtained
Probe depth—35 cm Sector depth—12–14 cm mpa—0–10⁰	Right side	Left side	Chamber enlargement LV Regional wall motion abnormalities—Anterolateral and inferoseptal wall Mitral and tricuspid valve disease Intra cardiac mass
	LA,LV,	R,RV,TV	

2. Mid esophageal mitral commissural (ME MC) view: The multiplanar angle is increased to 50^0–70^0 from the ME4C view to obtain ME MC view where the imaging plane bisects the two mitral commissures (Fig. 18.2).

Acquisition guide	Imaging structures		Information obtained
Probe depth—35 cm Sector depth—12–14 cm mpa—50^0–70^0	Right side	Left side	LV Regional wall motion abnormalities Mitral valve disease
	Posteromedial papillary muscle	Anterolateral papillary muscle	

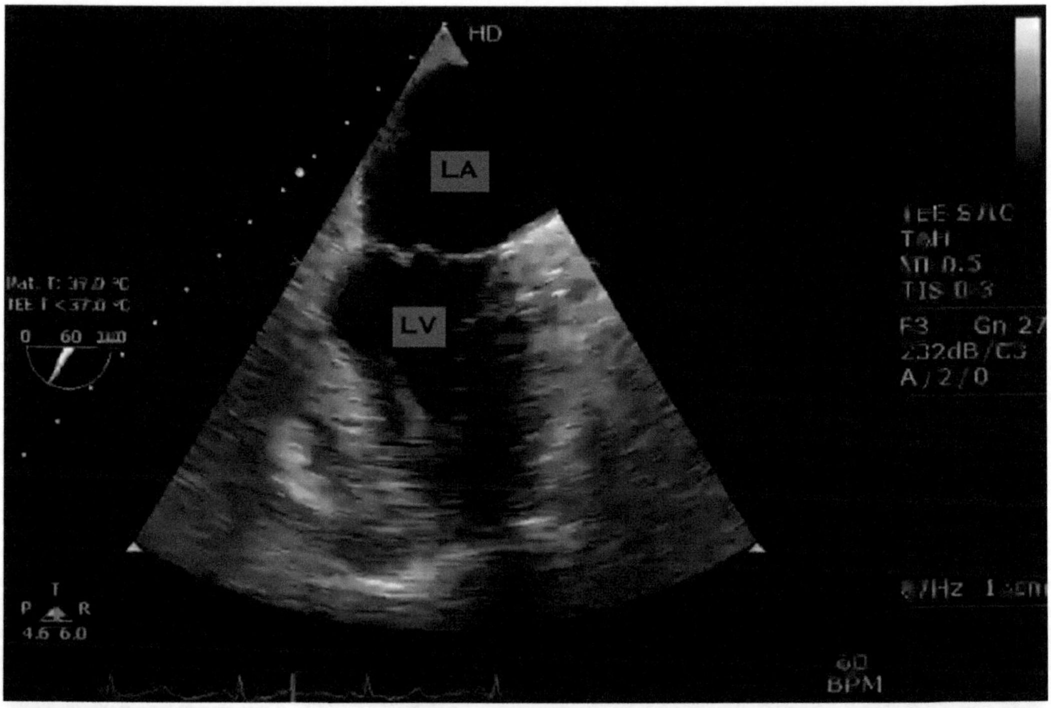

Fig. 18.2 Mid esophageal mitral commissural

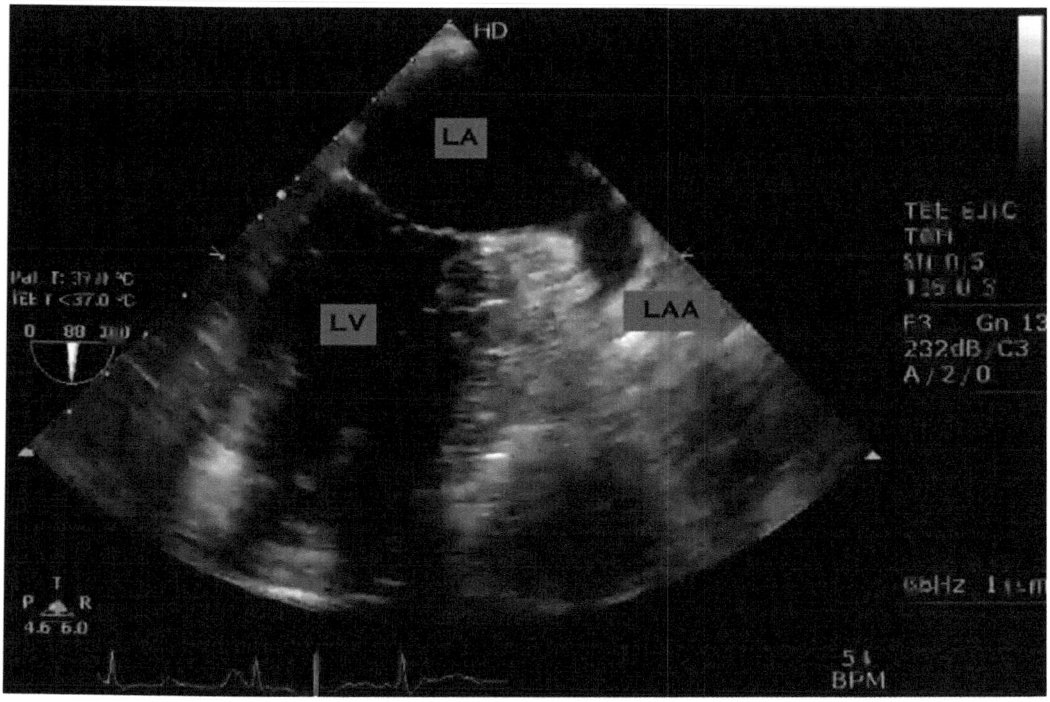

Fig. 18.3 Mid esophageal two chamber views

3. Mid esophageal two chamber (ME 2C) view: The multiplanar angle is increased to 80^0–100^0 from the ME MC view to obtain ME 2C view where the imaging plane bisects the LV (Fig. 18.3).

Acquisition guide	Imaging structures		Information obtained
Probe depth—35 cm Sector depth—12–14 cm mpa—80^0–100^0	Right side	Left side	LV Regional wall motion abnormalities— Anterior and inferior wall Miral valve disease LAA thrombus
	Inferior LV wall	LA appendage Anterior LV wall	

4. Mid esophageal Bicaval (ME BC) view: The probe is rotated to the right and optimize the image by increasing the multiplanar angle to 100^0–110^0 from the ME 2C view to obtain ME BC view, where the imaging plane bisects both the vena cavae (Fig. 18.4).

Acquisition guide	Imaging structures		Information obtained
Probe depth—35 cm Sector depth—10–12 cm Probe rotated to the right mpa—100^0–110^0	Right side	Left side	Atrial septal defect (ASD) Patent foramen ovale Sinus venosus type ASD Intra-atrial mass
	Inferior vena cava	Superior vena cava Left atrium posteriorly and right atrium at the bottom of the sector with interatrial septum in between them.	

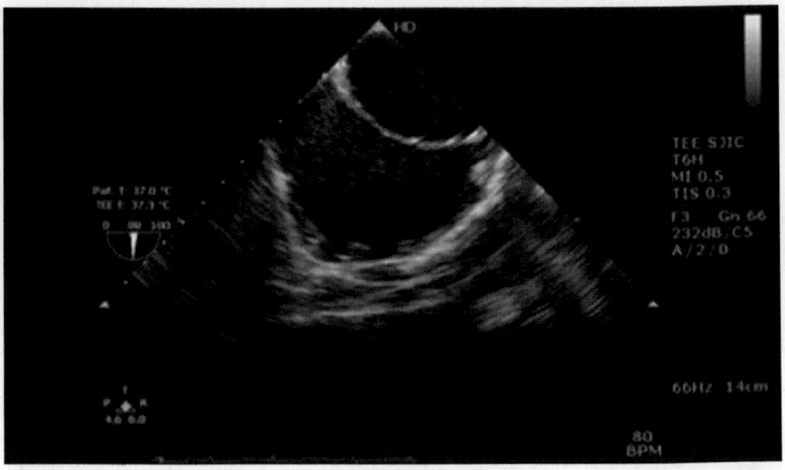

Fig. 18.4 Mid esophageal bicaval views

5. Mid esophageal LV long axis (ME LAX) view: The multiplanar angle is increased to 120^0–140^0 from the ME 2C view to obtain ME LAX view where the imaging plane bisects the mitral valve at A2 and P2 scallop (Fig. 18.5).

Acquisition guide	Imaging structures		Information obtained
	Right side	Left side	
Probe depth—35 cm Sector depth—12–14 cm mpa—120^0–140^0	Inferolateral LV wall Posterior mitral leaflet (P2)	Anteroseptal LV wall Anterior mitral leaflet (A2) Aortic valve RVOT	LV Regional wall motion abnormalities—Anteroseptal and Inferolateral wall Mitral valve disease Aortic valve disease

6. Mid esophageal aortic long axis (ME Ao LAX)view: The probe is slightly withdrawn without changing the multiplanar angle from ME LAX view to obtain ME Ao LAX view where the imaging plane displays the aortic valve in the long axis. Aortic measurements (aortic annulus, distance between sinus, sinotubular junction, ascending aorta) can be obtained in this view (Fig. 18.6).
7. Mid esophageal RV inflow outflow (ME RV outflow) view: The multiplanar angle is decreased to 50^0–70^0 from the ME Ao LAX view to obtain ME RV outflow view where the imaging plane displays the RV inflow (tricuspid valve) and outflow (pulmonary valve) wrapped around the aortic valve in the middle of the sector (Fig. 18.7).

Acquisition guide	Imaging stuctures	Information obtained
Probe depth—30 cm Sector depth—10–12 cm mpa—50^0–70^0	LA near to the probe Aortic valve RA Tricuspid valve RV RVOT Pulmonary valve	Tricuspid valve disease Aortic valve disease Pulmonary valve disease RVOT pathology (Tetralogy of Fallot) Ventricular septal defects

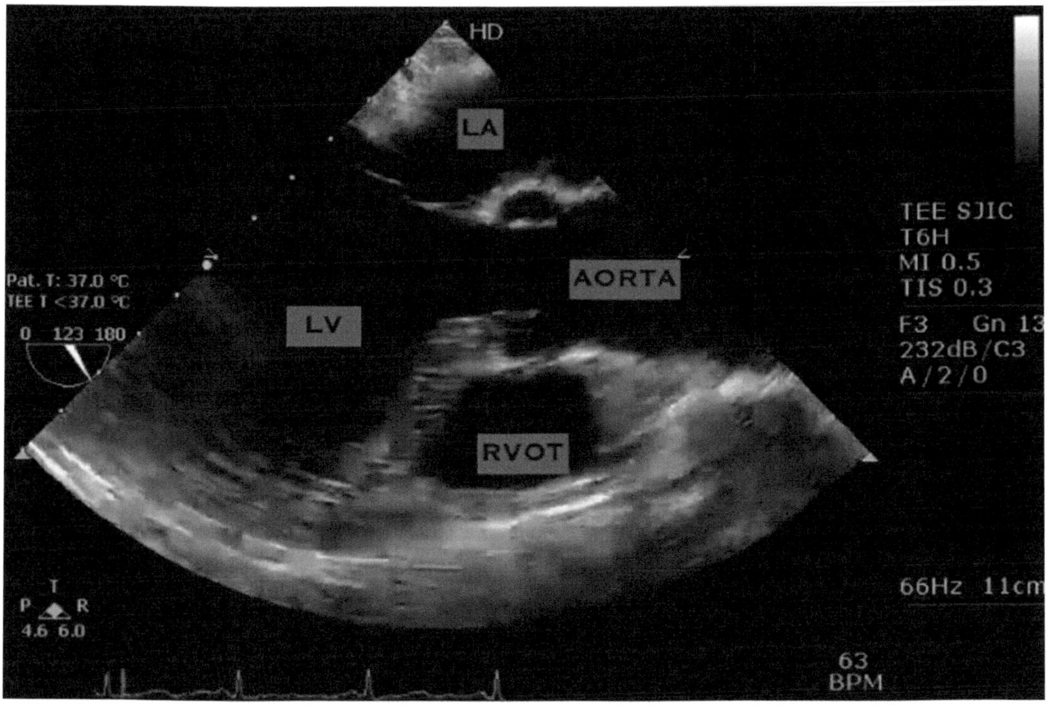

Fig. 18.5 Mid esophageal LV long axis view

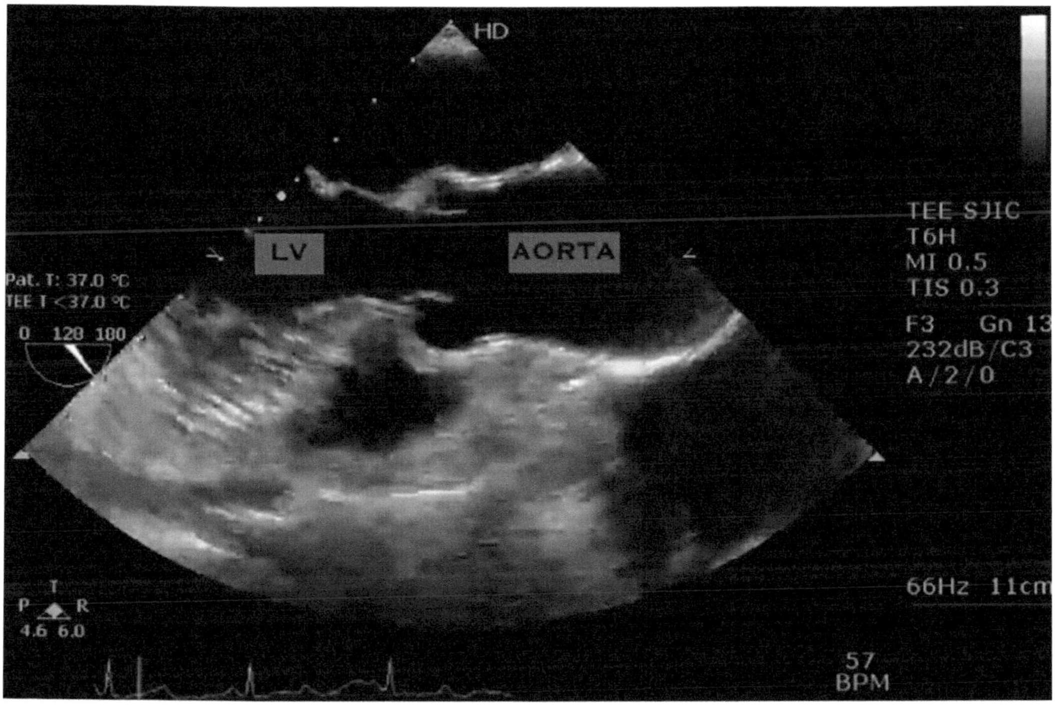

Fig. 18.6 Mid esophageal aortic long axis view

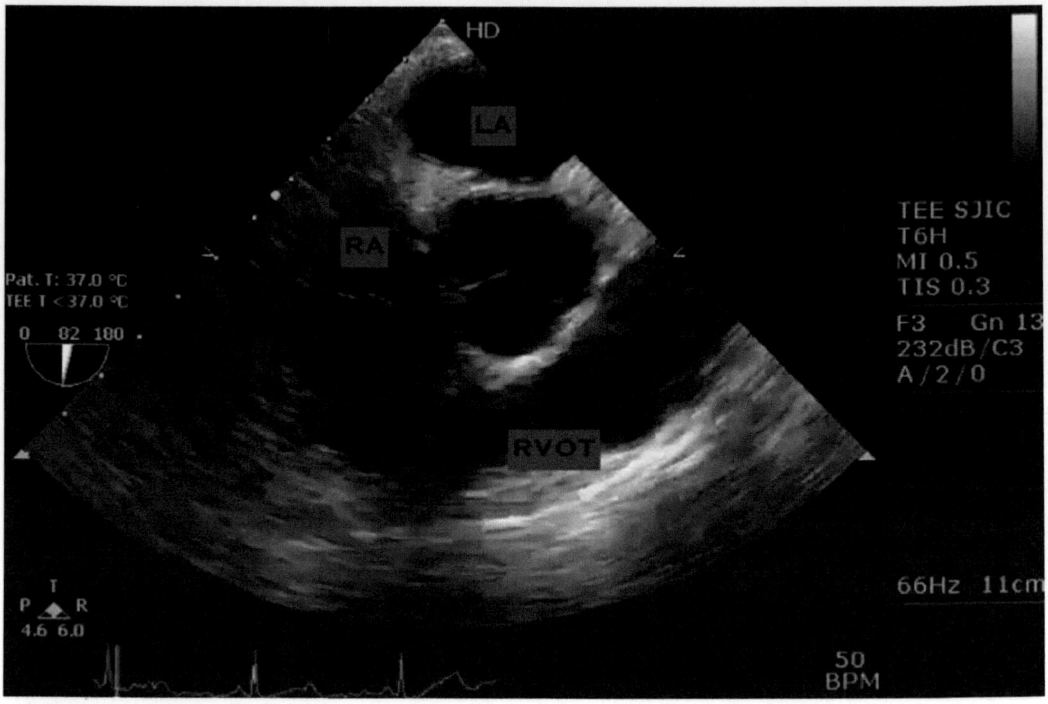

Fig. 18.7 Mid esophageal RV inflow outflow view

8. Mid esophageal aortic short axis (ME Ao SAX) view: The multiplanar angle is decreased to 20^0–40^0 from the ME RV outflow view to obtain ME Ao SAX view where the imaging plane displays the aortic valve leaflets in the centre of the imaging sector. Aortic valve area can be obtained in this view using planimetry (Fig. 18.8).
9. Mid esophageal ascending aortic short axis (ME AAo SAX) view: The probe is slightly withdrawn from ME Ao LAX view till the aortic valve leaflets disappear and slightly antevert the probe to visualize ascending aorta valve in short axis with main pulmonary artery to the left of the screen and SVC to the right of the screen. Ascending aortic aneurysms, dissection can be visualized in this view (Fig. 18.9).
10. Mid esophageal ascending aortic long axis (ME AAo LAX) view: The multiplanar angle is increased to 80^0–100^0 from the ME AAo SAX view to obtain ME AAo LAX view to visualize ascending aorta in long axis with right pulmonary artery in the short axis near to the probe (Fig. 18.10).
11. Mid esophageal descending aortic short axis (ME DAo SAX)view: The probe is rotated to the left from ME 4C view until descending aorta is seen. The sector depth has to be decreased to 6 cm approximately (Fig. 18.11).
12. Mid esophageal descending aortic long axis (ME DAo LAX) view: The multiplanar angle is increased to 80^0–100^0 from the DAo SAX view to obtain ME DAo LAX view to visualize descending aorta in long axis (Fig. 18.12).
13. Upper esophageal aortic arch long axis (UE AoArch LAX) view: The probe is withdrawn from ME DAo SAX view until circular aorta becomes oblong in shape. This would be the distal aortic arch in long axis (Fig. 18.13).

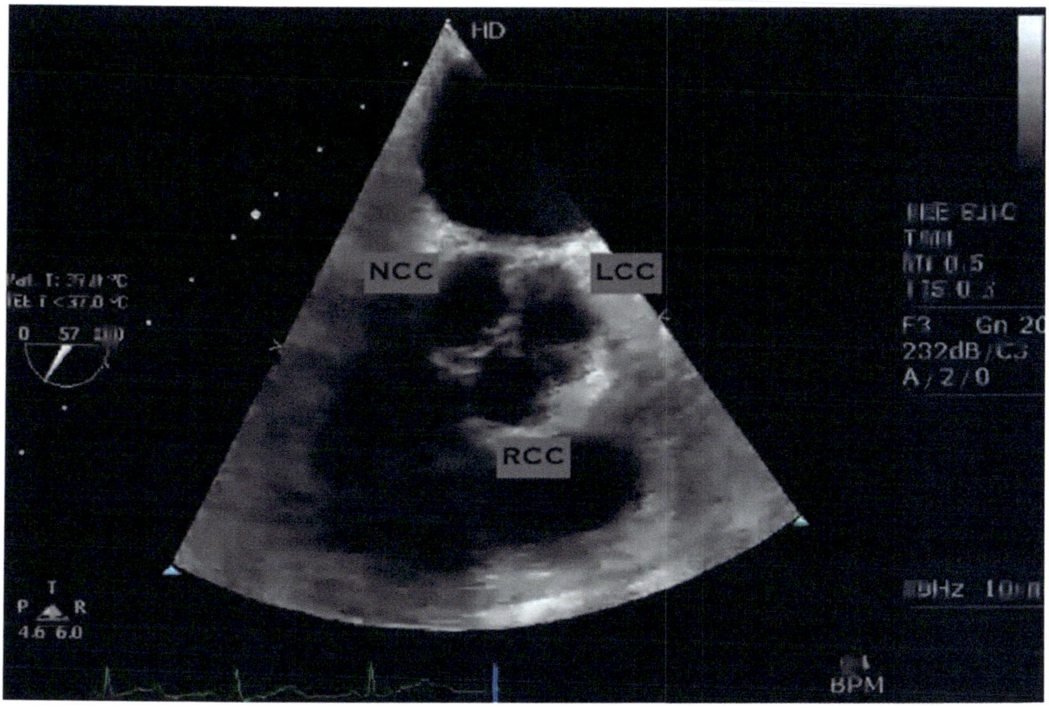

Fig. 18.8 Mid esophageal aortic short axis view

Fig. 18.9 Mid esophageal ascending aortic short axis view

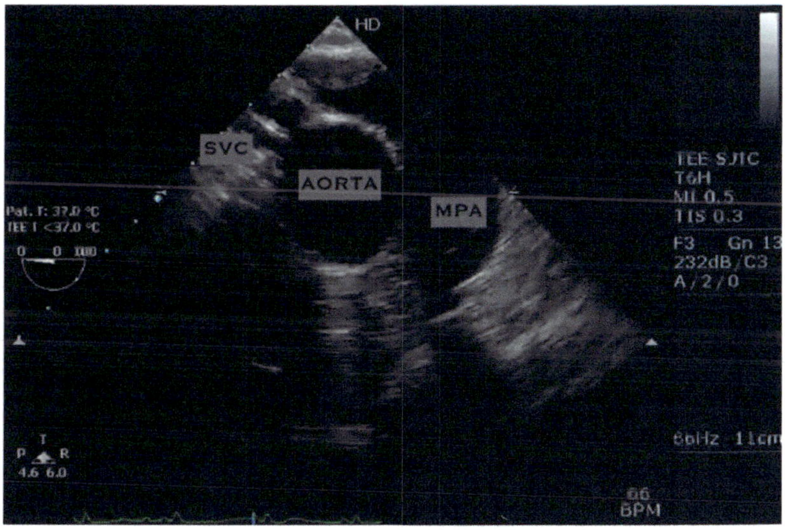

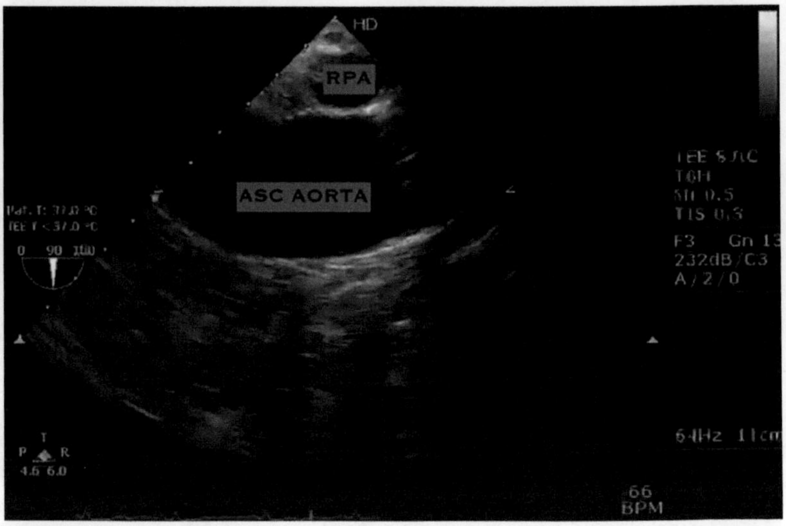

Fig. 18.10 Mid esophageal ascending aortic long axis view

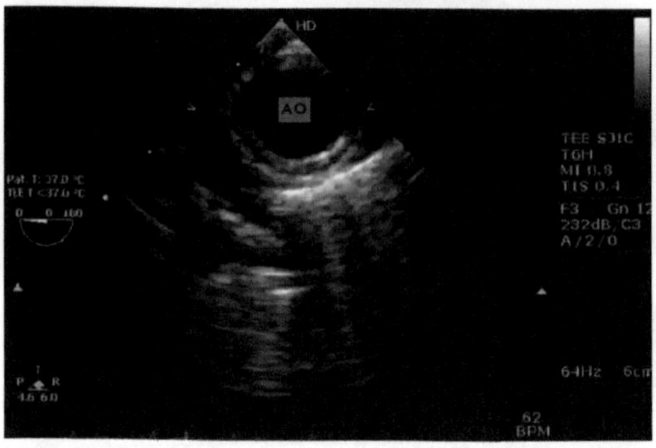

Fig. 18.11 Mid esophageal descending aortic short axis view

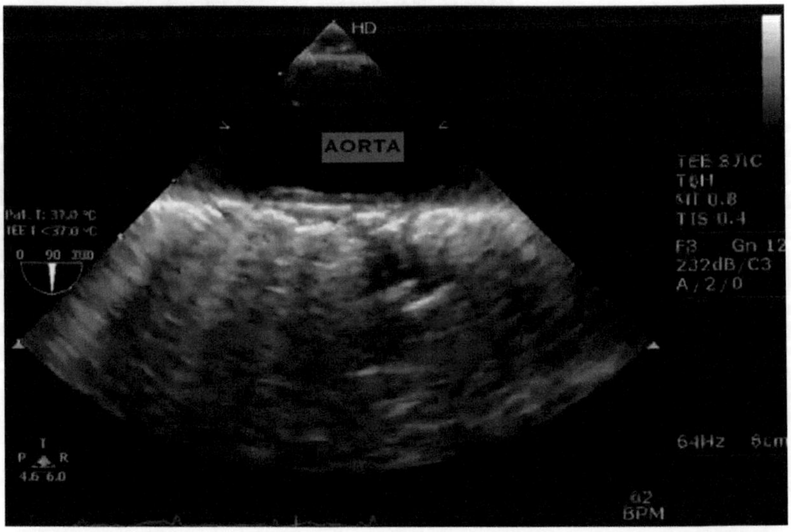

Fig. 18.12 Mid esophageal descending aortic long axis view

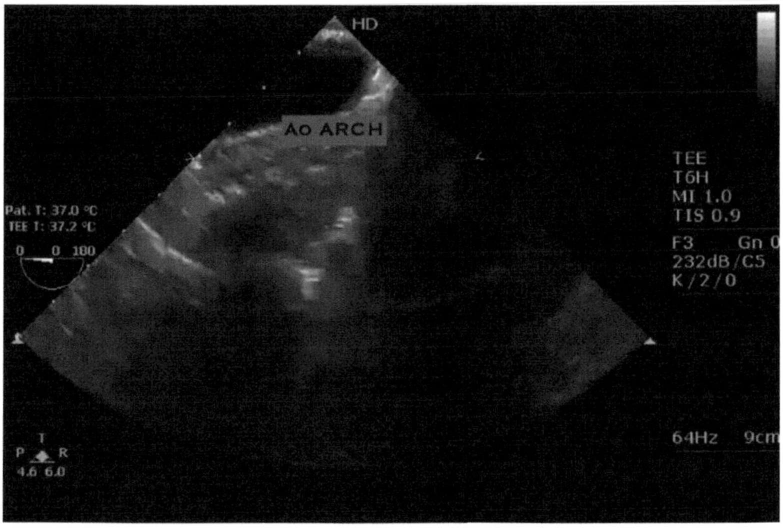

Fig. 18.13 Upper esophageal aortic arch long axis view

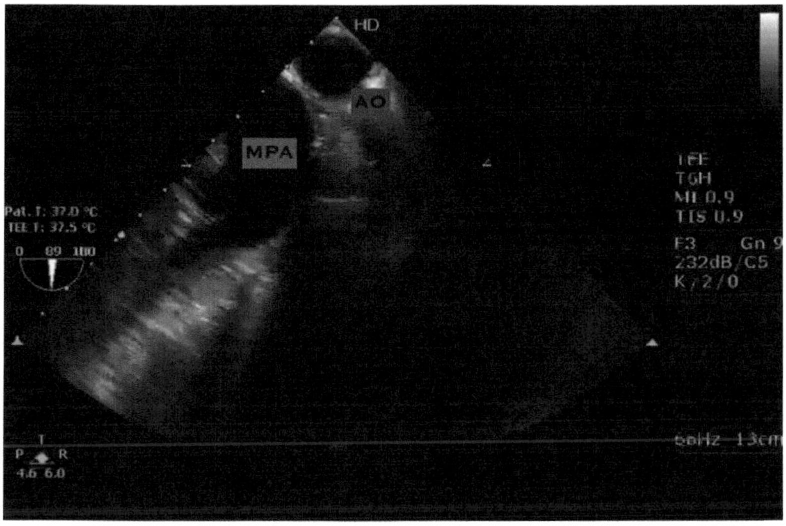

Fig. 18.14 Upper esophageal aortic arch short axis view

14. Upper esophageal aortic arch short axis (UE AoArch SAX) view: The multiplanar angle is increased to 80^0–100^0 from the UE AoArch LAX view to obtain UE AoArch SAX view to visualize aorta arch in short axis with left carotid artery visualized at 4° clock position (Fig. 18.14).
15. Transgastric basal short axis (TG basal) view: The probe is advanced into the stomach further from ME 4C view and anteverted optimize the image to visualize the LV along with mitral valve and crescent shaped RV in short axis. Mitral valve orifice can be obtained by planimetry in this view (Fig. 18.15).
16. Transgastric mid papillary (TG MID) view: The probe is advanced into the stomach slightly further from TG basal view or decrease the anteversion to visualize the LV along with the two papillary muscles and crescent shaped RV in short axis. Regional wall motion abnormalities can be assessed in this view (Fig. 18.16).

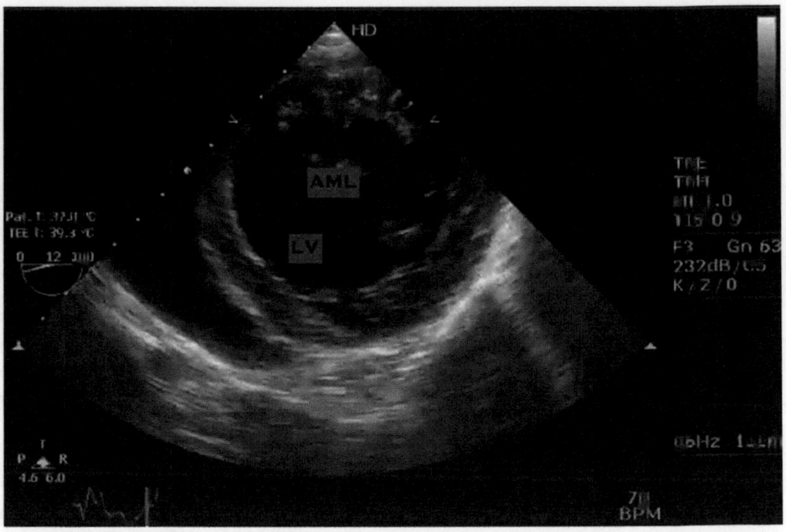

Fig. 18.15 Transgastric basal short axis view

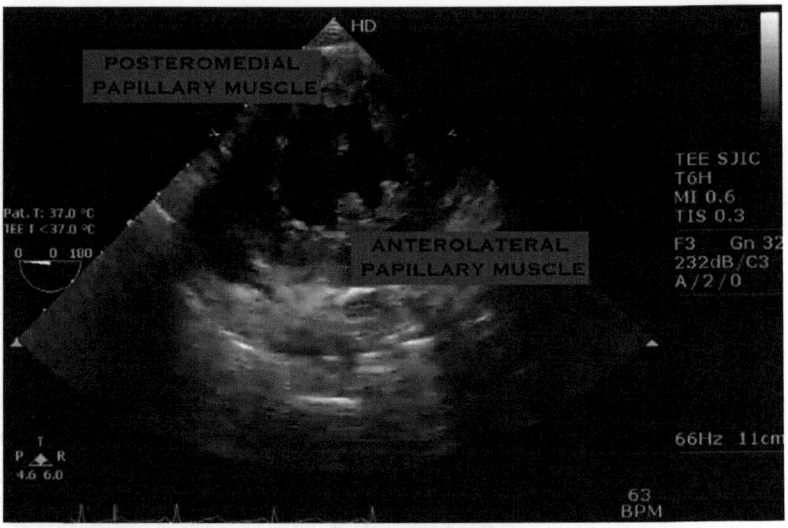

Fig. 18.16 Transgastric mid papillary view

17. Transgastric two chamber (TG 2C) view: The multiplanar angle is increased to 80^0–100^0 from TG MID view to visualize the LV along with the sub valvar apparatus in long axis (Fig. 18.17).
18. Transgastric long axis (TG LAX) view: The multiplanar angle is further increased to 110^0–130^0 from TG 2C view to visualize the LV along with the aortic valve in long axis. The aortic valve gradients can be obtained in this view as the doppler can be aligned parallel to the aortic flow (Fig. 18.18).
19. Transgastric RV inflow (TG RV inflow) view: The probe is rotated to the right from TG LAX view to visualize the RA and RV along with the tricuspid valve with its sub valvar apparatus in long axis (Fig. 18.19).
20. Deep trans-gastric long axis (DTG LAX) view: The probe is advanced into the stomach slightly further from TG MID view with probe in neutral position and then anteverted to visualise the LV from its apex in the long axis. LVOT gradients can be obtained in this view (Fig. 18.20).

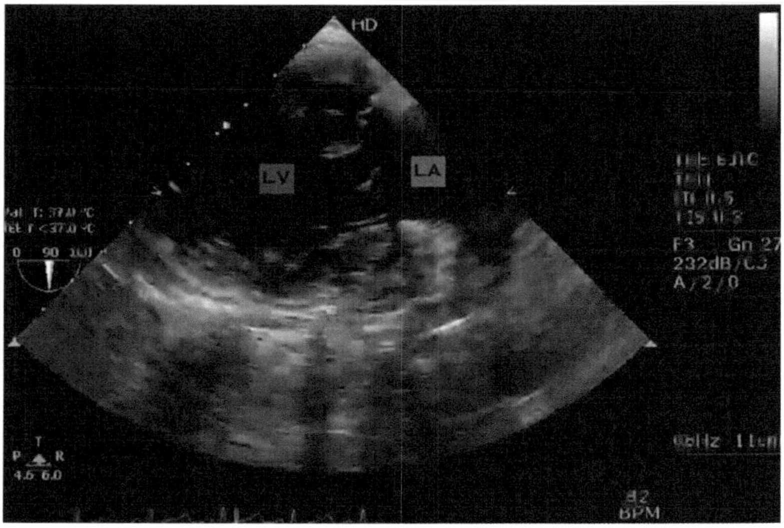

Fig. 18.17 Transgastric two chamber

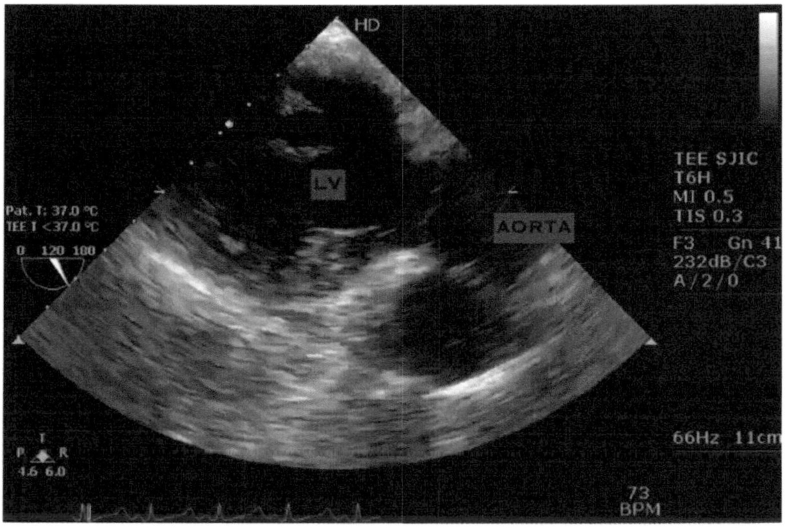

Fig. 18.18 Transgastric long axis view

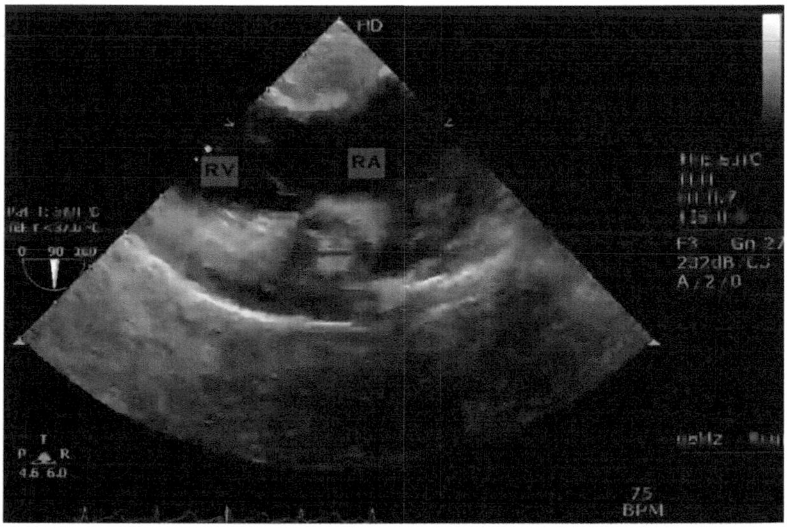

Fig. 18.19 Transgastric RV inflow view

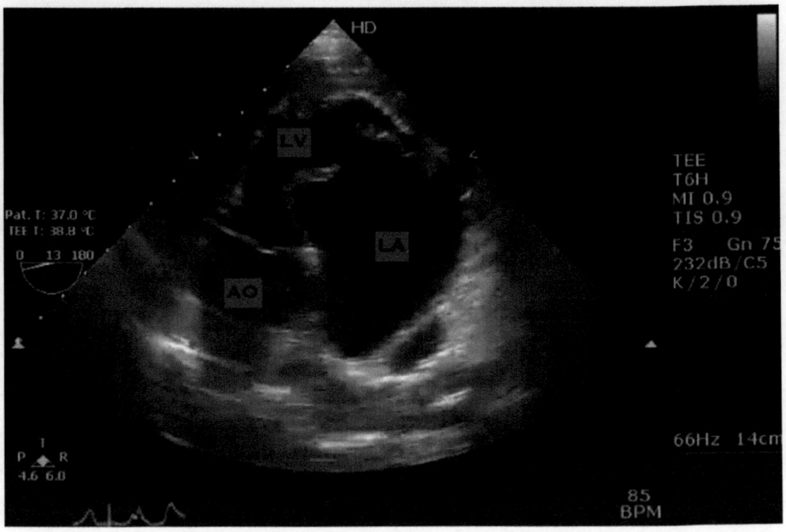

Fig. 18.20 Deep trans-gastric long axis view

18.6 Systolic Function

The estimation of systolic function is performed by global and regional indices.

Global LV function: The global systolic function of the left ventricle is limited by the preload and/ or afterload dependence. However, strain rate and end systolic elastance are exceptions for the same and are load independent indices. The load dependent indices are cardiac output, wall dimensions, LV thickness, ejection phase indices (ejection fraction, fractional shortening, velocity of circumferential fiber shortening, fractional area change), and isovolumetric phase indices (maximum dP/dt).

Linear dimensions: The change in the left ventricular dimensions and hypertrophy provides an early clue to the underlying pathology. LV dilation measured by major long axis in ME4C view from mitral annular plane to apical endocardium and minor short axis in TG MID view from medial to lateral endocardium. The normal LV end diastolic diameter for men is 42–58.4 mm and 37.8–52.2 for women [7]. The LV wall thickness is best measured in TG MID view. The normal range of inferior wall thickness for men is 6–10 mm and 6–9 mm for women.

Cardiac output can be obtained by continuity equation, which states that blood inflow across any of the normal mitral valve should be same across normal aortic valve if no intracardiac shunt exist. The LV outflow tract (LVOT) is usually used to measure cardiac output as LVOT is circular and relatively fixed. The stroke volume (SV) is given by the formula.

$$\mathrm{SV} = \mathrm{VTI}_{\mathrm{LVOT}} * \mathrm{LVOT\ area}$$

$$\mathrm{LVOT\ area} = 2\ \pi r^2 = 2\ \pi\ \left(d/2\right)^2$$

$\mathrm{VTI}_{\mathrm{LVOT}}$ can be obtained by applying pulsed wave doppler across LVOT in DTG LAX view.

LVOT diameter (*d*) can be measured in ME LAX view.

Cardiac output is obtained by multiplying SV with heart rate.

18.7 Ejection Phase Indices

These indices are volumetric indices.

Fractional shortening (FS): This is obtained by measuring the LV diameter in end systole and end diastole in TG MID view.

$$\mathrm{FS} = \frac{\left(\mathrm{LV\ end\ diastolic\ diameter} - \mathrm{LV\ end\ systolic\ diameter}\right)}{\mathrm{LV\ end\ diastolic\ diameter}} * 100$$

The normal FS is more than 25% in men and 27% in women.

Velocity of circumferential fiber shortening (Vcf) is derived from FS and is given by the formula. The lower limit of Vcf is 1.1 circumferences/second.

$$Vcf = FS / ET$$

ET is ejection time.

Fractional area change (FAC): The normal FAC should be more than 36%. This is given by the formula.

$$FAC = \frac{(\text{LV end diastolic area} - \text{LV end systolic area})}{\text{LV end diastolic area}} * 100$$

Ejection fraction (EF): This is obtained by modified Simpson rule method. The normal EF is 53%–73% [7].

$$EF = \frac{(\text{LV end diastolic volume} - \text{LV end systolic volume})}{\text{LV end diastolic volume}} * 100$$

18.8 Regional LV Function

The LV segmental function can be assessed semi quantitatively by wall motion score index. In a seventeen segment model [8], each segment is assigned a score from 1 to 4 (1 = normal, 2 = hypokinesia, 3 = akinesia, 4 = dyskinesia). Apart from this newer methods to assess LV function has been strain rate by speckle tracking.

18.9 Conclusion

Transesophageal echocardiography is an semi invasive real time perioperative monitoring tool and possessing the knowledge about the sequential assessment plays an important role in effective and optimal management of the patients.

Suggested Reading

1. Frazin L, Talano JV, Stephanidcs L, et al. Esophagcal echocardiography. Circulation. 1976;54:102–8.
2. Roclandt JR, Thomson IR, Vlertcr WB, et al. Multiplane uansesophageal echocardiography: latest evolution in an imaging revolution. J Am Soc Echocardiogr. 1992;5:361–7.
3. Practice guidelines for perioperative tranesophageal echocardiography. An updated report by the American Society of Anesthesiologists and the Society of Cardiovascular Anesthesiologists Task Force on Transesophageal Echocardiography. Anesthesiology. 2010;112:1084–96.
4. American College of Cardiology Foundation Appropriate Use Criteria Task F, American Society of E, American Heart A, et al. ACCF/ASEJAIWASNC/HFSAJHRS/SCAI/SCCM/SCCT/ SCMR 2011 Appropriate Use Criteria fur Echocardiography. A report of the American College of Cardiology Foundation Appropriate Use Criteria Task Force, American Society of Echocardiography, American Heart Association, American Society of Nuclear Cardiology, Heart Failure Society of America, Heart Rhythm Society, Society for Cardiovascular Angiography and Interventions, Society of Critical Care Medicine, Society of Cardiovascular Computed Tomography, Society for Cardiovascular Magnetic Resonance American College of Chest Physicians. J Am Soc Echocardiogr. 2011;24:229–67.
5. Hilberath JN, Oakes DA, Shernan SK, et al. Safety of transoesophageal echocardiography. JASE. 2010;23:1115–27.
6. Haln RT, Abraham T, Adams MS, et al. Guidelines for performing a comprehensive tansesophageal echocardiographic examination: recommendations from the American Society of Echocardiography and the

Society of Cardiovascular Anesthesiologists. J Am Soc Echocardiogr. 2013;26:921–64.

7. Lang RM, Badano LP, Mor-Avi V, et al. Recommendations for cardiac chamber quantification by echocardiography in adults: an update from the American Society of Echocardiography and the European Association of Cardiovascular Imaging. J Am Soc Echocardiogr. 2015;28(1):1–39.e14.

8. Cerqueira MD, Weissman NJ, Dilsizian V, et al. Standardized myocardial segmentation and nomenclature for tomographic imaging of the heart. A statement for healthcare professionals from the cardiac imaging Committee of the Council on Clinical Cardiology of the American Heart Association. Circulation. 2002;105(4):539–42.

Neuromuscular Monitoring

19

Kiran Mahendru, Nishkarsh Gupta,
and Anju Gupta

19.1 Introduction

Neuromuscular monitor devices were introduced into clinical practice in the 1970s. In 1979, Viby Mogensen et al. reported that 42% of patients administered a long acting neuromuscular blocking agent (NMBA) in the operating room arrived in the post anaesthesia care unit with objective evidence of postoperative residual neuromuscular block (defined as that time as train of four ratio [TOF] ratio < 0.7).

19.2 Rationale for Monitoring Neuromuscular Blockade

1. High incidence of incomplete neuromuscular recovery (residual blockade) of upto 40% (now defined as TOF < 0.9 with quantitative neuromuscular monitoring) even when intermediate acting muscle relaxants are used.
2. To optimize the use of nondepolarizing neuromuscular blocking drugs during perioperative period and in intensive care unit, to suit to individual patients needs and to titrate to the needs of surgery.
3. To choose the antagonist strategy. The choice of reversal agent, i.e., anticholinesterase or sugammadex along with the dosage and timing can be optimized by proper monitoring of neuromuscular blockade depth.

19.3 Complications and Consequences of Residual Neuromuscular Block

> Residual neuromuscular blockade cam lead to pharyngeal dysfunction, acute respiratory events like hypoxia, airway obstruction increased risk of aspiration, and may need to intubate the patient again. This may increase the length of stay in post anaesthesia care unit.

The neuromuscular monitoring should be done preferably in all patients. The need for close monitoring of the neuro muscular junction becomes especially important in certain high-risk groups highlighted in Table 19.1.

K. Mahendru
Department of Anaesthesiology, Dayanand Medical College and Hospital, Ludhiana, Punjab, India

N. Gupta (✉)
Department Onco-Anesthesiology and Palliative Medicine at DRBRAIRCH, All India Institute of Medical Sciences, New Delhi, Delhi, India

A. Gupta
Anesthesiology, Pain Medicine, Critical Care, All India Institute of Medical Sciences, New Delhi, Delhi, India

N. Gupta et al. (eds.), *Techniques in Anesthesia, Intensive Care and Emergency Medicine*,
https://doi.org/10.1007/978-981-96-1202-4_19

Table 19.1 Indications for neuromuscular monitoring

1. Prolonged infusions of NMBA or when long-acting drugs are used
2. Conditions wherein inadequate reversal is likely or can lead to adverse effects, for example, severe respiratory disease, morbid obesity
3. In conditions where administration of a reversal agent may cause harm, for example, tachyarrhythmias, cardiac failure
4. Liver or renal dysfunction when pharmacokinetics of muscular relaxants may be altered
5. Neuromuscular disorders such as myasthenia gravis or Eaton–Lambert syndrome
6. Day care surgery
7. Extremes of age
8. Use of special techniques like hypothermia, hypotensive anaesthesia
9. Surgical procedures requiring absolute immobility like aneurysm or other complex neurosurgery, microvascular surgery etc. to name a few.

19.4 Some Important Physiological Aspects of Neuromuscular Junction

1. The neuromuscular junction is responsible for chemical transmission of electrical impulses from nerve to muscle in order to generate an appropriate muscle contraction. A basic understanding of the physiology is necessary to understand the neuromuscular monitoring.
2. Neuromuscular junction has three distinct parts—.
   - Presynaptic part—Distal motor nerve ending.
   - Synaptic cleft.
   - Postsynaptic part—Muscle membrane.
3. Information from nerve to muscle is transmitted via release of acetylcholine (ACh) and activation of ligand gated, fast acting nicotinic acetylcholine receptors (nAChRs).
4. When an action potential arrives at the distal nerve terminal, voltage-gated calcium channels, open to generate a local inward calcium flux leading to increased intracellular calcium concentration.
5. The locally increased calcium concentration is sensed by specific vesicle membrane-associated synaptotagmins that mediate the formation of complexes of the three SNARE proteins. This leads to vesicle docking and fusion and subsequent release of acetylcholine into the synaptic cleft.
6. Under resting conditions (absence of a nerve action potential at the distal nerve terminal), small spontaneous endplate potentials can be recorded at the postsynaptic side of the NMJ termed as miniature end plate potentials (MEPP) caused by release of small number of ACh vesicles termed as quantal release.
7. When an action potential arrives at the nerve terminal, several hundred vesicles are released synchronously resulting in a summation of corresponding MEPPs to give an endplate potential.
8. An endplate potential large enough to depolarize the muscle cell triggers the propagation of the action potential along the postsynaptic membrane, ultimately leading to calcium release within the muscle and the actin–myosin interaction that results in muscle contraction.
9. The amount of Ach released by a stimulated nerve depends upon the levels of ionized calcium in extracellular fluid. If the extracellular calcium doubles, the quantal release increases by 16-folds. During tetanic stimulus, the calcium entering the nerve with every stimulus, doesn't get excreted and tends to accumulate. So, after tetanic stimuli, the nerve endings have more free calcium available and a stimulus applied to the nerve after tetanic stimulation releases much more acetylcholine (than with normal stimulation) which antagonizes the effect of non-depolarizing muscle relaxant and increases the size of the twitch (**post tetanic potentiation**).
10. If the tetanic stimulation is prolonged, the NMJ becomes refractory and is incapable of releasing enough quanta to maintain depolarization. This results in a **fade**.

19.5 Principles of Nerve Stimulation

(a) Typically, one nerve fiber will innervate between 5 and 2000 muscle fibers.
(b) The nerve chosen to be stimulated must fulfil the following criteria
- It must have a motor element
- It must be close to the skin
- Contraction in the muscle or muscle group which the nerve supplies must be visible or accessible to evoked response monitoring

(c) In order to stimulate the nerve electric current is applied transcutaneously using ECG electrodes.
(d) Generating an action potential in all of the nerve fibers in a motor nerve will require a current of sufficient magnitude and duration. Most nerve stimulators will apply a current for 0.1–0.3 ms, which is more than adequate.
(e) The current which generates a response through all nerve fibers and hence a maximal muscle contraction is termed a maximal stimulus.
(f) Traditionally, a current of 25% above the maximal stimulus is applied when stimulating a peripheral nerve: this is termed a *supra-maximal* stimulus.
(g) The degree of neuromuscular block can be assessed by applying a supramaximal stimulus to a peripheral nerve and measuring the associated muscular response.
(h) **Nerve stimulator**
1. It should be battery operated
2. Able to deliver a constant current upto 80 mA
3. Constant current stimulator is preferable to constant voltage stimulator as current will vary depending on the resistance of the skin according to Ohm's law V = IR (V = voltage, I = current and R = resistance) and current magnitude is the factor that determines whether a nerve depolarizes or not.
4. The pulse stimulus should last no longer than 0.3 ms and be of a monophasic, square wave type. This will ensure that a constant current is maintained throughout the stimulus.
5. The polarity of the electrode leads should be indicated

(i) **Electrodes**
1. Good electrical contact with the skin can be established using ECG electrodes of the silver/silver chloride variety.
2. It is recommended that the negative electrode be placed directly over the most superficial part of the nerve.
3. The positive electrode can then be placed in a position along the course of the nerve, usually proximally to avoid direct muscle stimulation.
4. Skin offers resistance to current flow and if skin resistance is high, the response at neuromuscular junction may not be adequate.
5. Skin resistance range from 0 Ω to 5 kΩ, and is affected by factors such as skin temperature, adequacy of electrode application, and disease state, for example, diabetes mellitus or chronic renal failure.
6. To minimize skin resistance remove greasiness, dry the skin, ensure good electrode contact and apply a conducting gel (silver/silver chloride).

(j) **Differential muscle sensitivity to neuromuscular blocking agents**
1. Muscle groups respond differently to neuromuscular blocking agents, such that the monitored twitch response may not accurately reflect neuromuscular transmission in clinically important muscles (e.g., airway muscles and diaphragm).
2. After neuromuscular blocking agent administration, block occurs faster in central muscles (e.g., larynx and diaphragm) than peripheral muscles (adductor pollicis, flexor hallucis), because of greater blood flow and drug delivery to the central muscles.

3. However, the diaphragm is also more resistant to the effects of nondepolarizing neuromuscular blockers, and recovers faster, because it has a higher density of nAChRs.
4. The response to stimulation at the corrugator supercilii muscle (at the eyebrow) correlates closely with neuromuscular block at the diaphragm and larynx, whereas stimulation at the orbicularis oculi correlates closely with the adductor pollicis muscle. However, in practice it is difficult to separate the responses of these two muscles, and therefore facial nerve stimulation may overestimate the degree of recovery from neuromuscular block.
5. The sequence of recovery of various muscles after nondepolarizing neuromuscular blockade is as follows (fastest to slowest): diaphragm > laryngeal muscles > corrugator supercilii > abdominal muscles > orbicularis oculi > geniohyoid muscle (upper airway) > adductor pollicis muscle.

19.6 Clinical Implications of Differential Muscle Sensitivity

- During intubation if deep neuromuscular blockade is confirmed by monitoring adductor pollicis or flexor hallucis stimulation, pharyngeal muscles are usually blocked as well, and optimal intubating conditions are achieved.
- During surgery, the absence of a twitch at the adductor pollicis muscle does not guarantee that the diaphragm will be paralyzed. A post-tetanic count of 1 or 2 at the adductor pollicis indicates deep block, but diaphragm movement is still possible.
- During recovery from neuromuscular block, a train-of-four ratio >0.9 at the adductor pollicis represents full recovery; the airway muscles and diaphragm have recovered fully.
- Monitoring facial muscles will overestimate the degree of recovery. If the arms are not accessible due to surgical positioning, monitor the facial muscles but transition to the arms once they become available.

(k) **Sites of stimulation:** Any superficial peripheral nerve can be used for neuromuscular monitoring.

Ulnar Nerve

1. The ulnar nerve is the preferred because
   - It is easy to locate
   - Single nerve supplies a single muscle, i.e., adductor pollicis longus
   - The response is assessed by monitoring adduction of the thumb
   - Chances of direct muscle stimulation are less (the muscle is opposite to the site of stimulation)

2. Maximal neuronal stimulation and muscular response are achieved by placing the negative electrode one centimeter proximal to the wrist crease, with the positive electrode four to five centimeters proximally along the ulnar surface of the volar forearm.

Facial Nerve

1. If surgical positioning limit access to the hands, facial nerve can be used for monitoring.
2. It is less accurate than ulnar nerve stimulation.
3. Facial nerve electrodes are placed on the mastoid process and just anterior to the tragus of the ear, to minimize the risk of direct muscle stimulation.
4. Contraction of the orbicularis oculi (at the eyelid) or the corrugator supercilli muscle (at the eyebrow) is assessed.
5. Recovery of the stimulation response at the muscles around the eye may not reflect a degree of recovery in other muscles that would allow safe extubation.
6. If facial nerve monitoring is used during surgery, ulnar nerve stimulation should be used to confirm adequate reversal of neuromuscular block before extubation, preferably by objective means.

Posterior Tibial Nerve

1. Stimulated by placing electrode superior to medial malleolus.
2. Response is flexion of the great toe.

19.7 Stimulation Pattern and Their Uses

Degree of neuromuscular block can be assessed objectively by recording the response to stimulation of a motor nerve. The different patterns of stimulation include:

(a) **Single twitch stimulation:** Single square wave supramaximal stimulus is applied to peripheral nerve for period of 0.2 msec at regular intervals and evoked response is observed (Fig. 19.1).

The most useful time to apply the single twitch pattern of nerve stimulation is at the onset of neuromuscular block. Using a single twitch at 1 Hz (1 twitch every second), it is possible to establish the level at which a supramaximal stimulus is obtained. The onset of neuromuscular block can then be observed, using a single twitch at 0.1 Hz (1 twitch every 10 s). The onset and recovery from depolarizing and non-depolarizing block monitored using single twitches have a similar pattern, differing only in timescale.

The major limitation to this technique is the need to measure a control twitch before administering the neuromuscular blocking agent.

(b) **Train-of-stimulation:** Developed in 1970 by Ali and colleagues. The pattern involved stimulating the ulnar nerve with a TOF supramaximal twitch stimuli, with a frequency of 2 Hz, that is, four stimuli each separated by 0.5 s. The TOF is then repeated every 10 s (train frequency of 0.1 Hz). As well as enabling the observer to compare T1 (first twitch of the TOF) to T0 (control), it also enables comparison of T4 (fourth twitch of the TOF) to T1. This is known as the *TOF ratio (T4/T1)*.

When a **non-depolarizing agent** is given, there is a reduction in the amplitude of the evoked responses, with T4 affected first, then T3, followed by T2, and finally T1. This decrement in twitch height is known as ***fade***. As the non-depolarizing block becomes more intense, T4 disappears followed by T3, T2, and finally T1. The reverse is true during recovery from non-depolarizing block: T1 reappears first followed by T2, T3, and finally, T4.

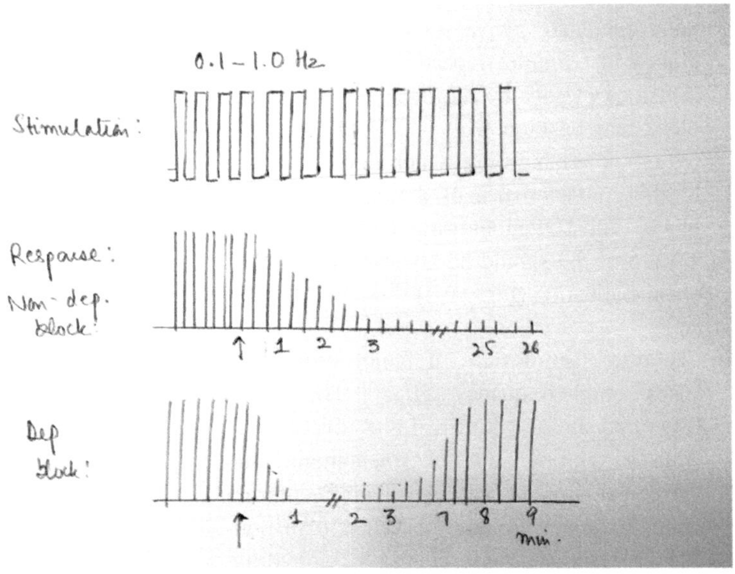

Fig. 19.1 Pattern of electrical stimulation and evoked muscle responses to single twitch nerve stimulation

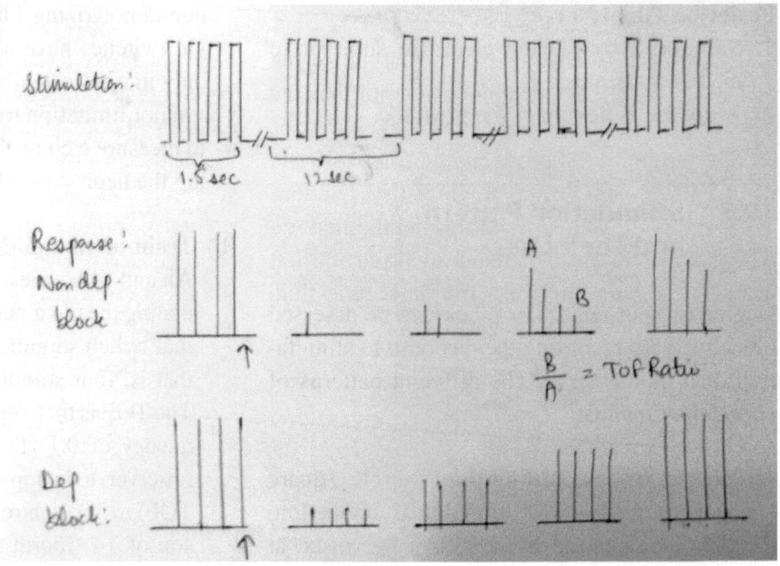

Fig. 19.2 Pattern of electrical stimulation and evoked muscle responses to Train of Four nerve stimulation

During partial non-depolarizing block, the number of twitches (*TOF count*) correlates with the degree of neuromuscular block. Twitch suppression of 90% would equate to a TOF count of 1 or less. Reversal of residual neuromuscular block can safely be achieved when the TOF count is 3 or greater.

The TOF pattern is less useful in monitoring **depolarizing neuromuscular block**. During onset of depolarizing block, each of the four twitches is decreased equally in size, that is, there is no fade. This is also observed during recovery. However, if larger doses of depolarizing agent are given, for example in techniques that require repeated bolus doses or infusions of succinylcholine, then a Phase 2 block may develop. This is a block produced by a depolarizing drug which develops some of the characteristics of a non-depolarizing block. With TOF monitoring, fade is observed.

TOF ratio of 0.9 should be achieved before tracheal extubation (Fig. 19.2).

(c) **Tetanic stimulation:** Tetanic stimulation uses a high frequency (50–200 Hz) supramaximal stimulus for 5 s. In healthy skeletal muscle during normal movement, the response is maintained as a tetanic contraction. However, on administration of a non-depolarizing neuromuscular blocking drug, the muscle, depending on the degree of block, will show signs of fade, that is, the stimulated muscle will be unable to sustain a muscular contraction. At higher frequencies (100–200 Hz) muscular fatigue may develop, but at a stimulation frequency of 50 Hz this should not occur, and the degree of fade will correspond more closely to the degree of neuromuscular block. This pattern of stimulation is very sensitive and can elicit minor degrees of neuromuscular block, which is potentially useful in the postoperative recovery room.

During partial depolarizing block, fade is not observed in response to tetanic stimulation. The amplitude of the evoked response will be lower but the tetanic contraction will be maintained.

However, its use is limited by the fact that tetanic stimulation is extremely painful.

(d) **Post-tetanic count:** During profound non-depolarizing neuromuscular block, there may be no response to TOF or single twitch stimulation. In such circumstances, a post-tetanic count (PTC) may be useful. If a 5 s tetanic stimulus at 50 Hz is administered, after no twitch response has been elicited, followed 3 s later by further single twitches

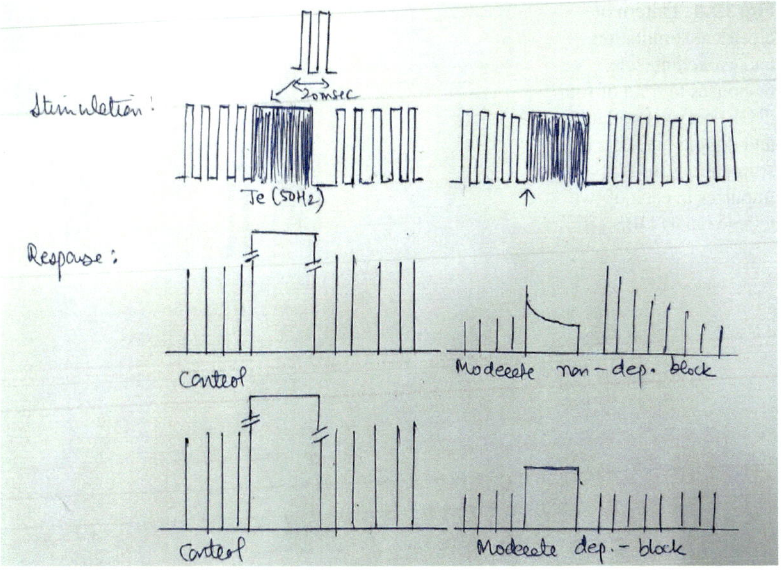

Fig. 19.3 Pattern of electrical stimulation and evoked muscle responses to Tetanic (50 Hz) nerve stimulation for 5 seconds (Te) and post-tetanic twitch stimulation (1 Hz)

at 1 Hz, there may be a response to single twitch stimulation. Although this pattern will not be seen during very profound block, a response will be seen in the early stages of recovery, before the TOF reappears. This is known as *post-tetanic facilitation*.

On completion of a tetanic stimulus, acetylcholine synthesis and mobilization continue for a short period. As a result there is an increased, immediately available store of acetylcholine which causes an enhanced response to subsequent single twitch stimulation. The number of post-tetanic twitches is an indication of when the first twitch of the TOF will reappear. For instance, the first twitch of the TOF generally returns with a PTC of 9 when using atracurium or vecuronium.

The main use of PTC is when profound neuromuscular block is required, for example, during retinal surgery, when movement or coughing could have devastating effects.

It should be remembered that a tetanic stimulus, by mobilizing acetylcholine, might affect the neuromuscular junction of a stimulated nerve for a significant time. If two PTCs are administered in quick succession, the degree of neuromuscular block will be underestimated. It is recommended that tetanic stimulation should not be repeated for a period of 6 min (Fig. 19.3).

(e) **Double burst stimulation:** DBS was developed to enable the anaesthetist to detect even small degrees of neuromuscular block clinically.

In DBS, two short bursts of tetanus at 50 Hz at a supramaximal current are applied to a nerve. Each burst will have three impulses lasting 0.2 msec. Each impulse is delivered every 20 msec and the two bursts are separated by 750 msec.

In unparalysed muscle, two separate muscle contractions of equal intensity will occur. In muscle partially paralysed with a non-depolarizing agent, the response to the second burst is reduced. This is the phenomenon of fade. The ratio of the magnitude of the second stimulus to the first is known as the *DBS ratio*.

Tactile evaluation of the DBS ratio has been shown to be more accurate than tactile evaluation of the TOF ratio (Fig. 19.4).

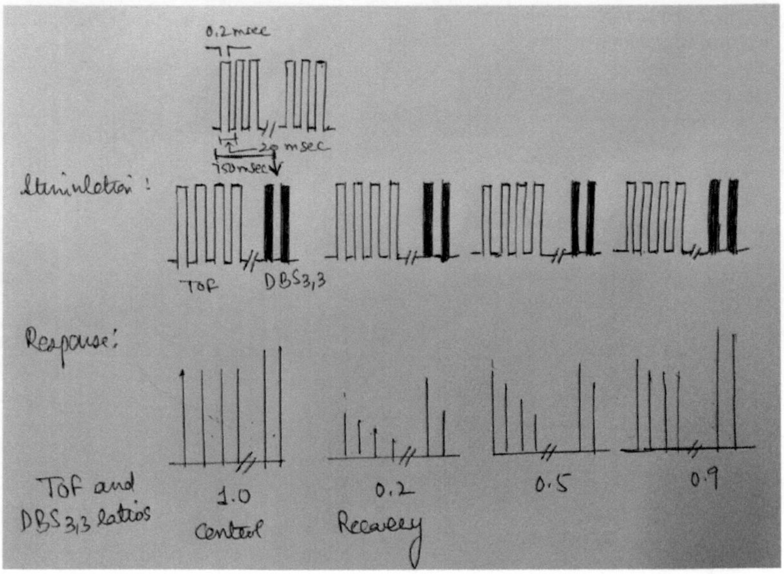

Fig. 19.4 Pattern of electrical stimulation and evoked muscle responses to train of four (TOF) nerve stimulation and double-burst nerve stimulation (three impulses in each of two tetanic bursts DBS $_{3,3}$)

19.8 Methods of Neuromuscular Monitoring (Tables 19.2, 19.3, and 19.4)

1. **Clinical tests**—It depends on the ability of the patient to perform certain tasks on stimulation. After administering NMBDs one can observe the following clinical signs:
   - Weakness of extra-ocular muscles, diplopia
   - Feeling of weakness or heaviness, poor grip strength
   - Swallowing difficulty
   - Patient may not be able to sustain head lift, decreased peak inspiratory force
   - Decreased vital capacity
   - Jerky respiration, respiratory failure
   - Diaphragmatic paralysis

The following tests may be used to determine the adequate recovery from neuromuscular blocking agents:

(i) Patient opens eyes widely to command and denies diplopia
(ii) Sustained tongue protrusion
(iii) Effective swallowing
(iv) Sustained head/leg lift for 5 seconds
(v) Sustained firm hand grip
(vi) Effective cough
(vii) A vital capacity of at least 15 ml/kg
(viii) Ability to generate an inspiratory force of at least −30 cmH_2O

But all of these are not always enough because they depend upon the degree of consciousness, need patient cooperation and there is interindividual variation in the response.

2. **Qualitative evaluation using peripheral nerve stimulator**—To assess visually or tactilely the response of the stimulated muscle. A standard PNS can provide several patterns of nerve stimulation such as train of four, double burst, tetanic and post tetanic count. Although they are more reliable than clinical tests, does not eliminate the risk of post-operative residual curarization. Out of all, Double burst stimulation is most sensitive to assess visually or tactilely the response to muscle stimulation.
3. **Quantitative monitoring using neuromuscular monitors**—includes devices that stimulate the peripheral nerve while also recording, quantifying, and displaying numerically the evoked responses. Multiple techniques used with its advantages and limitations given in the following table:

Table 19.2 Preferred simulation pattern during anesthesia and surgery

S. No	Phase	Stimulation pattern	Level
1	Induction/ intubation	TOF	0
2	Surgical paralysis	TOF	1/2
3	Intense NM blockade	PTC	0
4	Timing reversal	DBS >> > TOF	TOF 2/3, presence of 2nd response on DBS
5	Adequate recovery	TOF ratio	>0.9 preferably 1

Table 19.3 Summary of patterns of neuromuscular stimulation

	ST	TOF	Tetanus	DBS	PTC
Current strength	Supra-maximal	Supra or submaximal	Supra or submaximal	Supra or submaximal	Supra or submaximal
Frequency/description	0.1 to 1 Hz	2 Hz four stimuli	30 to 50 Hz for 5 seconds	3 impulses at 50 Hz repeated after 750 msec	30 Hz for 5 sec, 3 sec later ST at 1 Hz
Pre-relaxant control	Needed	Not needed	Not needed	Not needed	Not needed
Pain on stimulation	–	–/+	++	+	++
Sensitivity of manual Detection (visual/tactile)	Not sensitive	Not sensitive at TOF ratio of 0.4–0.7	Sensitive	Highly sensitive	Sensitive
Alteration of subsequent responses	Not altered	Not altered	Altered (post- tetanic facilitation)	Not altered	Altered
Interval between successive stimuli	5 sec	12 sec	6 min	12–15 sec	6 min
Receptor occupancy detection	75–90%	70–90%	70–90%	70–90%	>90% also
Sensitivity for detection of subtle block	Not sensitive	Sensitive	Sensitive	Sensitive	Not applicable
Monitoring of profound block	Not useful	Not useful	Not useful	Not useful	Useful

ST single twitch, *TOF* train of four, *DBS* double burst stimulation, *PTC* post tetanic count

Table 19.4 Techniques for quantitative neuromuscular monitoring

Monitoring technique	Description	Devices for clinical use	Advantages	Limitations
Mechanomyography (MMG)	Measurement of evoked mechanical response	None	Precise Reproducible Gold standard	Cumbersome setup
Electromyography (EMG)	Measurement of muscle action potential following nerve stimulation	Datex Ohmeda NMT ElectroSensor	Best indicator of pure neuromuscular function Comparable with MMG but more consistent with time Available for many sites Free muscle movement not required	Influenced by other electronic devices in the operating room (diathermy) or local temperature

(continued)

Table 19.4 (continued)

Monitoring technique	Description	Devices for clinical use	Advantages	Limitations
Acceleromyography (AMG) Standard of clinical care (Fig. 19.5)	Measurement of the acceleration of the stimulated muscle with piezoelectric sensor	TOF watch	Easy to handle Suitable for any free moving muscle	Not interchangeable with EMG/MMG TOF ratio overestimation by at least 0.15 Baseline TOF ratio > 1.0
Kinemyography (KMG) (Fig. 19.6)	Measurement of electrical signal generated by the bending of the piezoelectric sensor strip placed between thumb and the index finger	Datex Ohmeda NMT MechanoSensor	Easy to use	Available only for ulnar nerve Free thumb movement required Good strip placement between fingers required
Phonomyography (PMG)	Measurement of low frequency sounds evoked by muscle contraction	None	Easy to apply Usable for many sites Good correlation with AMG,EMG, MMG	
Compressomyography (CMG)	Modified non invasive blood pressure cuff measuring the block depth by brachial plexus stimulation through electrodes attached on its inner surface	TOF-cuff	No need for free arm movement	Not interchangeable with MMG, but a TOF-cuff TOF ratio > 0.9 correlates with a MMG TOF ratio > 0.7

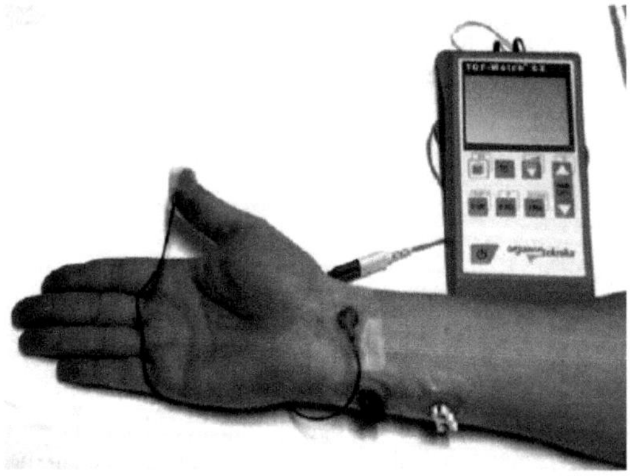

Fig. 19.5 Acceleromyography

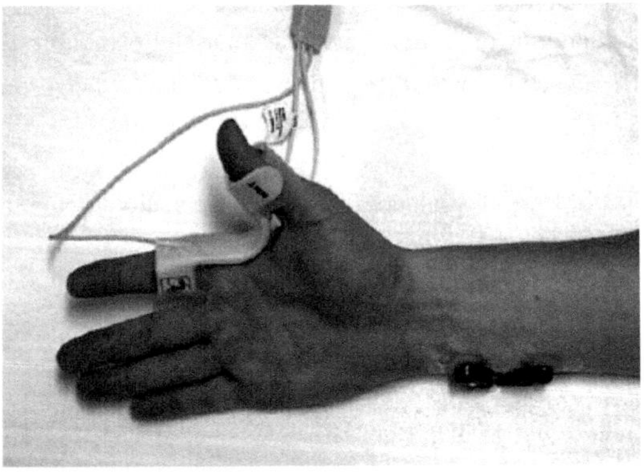

Fig. 19.6 Kinemyography

19.9 Conclusion

The onset, peak, and recovery from the effect of neuromuscular blocking drug are variable between patients and so it mandatory for us to use objective neuromuscular monitoring. There is no ideal neuromuscular monitor available but at present, mechanomyograpgy is the gold standard for research but acceleromyography is the most versatile technique to monitor neuromuscular function in clinical settings. The concept of "site-related" neuromuscular block should be used to ensure accurate monitoring of neuromuscular function, drug titration, and optimal block at the surgical site. A Train of Four ratio > 0.9 should be targeted before awakening the patient.

Suggested Reading

1. Viby-Mogensen J, Jorgensen BC, Ording H. Residual curarization in the recovery room. Anesthesiology. 1979;50:539–41.
2. Dutu M, Ivascu R, Tudorache O, Morlova D, Stanca A, Negoita S, et al. Neuromuscular monitoring: an update. Rom J Anaesth Intensive Care. 2018;25(1):55–60.
3. Viby-Mogensen. Neuromuscular monitoring. In: Miller RD, editor. Anesthesia. 5th ed. New York: Churchill Livingstone; 2000. p. 1351–66.
4. Fagerlund MJ, Eriksson LI. Current concepts in neuromuscular transmission. Br J Anaesth. 2009;103:108–14.
5. McGrath CD, Hunter JM. Monitoring of neuromuscular block. Br J Anaesth CEPD Rev. 2006;6:7–12.
6. Wright PM, Caldwell JE, Miller RD. Onset and duration of rocuronium and succinylcholine at the adductor pollicis and laryngeal adductor muscles in anesthetized humans. Anesthesiology. 1994;81:1110.
7. Meistelman C, Plaud B, Donati F. Neuromuscular effects of succinylcholine on the vocal cords and adductor pollicis muscles. Anesth Analg. 1991;73:278.
8. Donati F, Meistelman C, Plaud B. Vecuronium neuromuscular blockade at the adductor muscles of the larynx and adductor pollicis. Anesthesiology. 1991;74:833.
9. Hemmerling TM, Schmidt J, Hanusa C, et al. Simultaneous determination of neuromuscular block at the larynx, diaphragm, adductor pollicis, orbicularis oculi and corrugator supercilii muscles. Br J Anaesth. 2000;85:856.
10. Padmaja D, Mantha S. Monitoring of neuromuscular junction. Ind J Anaesth. 2002;46:279–88.

20 Defibrillation, Cardioversion and Pacing

Arindam Choudhury and Raj Mohan

Key Points

- Electrical therapy is one of the most important armamentaria for treating rhythm disorders. A thorough knowledge about the principles of defibrillation and pacing is necessary before their practical applications to those patients who are frequently in the brink of life and death situation.
- Essential difference between cardioversion and defibrillation is that the electrical therapy in the former is always delivered in synchrony with patients R wave of patients QRS complex. Typically, the energy required is lower in comparison to defibrillation as the later always cater to the ventricular arrythmias which are potentially fatal.
- Pacemakers are wonderful cardiac rhythm management devices (CRMD) whose invention was really "God sent" as millions of patients are benefitted today for their non-invasive deployments and widespread success in treating hemodynamically significant bradycardias without which sustenance of life would be impossible for them.
- ICDs are another lifesaving device whose role in terminating malignant VT/VFs and preventing SCDs are well proven. Millions of patients are benefitted since their inception. Special considerations apply while evaluating and caring for patients undergoing surgery with either of these devices during perioperative period.
- A special relationship exists between pacemaker/ICDs and Magnet (depending on the manufacturer) as basic as relationship between electricity and magnetism. Magnets can induce certain predetermined changes in the CRMD behaviors which can be utilized intraoperatively for the benefit of the patient with one of these devices undergoing modern day surgery (utilizing ESUs).

20.1 Introduction

Electrical therapies are among the most definitive and advanced therapeutics for cardiac ailments manifesting as rhythm disturbances or dysrhythmias. They are of different nature and each one of them require a different approach of manage-

A. Choudhury (✉) · R. Mohan
Department of Cardiac-Anaesthesia and Intensive care, AIIMS, Delhi, India

N. Gupta et al. (eds.), *Techniques in Anesthesia, Intensive Care and Emergency Medicine*,
https://doi.org/10.1007/978-981-96-1202-4_20

ment. In general, bradyarrhythmias need electrical pacing while tachyarrhythmias require electrical cardioversion and/or defibrillation.

Ventricular fibrillation (VF) is a life-threatening arrhythmia that can be fatal if not terminated promptly with electrical therapy better known as defibrillation. The incidence of cardiac arrhythmias in critically ill patients is anything between 50% and 90% depending on the etiology of the hospital/ICU admission. In the ICU, the most common arrhythmias are atrial fibrillation (AF) and ventricular tachycardia (VT). Rapid diagnosis and prompt management of these arrhythmias are important as they potentially cause hemodynamic instability, prolonged hospital stay, increased morbidity, and mortality.

For almost a hundred years now, electric shocks are used to terminate all chaotic and bizarre ventricular rhythms such as VF. As ideas about the mechanism by which an electric shock halts VF changed, so did the technology change over time to deliver effective shock with minimal damage to the cardiac tissue. Today, defibrillation is an important component of any advanced cardiac life support (ACLS) algorithms for pulseless VT/VF. The delivery of electrical shock therapy results in depolarization of the entire myocardium rendering the heart refractory to the ongoing chaotic electrical discharges. This leads to interruption of the abnormal rhythm and re-establishment of normal heart rhythm. This is discussed in greater details in the following section.

20.2 Mechanism of Action

Cardioversion terminates arrhythmias by delivering a shock that depolarizes the myocardial tissue involved in a re-entrant circuit. By depolarizing all excitable tissue (circuit) and making them refractory and they are no longer available for impulse conduction or re-entry. As a result, cardioversion terminates all arrhythmias resulting from a single reentrant circuit, like AVNRT, atrial flutter and monomorphic VT.

In contrast to pacing, defibrillation is carried out using electrodes with large surface area (35–70 cm^2 for a cutaneous or epicardial electrodes) separated by 10–40 cm. This creates sufficient "global" electrical field for a successful cardioversion/defibrillation. In humans, the minimum global field required to terminate a VF is 3–4 V/cm (using biphasic shock) and 5–6 V/cm (using monophasic shock). Although the field strength required for successful defibrillation is 8–10 times that of pacing, the former requires generation of field strengths across both ventricles (hence, global), whereas the later needs achieving them only locally within a few millimeters of the tip of the pacing wire.

Despite widespread use, controversy remains regarding the electro-physiologic mechanisms behind defibrillation and cardioversion. Most investigators agree that defibrillation occurs when a certain amount of current density reaches the heart. At the cellular level, the delivered current passes through the myocardial cells resulting in alteration of the transmembrane potential. At the organ level, there is still no clarity and concurrence amongst the investigators.

Two theories have been proposed, viz. **critical mass hypothesis** and the **upper limit of vulnerability**, both of which are not mutually exclusive.

(a) **Critical mass hypothesis:** It is now known that fibrillary activity can be terminated with a high defibrillation energy level. According to critical mass hypothesis, a certain amount of myocardium must be available to sustain atrial or ventricular fibrillation and the entire myocardium must be uniformly depolarized in order to terminate arrhythmia. Defibrillation was successful only when fibrillatory activity was terminated at all sites.
(b) **Upper limit of vulnerability:** According to this hypothesis, fibrillation can be induced with limited energy shocks where any further increases in energy do not induce any rhythm disturbances, and the largest socks that are unable to induce fibrillation are slightly weaker than necessary for defibrillation. Although these shocks abolish small areas of localized reentry during ventricular fibrilla-

tion (VF), shocks at strengths lower than the upper limit of vulnerability stimulates other regions of myocardium during their vulnerable period, giving rise to new areas of reentry initiating fresh VF. Therefore, to successfully terminate a VF, the optimum shock energy must be greater than the largest shock that reinitiates fibrillation (the upper limit of vulnerability).

20.3 Thresholds for Defibrillation

One important factor in the response of tissue to a certain stimulus is the state of the tissue immediately prior to the stimulus. Depending on its state of the cardiac myocyte, and the strength of the stimulus (in this case a shock), it can (a) illicit a new action potential, (b) shorten the action potential (AP), (c) prolong the AP or (d) have no effect on the existing AP. Electrical and optical mapping studies have shown that shocks that are well below the defibrillation threshold (DFT) do not terminate a VF wave front. Monophasic shock that are slightly below the DFT may halt the fibrillation wave fronts, but it may also create a virtual anode and cathodes that can reinitiate VF. With DFT appropriate shocks, a period of electrical inactivity (typically 30–90 ms) known as isoelectric window (IW) is observed. After a near-DFT level shock, three outcomes are seen: (a) type A success (IW >130 ms); (b) type B success (IW <130 ms); or (c) failure.

20.4 Waveforms

Modern defibrillators deliver energy or current in "waveforms." The waveform of an electrical impulse is the temporal signature of its amplitude measured in terms of voltage/current. According to Ohm's law, current is linearly related to voltage ($E = I \times R$, where E is voltage, I is current and R is the resistance). Waveform duration is critical because the electrical shock interacts with the heart for about the same duration. Defibrillation pulses are capacitive discharge, truncated exponential waveforms. It has been observed that biphasic waveforms defibrillate more efficiently (requiring lower voltage) than monophasic waveforms. Modern defibrillators are all moving towards biphasic waveform technology gradually replacing older units that used to deliver monophasic shocks. Monophasic waveforms deliver current in one direction and could vary the speed and amount of decline in energy and the return to zero. If the monophasic waveform falls to zero gradually, the term "damped sinusoidal waveform" is used. If the waveform falls instantaneously, the term "truncated exponential" is used. On the contrary, biphasic waveform delivers current first in the positive direction for a specific duration which is followed by current flow in negative direction. Typically, they are called "biphasic truncated exponential waveform." Triphasic waveform are also used, albeit experimentally but data are not sufficient for routine clinical use.

20.5 Defibrillator Types

There are three broad types of defibrillators, viz. (a) Public access defibrillator and AED, (b) Manual defibrillators with vital monitor, (c) Implantable cardioverter defibrillators (ICD).

Public access defibrillator (PAD) got a boost in USA during the late 90s because of their successful deployment in airports. Early defibrillation by first rescuers and trained early responders reversing SCA due to VF were documented in number of small case series (American airlines, QANTAS air and Chicago's O'Hare airport) during 1990s. This is partly because of the concept that earlier the defibrillation is performed, better is the rate of survival to hospital discharge. For, more than a decade beginning 1991, the American Heart Association (AHA) has promoted ambulances be equipped with defibrillator and personnel trained in defibrillation. ICDs have been discussed with pacemakers (see below).

In hospital settings, defibrillation is carried out with devices with facilities for energy selection. They also have capability to deliver synchronized shocks for cardioversion.

20.6 Energy Requirements for Defibrillation

Defibrillation depends on successful selection of energy and most defibrillators are energy based, meaning thereby the device charges a capacitor to the selected voltage and discharges a prespecified energy in joules. The amount of energy passes through the heart is dependent on the energy selected and the transthoracic impedance which varies between patients. As mentioned earlier, defibrillators are capable of delivering energy in a variety of waveforms. For example, biphasic waveforms have replaced monophasic ones as the former effectively terminates arrhythmias consistently at lower energy levels.

20.7 Factors Affecting Success of Defibrillation

A number of equipment and patient related factors will influence the chances of successful defibrillation or cardioversion. The equipment related factors include (1) Electrode related (e.g., position, size), (2) Type of Paddle related (e.g., hand held versus self-adhesive patches) and (3) energy delivery related (number of joules, type of waveform) while the patient related variables are (a) thoracic impedance related (obesity, excessive hair), (b) abnormal conductance related (wet skin).

20.8 Equipment-Related Variables

1. Electrodes or Paddle: A number of electrode and paddle characteristics can affect the outcomes of defibrillation. They include paddle position, paddle size and hand held versus self-adhesive pads (or patches) (Fig. 20.1).
   (a) Paddle position: The paddle placement determines current pathways traversing the myocardium. Conventionally, the two recommended positions are:
      - Antero-lateral placement (right subclavicular and apical orientation) and,
      - Antero-posterior placement (over the thoracic midline)

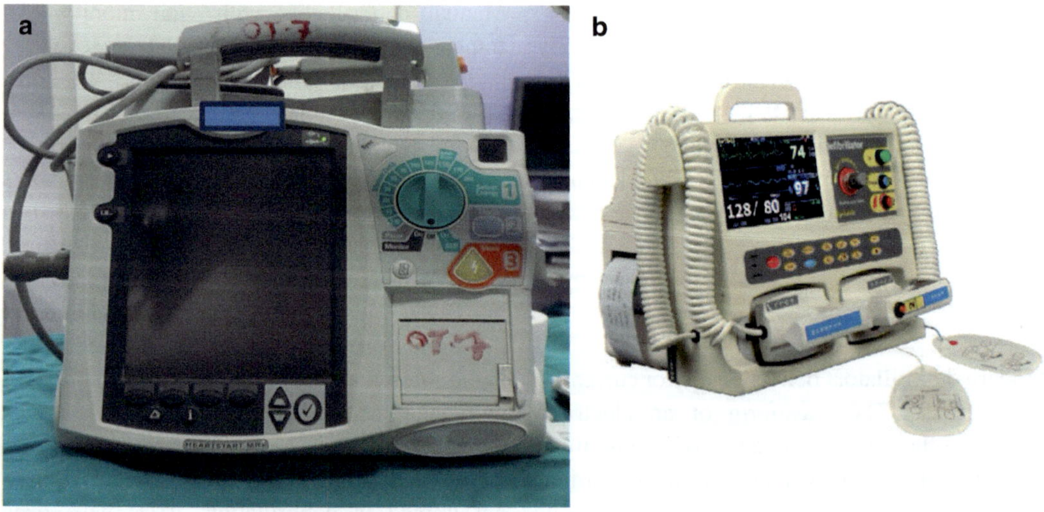

Fig. 20.1 Defibrillator

(b) In some patients, one of the two position may be appropriate. This is especially true when there is contraindication of the former due to pre-existing presence of CIED (e.g., a pacemaker) overlying the paddle placement site. Also, if initial attempts at cardioversion/de-fibrillation fails, the alternate paddle/patch position can be used for repeat attempts at defibrillation/cardioversion.

(c) Paddle size: The Paddle/pad/patch size is an important determinant of the flow of energy during external (surface application) defibrillation. Larger paddle/pad size is associated with decreased impedance and increased current flow with (probably) less myocardial injury. However, there appear to be an optimal paddle size (12.8 cm in diameter) above which any increase in paddle surface area leads to a decrease in current density.

2. Type of paddle (i.e., hand held versus self-adhesive pads/patches):

Steps of Defibrillation

(a) Apply electrodes and connect ECG leads to the patient/victim and select the limb lead you want to monitor. If no ECG electrodes/leads available, select "Paddle" as the monitored lead and confirm the rhythm (whether shockable or un-shockable)
(b) Apply conductive (defibrillator jelly only) gel on both paddles thoroughly
(c) Firmly press both the paddles over the chest wall on the recommended area
(d) Select energy to be delivered (press "sync" button if needed)
(e) Stay "clear" of the patient (announce loudly and ensure clearance by all before shock delivery)
(f) Deliver shock after ensuring other necessary precautions exercised.
(g) Resume CPR and do not waste time assessing pulse after every shock delivered.

20.9 Indications of Defibrillation

Defibrillation is indicated in patients with pulse less VT, unstable polymorphic VT or frank VF where synchronized cardioversion is not possible. As mentioned, these are fatal dys-rrhythmias that require prompt recognition and early intervention in the form of electrical shock. This takes precedence over all other therapy or procedures being performed in the setting of emergency cardiac care (ECC) except initial few cycles of chest compressions before shock delivery per ACLS protocol. The following are the shockable fatal rhythms that need prompt recognition and defibrillation:

1. Ventricular fibrillation (VF).
2. Pulseless ventricular tachycardia (VT).

20.10 Other Uses of a Defibrillator

1. Synchronized cardioversion.
2. Transcutaneous pacing.

20.11 Synchronized Cardioversion

Synchronized cardioversion is utilized for reversing persistent unstable tachyarrhythmia in patients with a pulse. It is a procedure similar to electrical defibrillation with certain special considerations. Unlike defibrillation, it is used for treatment of hemodynamically unstable ventricular as well as supraventricular rhythms. Cardioversion is the delivery of a lower energy shock that is synchronized to the R wave of the QRS complex.

Supraventricular Tachycardia (SVT) refers to a cardiac rhythm greater than 100 beats per minute, which originates above the bundle of His. Any tachycardia that does not originate in the ventricles is referred to as SVT. This includes sinus tachycardia, junctional tachycardia, reentrant tachycardias, multiple atrial tachycardia (MAT), atrial fibrillation, and atrial flutter. Although different supraventricular rhythms precipitate SVT, clinically, they are all treated with the same approach.

20.12 Indications for Cardioversion

(a) Emergency DC cardioversion is indicated for any broad or narrow QRS complex tachyarrhythmia that causes hemodynamic decompensation.
(b) Relatively urgent cardioversion is indicated for supra ventricular tachycardias (SVTs) and monomorphic ventricular tachycardias that have not responded to a trial of drug therapy.
(c) Routine cardioversion is still frequently indicated in the management of atrial fibrillation (AF) when a rhythm rather than rate control strategy is employed.
(d) Indications for a rhythm strategy include a reversible cause of the AF, heart failure primarily caused by the AF, and/or new onset AF.

20.13 Procedural Considerations

1. **Location of procedure:**
   (a) DC cardioversion is performed in a variety of locations.
   (b) It is mandatory that skilled assistance and full resuscitation equipment are available.
   (c) Following cardioversion, the patient must also be managed in an area with facilities for suction and oxygen administration.
   (d) Full resuscitation facilities should be readily available and appropriately trained staff in attendance until the patient has fully recovered from the effects of anaesthesia.
   (e) For AF an initial shock at 120–150 J escalating to 200 J is appropriate.
   (f) Atrial Flutter and paroxysmal SVT convert more easily with initial energy settings of 70–120 J usually proving adequate cardioversion.
2. **Precautions**:
   (a) Check the defibrillator possesses a backup external pacing function.
   (b) Ensure that the defibrillator is set to sync. Mode.
   (c) Remember to disable sync. Mode if VF occurs and defibrillation is required.
   (d) Make sure all staff avoid direct contact with the patient during shock delivery.
   (e) Face mask oxygen should be moved at least 1 m away from the patient's chest prior to shock delivery.
3. **Pre-oxygenation and airway management:**
   (a) All patients should be fully preoxygenated for at least 3 min prior to cardioversion.
   (b) This buys valuable time if unanticipated airway difficulty or apnoea occurs.
   (c) Spontaneous ventilation can usually be maintained using a Hudson's facemask.
   (d) Assistance of ventilation by manual ventilation or insertion of a Guedel airway/laryngeal mask rarely proves necessary.
4. **Sedation**:
   (a) No or minimal sedation can be associated with serious psychological sequela, whereas increasing anesthetic depth increases the risk of significant cardiorespiratory depression.
   (b) Deep sedation describes a level of sedation at which an individual cannot be easily aroused, but responds purposefully to repeated or painful stimulation.
   (c) It may require airway intervention and respiratory support, but cardiovascular function is usually maintained.
   (d) Although most anaesthetists prefer utilizing a conventional depth of anaesthesia, deep sedation seems perfectly acceptable to most patients.

(e) This level of sedation can readily be attained by administration of a slow bolus dose of propofol (0.5–1 mg kg^{-1}), with further top up doses (0.25 mg kg^{-1}) as required.

5. **Analgesia:**
   (a) Cardioversion is an intensely painful and stimulating procedure, but patients rarely experience pain following the procedure.
   (b) The co-administration of opioids is therefore unnecessary and potentially increases the risk of apnoea and post procedural nausea and vomiting.

20.13.1 Complications of Defibrillation

(a) Cutaneous burns or irritation at the paddle site.
(b) Electrocution of by-standers.
(c) Fire accidents.
(d) Ischemia and pulmonary edema.
(e) Myocardial necrosis, skeletal muscle injury, rhabdomyolysis, and renal failure have been reported as complications.

20.13.2 Pacemakers

Pacemakers are devices that are implanted in a symptomatic bradycardia patient with slower heart rate and millions of patients must have received these devices by now. There are considerable confusions regarding the behavior of pacemakers and also the perioperative care of a patient with such a device. The reasons could be anything from lack of evidence based literatures, incorrect and irrelevant data to inability to keep pace with the fast paced technological advancements. Most patients with a pulse generator can have significant co-morbidities. Care of these cohort requires clearer understanding of their medical and psycho-social status as well as the status of the pulse-generators within them. Whether or not a patient with a pacemaker is at increased perioperative risk is not well-known, but a couple of reports suggest that they deserve extra attentions.

20.13.3 Technology Behind a "Pacemaker"

A pacemaker functions seamlessly due to closed interactions between four important elements like a symphony:

1. The pulse generator (PGR) or the implantable "pacemaker" device.
2. The lead system that establishes connections between the PGR and the heart.
3. A programming device (viz., a PC) that can communicate with the implanted PGR.
4. The "needy" patient.

The optimal function of a PGR is also dependent on a well performing battery. In fact, the battery is the largest single element inside the device, taking up as much as 50% of the total volume of the device. Most PGR have a low voltage battery (about 2.8 V). Often PGR have to deliver output pulses more than 2.8 V, they have to depend on a circuit, called voltage amplifier to amplify the voltage output. The size of the output pulse is the biggest controllable factor in device longevity. However, the single most important element in device longevity is the pacing itself (e.g., how often the device delivers output and how much energy is delivered per output). The pacing output pulse is defined by two programmable variables: the pulse amplitude (measured in millivolts) and the pulse width or pulse duration (measured in milliseconds). Of these two variables, pulse amplitude or voltage settings determines the major share of how much energy is spent to produce an output pulse. Since, the output is such a crucial factor in device longevity, clinicians have to be very careful in programming the output setting as low as possible, but not so low that they fail to "capture" the heart, i.e., to cause the heart to contract. The goal is to find the "pacing threshold," the minimum amount of energy necessary to reliably and consistently capture the heart. Below it, the output pulse will not produce myocardial contraction.

The problem with the pacing threshold is that it is an imprecise and individualized setting. It varies from patient to patient. Moreover, pacing threshold changes over the course of the day and can change significantly over time. Many factors such as drugs and disease progression are more common determinants of fluctuating pacing thresholds in cardiac patients than the general population. If a particular pacing threshold was taken at the "low point" of the day, it may not work well when patient experiences diurnal circadian changes in his pacing threshold. To overcome these issues, clinicians have adopted a simple measure to accommodate these threshold variations called a "safety margins." As a "rule of thumb," after determining the pacing threshold, clinicians just doubles it to remain safe. Some clinicians can chart a strength-duration curve and mark a specific on it—the "rheobase"—which marks the individual pacing threshold of the patient. The rheobase is then doubled to arrive at a point called "chronaxie" within the limits of the strength-duration curve (Fig. 20.2). When pacemaker lead is implanted on the heart, the pacing threshold is measured intraoperatively, i.e., what is the lowest amount of energy required to consistently produce depolarization of the heart. From there on and several weeks thereafter, the lead

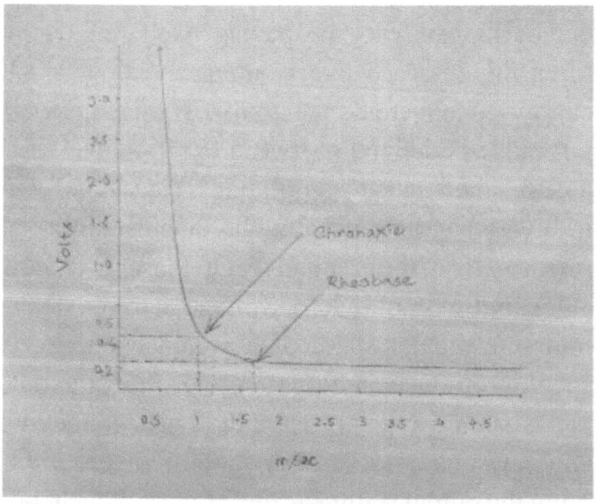

Fig. 20.2 The "strength-duration curve" depicts how much energy is needed to capture or depolarize the heart. At short pulse durations, it takes more voltage; while at longer pulse durations less voltage is needed. At point 1.5 ms the curve plateaus. The rheobase is the point at which plateau begins and it roughly correlates with the minimum voltage required to capture the heart. The point at which twice the rheobase voltage value meets the curve is defined as chronaxie. Setting the output of a pulse generator to the chronaxie value provides a safety margin for capture (see text)

goes through an acute on chronic threshold change. The increase in the threshold is directly related to lead maturation and encapsulation at the myocardium-lead interface. Although, this increase was reported to be five to ten folds (historically), with newer lead technology (steroid-eluting leads), this threshold changes are likely to be up to two to threefold. This is the rationale behind the "thumb rule" of keeping the pacing output at twice the threshold after carefully determining the latter. The idea is that it is better to err on the side of safety than to accept serious consequences due to pacemaker failure. By setting this high safety margin, physicians remained confident that their patients' heart will be paced—but considerable amount of energy was wasted in this process. However, new algorithms incorporated in most pacemakers today assess this changing pacing threshold regularly and then deliver large output impulses commensurate with the higher or lower threshold to successfully capture the heart. These algorithms have added many years of longevity to the average pulse generators. In fact, today's pacemakers are smaller in size than ever before but their battery last much longer! Nowadays, it is not unusual to get projected longevity of pacemakers as high as 10 years or more.

Any discussion on pacemaker is incomplete unless a mention of generic pacing codes [(NBG)] is not made to the extent described by the North American Society of Pacing and Electrophysiology (NASPE)/British Pacing and Electro-Physiology Group (BPEG) updated and revised in 2002 (originally described in 1983). The position 1 describes pacing chamber, II describes sensing chamber and position V describes multisite pacing as O = none, A = atrium, V = ventricle and D = dual i.e. both atria and ventricle. Position III is for response setting (O = none; I = inhibitory; T = triggered and D = dual inhibitory and triggered) whereas position IV describes programmability (O = none and R = rate modulation).

There are three basic selector switches that needs to be operated and appropriate modes need to be activated once it is decided to pace after reviewing the indications of pacing for a particular patient. A detailed principle of operation and technical nitty gritty of pacing is provided below. Pacemakers are also associated with various terminologies which are generally unfamiliar to the anesthesiologists, many of them will be also explained towards the end of this chapter.

20.13.4 Indications for Pacing

In the perioperative scenario or otherwise, pacing can be temporary or permanent. We offer temporary pacing when we know that the bradycardia is iatrogenic and normal heart rate (HR) will establish after a known therapeutic course and restoration of altered physiology (e.g., gradual rewarding of heart after releasing of aortic cross clamp following a period of cold cardioplegic arrest state). Temporary pacing (Box 20.1 for indication) usually is done utilizing epicardial pacing leads implanted over the target epicardium using special sutures to be removed afterwards. On the other hand, permanent pacing is established using pacing leads (wires) inserted through a trans-venous routes in suitably placed puncture sites closest to the dermal pockets where the pulse generator is seated. The most common indications for permanent pacing are symptomatic sinus node dysfunction and AV node disease (complete heart block, second degree block etc), Long QT syndrome, hypertrophic-obstructive and dilated cardiomyopathy (Multi-site pacing) (Box 20.2).

20.13.5 Various Types of Pacing

Permanent or temporary pacing can be established once the leads are connected to the pulse generator in the appropriate terminals. Usually, there is a anode and a cathode terminal indicated be a "+" and "–" symbol near the terminals. The terminals of the temporary pulse generators (which are usually bigger in size) are generally color coded so that the pacing cables acting as an extension for those terminals can be easily identified. The various knobs available in a temporary pulse generator are shown in Fig. 20.1. Pacing can be single, double/dual and triple (multi-site) chambered depending on the number of heart chamber paced by a pulse generator. The dual chamber pacing (i.e., atrio-ventricular) as opposed to single chamber ventricular pacing is more physiological if we can match the **AV delay**. This is frequently referred to as A-V sequential pacing. In the perioperative period, we often utilize single chamber (atrial) pacing (and sometimes **over-drive** pacing) which is physiologically and hemodynamically much better than ventricular pacing. Many devices are approved by the US-FDA for triple chamber pacing (right atrium, both ventricles) or bi-ventricular pacing (BiV) for treating dilated cardio-myopathy. This is popularly known as cardiac re-synchronization therapy (CRT) where ventricle is paced 100% of the time and they require careful attention towards pacemaker programming. Recently, FDA has approved multi-site atrial pacing for Atrial arrhythmia prevention trial (Atrial septal pacing efficacy or ASPECT clinical trial).

20.13.6 Pacing Modes

Once the diagnosis has been established as conduction anomaly, the ensuing bradycardia warrants pacing, and the most appropriate mode of pacing for the patient must be selected. To facilitate the ease of use and understanding of pacing technology, a standardized (generic) classification code has been developed. Majority of the patients can be managed with two or three common modes (AAI, VVI, DVI, or DDD) with or without rate modulation/responsiveness.

The first position always indicates chamber paced, the second position is for chamber sensed and the third position in the above modes responds to sensing. Here, in all top three modes, the response to sensing is inhibition of the respective chamber. Only, in the fourth mode, the response to sensing is triggering of the downstream chamber with a rate appropriate AV delay. The first three-letter of the five position NBG codes described above enumerates the basic pacing systems first proposed in 1974 by the then combined task force of AHA/ACC/HRS. Today, when a code only includes three or four character, it can be assumed that the position not mentioned are either "O" or absent.

20.13.7 Pacemaker Settings

Every pulse generator has a few knobs/controls to set the desired heart rate, intensity of current output (in milliampere or mA), and sensitivity of the sensing lead (millivolts or mV). These days, pacemaker with touch screen function may have no physical button at all, yet they can perform all the basic functions of a simple single chamber pace maker. It is easy to learn the basic functionalities of a pacemaker on a single chamber temporary pulse generator (Fig. 20.1). Much of these functions are set by telemetry from an external programming device kept in close proximity over the pulse generator in case of a permanent pacemaker. Before setting up temporary pacing, it is essential to know whether we are going for **asynchronous** or **demand pacing**. Also, it is essential to have a knowledge of two fundamentals of pacing: **capture** (depolarization of myocardium following a stimulus) and **sensing** (meaning "seeing" the heart's own intrinsic signal). Simply put, sensing is the ability of the pacing device to recognize the intrinsic activity of the Heart. Pacemakers sense through the electrodes implanted on the endocardium and when the heart depolarize, it picks up the electrical signal so created and relays it back to the pacemaker. Capture can be explained as the depolarization of the heart that occurs in response to the electrical stimulus from the pulse generator (evident on an ECG strip as the pacing spikes) as shown in the following ECG strips (Figs. 20.3 and 20.4).

Another factor for successful pacing (capture) is the pacing **threshold**. It is the amount of current required to initiate a phase of depolarization, i.e., for the myocytes to receive the stimulus and depolarize. It is expressed in mA and is influenced by myocardial ischemia, drugs, electrolyte imbalance, and pacing lead contact and placement.

20.13.8 Practical Tips for Temporary Pacing

Step 1: First determine the appropriate heart rate for the patient (according to age and desired cardiac. Index) and then set the heart rate accordingly.

Step 2: Then, decide whether going for demand or asynchronous pacing. In case of asynchronous (fixed) pacing, the pacemaker need not sense intrinsic cardiac electrical activity and starts its output at the preset rate regardless of patient's cardiac activity. If fixed rate is used and the patient has an underlying rhythm, the rate must be set higher (typically 800 bpm) than the patient's own rate to avoid competition. This is sometimes also referred to as **over-drive pacing**. However, there is a slight risk of **R-on-T** phenomenon with asynchronous pacing (theoretical).

In **demand** (synchronous) **mode**, the pulse generator senses for the intrinsic rate and rhythm of the heart and generates stimulus when

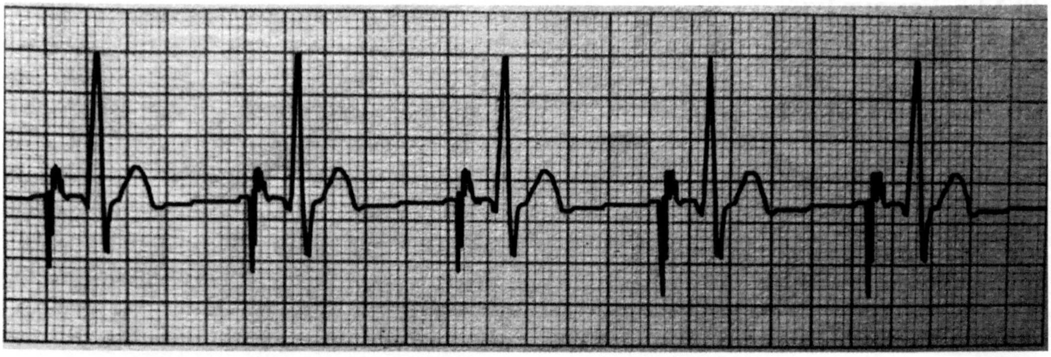

Fig. 20.3 Typical ECG tracing of atrial capture in AAI mode. Note downward pacing spikes are followed by "P" waves or atrial depolarizations

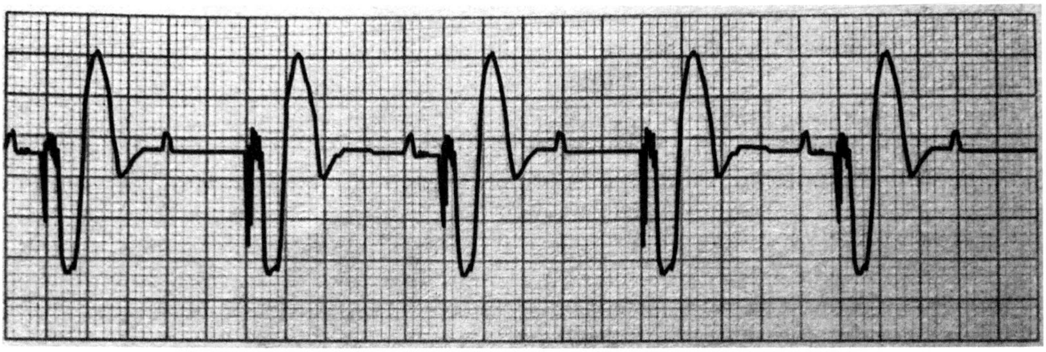

Fig. 20.4 Typical ECG tracing of ventricular capture in VVI mode. Note downward pacing spikes are followed by wide "QRS" complexes of ventricular depolarization

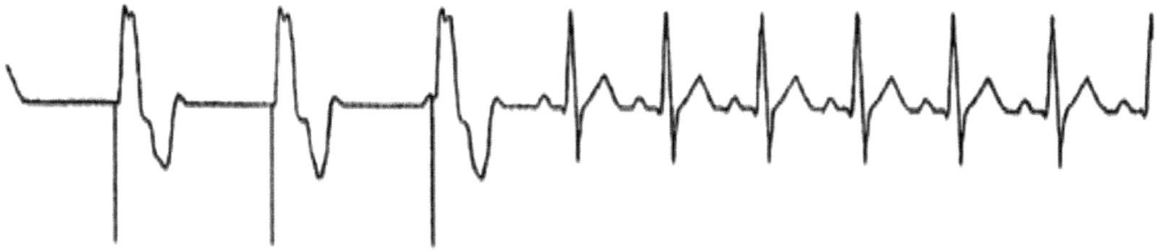

Fig. 20.5 In demand or synchronous pacing, pacemaker will emit an output only when there is no intrinsic activity or the rate of the intrinsic activity is less than a desired (set) threshold

patients' own HR drops below the preset heart rate. That is, if you have set the rate of pace-makers at 60 bpm, it won't pace until patient's heart rate drops below 60 bpm. It becomes absolutely essential for the pacer to have adequate or good sensing capability for the demand mode to work without fail. Otherwise, serious consequences of symptomatic bradycardia may go unnoticed due to the false presumption of an active pacemaker support (Fig. 20.5).

Step: 3: Thus, it is imperative to set the "sensitivity" of the pacer to the maximum, (so that it doesn't miss any intrinsic activity) and it will emit an output after the escape interval, following the last sensed intrinsic activity. Sensitivity refers to pace-makers ability to "see" the intrinsic electrical activity of the patients' heart to prevent any competition with the hearts electrical activity. The energy coming out of the heart is measured in millivolts (mV). We can measure the electrical energy emanating from the heart by calculating height in mm on the *y*-axis on ECG strips. Each mm of height corresponds to 0.1 mV for a particular ECG wave (Fig. 20.6). We set the sensitivity of the pulse generator to see even the smallest electrical activity or in "demand" zone in dial settings (in some pulse generators) so that it does not pace inappropriately. We set the sensitivity dial setting to the lowest number (mV) so that it will detect even the smallest amount of electricity produced by the heart (Fig. 20.7).

As such, the sensitivity threshold can be determined by increasing the dial setting up to the minimum R wave amplitude (in case of VVI mode) needed to be detected by the pacer (as you dial up the sensitivity, the pacer will start firing inappropriately). Thus, by determining the minimum R amplitude, the sensitivity is adjusted and set 2–3 times lower than the sen-

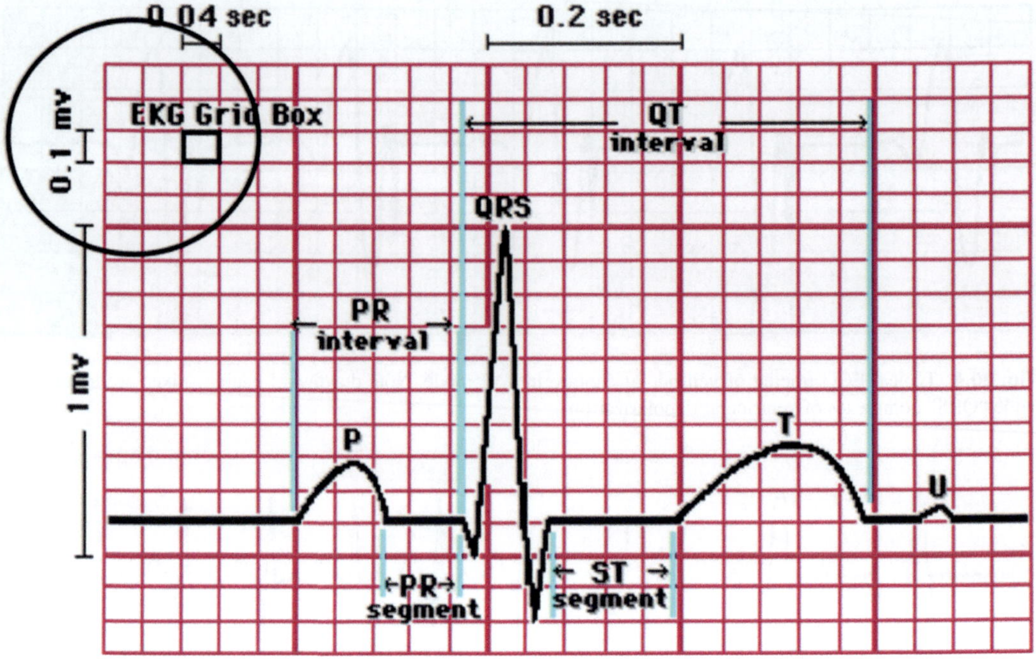

Fig. 20.6 ECG paper-strip explaining the significance of each small squares in terms of measurement of electrical energy (in mV) in *y*-axis and time intervals (in ms) in the *x*-axis

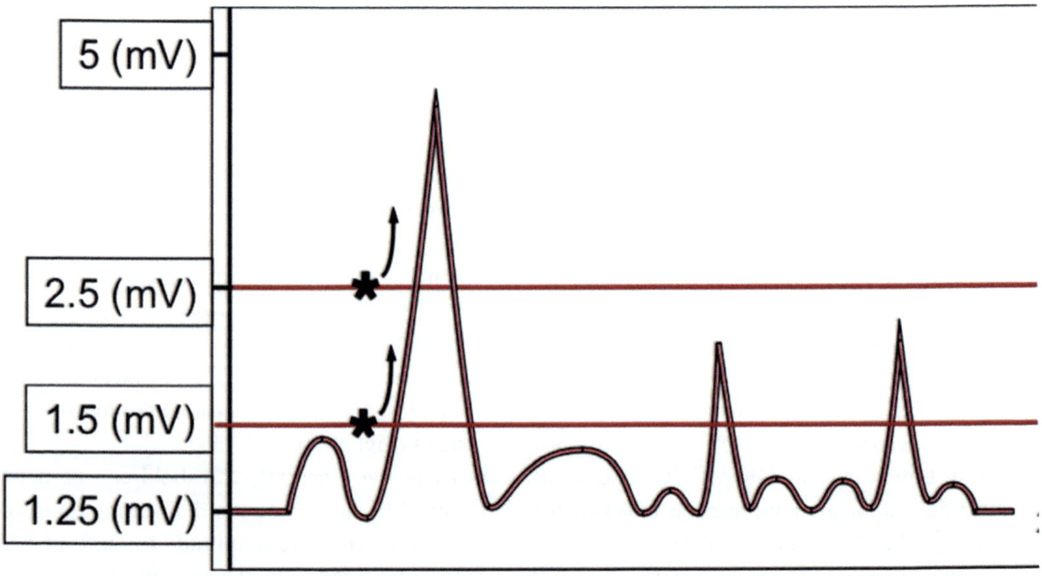

Fig. 20.7 The sensitivity represented in the *y*-axis represents each level and the corresponding dial setting only above which any activity produced is detected

sitivity threshold. Remember: lower the setting the more sensitive is the pacer to intra-cardiac electro gram (EGM).

Also it is worth remembering a golden rule w.r.t. pacer sensitivity:

Over-sensing leads to under pacing.

Under-sensing leads to over pacing.

Step 4: Finally, it's time to determine the minimum amount of pacer output that is necessary for effective pacing. In case of permanent pacing, this is important because the battery life is inversely related to the pacer output (mA). In case of temporary pacing, even though conservation of battery is important, it is not a big hassle to change the battery vis-a-vis replacement of depleted battery of a permanent pacemaker. Thus, selecting an optimum mA is necessary for proper functioning of a permanent as well as a temporary pace maker with a reasonable working life. The usual methodology is to start with a higher mA so that a definitive "capture" happens (with less ambiguity) and then, the mA is gradually reduced till the lowest possible mA at which the myocardium loses its capture, i.e., it fails to respond to the pacer stimuli. At that point, the output (mA reading) is noted and the final output is set at 2–3 times this value. In the peri-operative scenario, the mA set is much higher (up to 10 times after cardiac surgery) than this value as the myocardium is recovering from the insult of hypothermic/ischemia-reperfusion injury or direct handling of the tissue produces edema and other electro-chemical changes of the myocardial cell. This probably raises the capture threshold much higher than normal ultimately forcing us to set a higher mA output until the myocardium recovers completely. Moreover, indications for perioperative (post cardiac surgery) pacing are frequently temporary as they are partly because a permanent endocardial pacing is not possible during operation or partly because the conditions are self-mitigating (e.g., bradycardia) (Boxes 20.1 and 20.2).

Box 20.1 Indications for Temporary Pacing

Patient condition	Event requiring temporary pacing
Prophylactic	Pulmonary artery catheterization with LBBB Cardioversion with sick-sinus syndrome Post defibrillation bradycardia New AV block or bundle branch block following aIE Post cardiac surgery for prophylaxis against AF Postorthotopic heart transplantation Counteract perioperative pharmacologic treatments and electrolyte abnormalities causing hemodynamically significant bradycardia
Acute myocardial infarction	Symptomatic bradycardia (refractory to medicine) New bundle branch block with transient CHB Complete heart block Postoperative complete heart block Mobitz II with anterior myocardial infarction New bifascicular block Bilateral bundle branch block and 1° AV block Symptomatic alternating Wenckebach block Symptomatic alternating bundle branch block
Tachycardia treatment or prevention	Bradycardia-dependent VT Torsade de pointes Long QT syndrome Treatment of recurrent SVT or VT

AF, atrial fibrillation; aIE, acute infective endocarditis; AV, atrio-ventricular; SVT, supraventricular tachycardia; VT, ventricular tachycardia.

Box 20.2 Indications for Permanent Pacing

Symptomatic sinus node dysfunction
Symptomatic atrioventricular node disease
Long QT syndrome
Hypertrophic obstructive cardiomyopathy
Dilated cardiomyopathy (due to AV conduction abnormality mostly due to amyloid deposition)

20.13.9 Pacemaker and Magnets

Despite common beliefs, most pacemaker manufacturers categorically state that magnets were never intended to treat pacer emergencies or electro surgical unit interferences. In fact, magnets activate switches within the pacemaker such as mechanical (Reed switch) and electronic (Hall-effect sensors) switches to demonstrate remaining battery life, reveal and produce pacing behavior or to alter pacing threshold safety factors.

Placing a magnet directly over the pulse generator might not produce any effect in pacing as not all pacemaker switch to asynchronous mode. Also, all models from a particular brand do not behave similarly when a magnet is placed over them. Although, more than 90% of pulse generators discharges at 80–100 beats/min asynchronously on magnet application, some respond with only a brief period of asynchronous pacing while others switch to asynchronous pacing at programmed rate. In many devices, magnet behavior can be altered via a pacemaker programming device. Other possible effects of magnet placement are shown in Box 20.3. For all generators, calling the manufacturer or visiting their website remains the most reliable method for determining magnet behavior and using this magnet response to estimate the remaining battery life.

Box 20.3 Pacemaker Response to Magnet Application

Asynchronous pacing without rate responsiveness (possibly not in patient's best interest)—this is the most common behavior, although pacemakers manufactured by Biotronik, Boston Scientific, and St. Jude Medical have programmable magnet behavior

Unexpected behavior (e.g., VOO in Medtronic or VDD in Biotronik dual-chamber pacemaker) suggests elective replacement has been reached and the pacemaker should be interrogated promptly

No apparent rhythm or rate change

Magnet mode disabled permanently by programming (possibly with Biotronik, Boston Scientific, St. Jude Medical) or temporarily suspended (see Medtronic)

Program rate pacing in already paced patient (many older pacemakers)

Improper monitor settings with pacing near the current heart rate (pace filter on)

No magnet sensor (some pre-1985 Cordis, Telectronics models)

Brief (10–100 beats) asynchronous pacing, then return to program values (most Biotronik and Intermedics pacemakers)

Continuous or transient loss of pacing

Discharged battery (some pre-1990 devices)

Pacer enters diagnostic "Threshold Test Mode" (some Intermedic, Medtronic, St. Jude Medical devices, depending on model and programming)

For pulse generators with programmable magnet behavior (such as Biotronik, Boston scientific and St. Jude Medical), only an interaction with the programmer can reveal current settings. Although, most manufacturers publish a reference guide, it is not necessary that all of these guides enlists all magnet behaviors.

20.14 Pre-anesthestic Considerations

Preoperative management of patients with a pacemaker necessitates an evaluation and optimization of his or her co-existing disease(s). No additional tests or laboratory investigation is indicated in a conscious, oriented and co-operative adult patient with a pacemaker. However, in a critically ill, unconscious especially pediatric age group patient, a skiagram often reveals a pulse generator in unusual sites which may not be apparent on general physical examination, but it is worth remembering that, X-rays are also very insensitive in determining any pacemaker lead issues. Sometimes, a chest

X-ray (CXR) may be useful in documenting the position of the coronary sinus lead in a patient with Bi-ventricular pacing or AICD in situ, especially, if central venous catheter insertion is contemplated in such a patient as there is a high risk of spontaneous lead displacement [Europace 3:60–63, 2001]. A CXR is also indicated in a patient with a device malfunction discovered during his or her pacemaker evaluation.

The diligent anesthesiologist will thoroughly review the patient's pacemaker history and check-up and follow-up schedule. The NASPE and the HRS recommends pacemakers should be evaluated for battery health every 3 months. It also advocates a comprehensive evaluation (telemetric interrogation) every year. A recent pre-operative interrogation remains an important advisory from the American college of cardiology (ACC) guidelines. Important features to be evaluated during a pre-anesthetic visit are summarized in Box 20.4. In counties, where pacemakers are re-used, battery performance might not be related to length of implantation in the current patient. Although, battery life is an important concern during the PAC, the clinician should remember that in a registry of 345 pacemaker malfunction, 7% of failures were not related to battery depletion.

Box 20.4 Pre-anaesthestic Evaluation of CRMD (e.g., Pacemakers, AICDs)

Determining the indications for and date of initial device placement
Identifying the number and types of leads
Determining the last generator test date and battery status
Obtaining the current program information (device interrogation)
Obtaining a history of generator events (if any)
Ensuring that the magnet detection feature is enabled
Ensuring that generator discharges become mechanical systoles with adequate safety margins
Determining whether the pacing mode should be reprogrammed

Sometimes, pacemaker reprogramming may be necessary (see Box 20.5). Appropriate reprogramming may be the only safest way to avoid any intraoperative pacemaker malfunction, especially if a unipolar ESU is used during the operation. Most cardiac rhythm management device (CRMD) manufacturer has a separate service to cater to this need (refer to company's customer care numbers). Reprogramming a pacer to asynchronous mode at a rate higher than the patients intrinsic rate will ensure that no over or under-sensing will happen during any intraoperative electro-magnetic interference (EMI), thus protecting the patient. However, reprogramming advice will not save it from internal damage or CRMD reset caused by EMI.

Box 20.5 Probable Indications for Reprogramming a Pacemaker

Any rate-responsive device
Special pacing indications
- Hypertrophic obstructive cardiomyopathy
- Dilated cardiomyopathy
- Pediatric patients

Major procedures of the chest or abdomen
Special procedures (see Box 20.6)

In general, rate responsiveness and other functions (hysteresis, sleep rate, AV search etc) should be disabled by pre-operative programming because many of these features can potentially mimic pacer malfunction. Also, it is noteworthy that some pacemaker (e.g., Boston scientific) physician's manual recommends temporarily increasing the pacing output to 5 mV or higher to circumvent the EMI from mono-polar electrocautery, if used during surgery. Special attention must be given to pacer with minute ventilation (bio-impedance) sensors, because inappropriate tachycardia have been observed secondary to mechanical ventilation, mono-polar electrocautery use and connecting to an ECG monitor with respiratory rate counter.

Box 20.6 Special Procedures and Their Implications in Patients with CRMD

MRI	Absolutely contraindicated, by most generator manufacturers, and deaths have been reported [..], however, with appropriate precautions MRI is possible in some patients
ECT	Requires asynchronous (non-sensing) mode
Nerve stimulator use	Inappropriate detection of transcutaneous electrical nerve stimulation (TENS), neuromuscular stimulation as VTech and VF has been reported [..]
Lithotripsy	Acceptable with precautions to protect the pulse generator
TUR and Hysteroscopy	Procedures using monopolar electrocautery that can be easily performed after appropriate device reprogramming

20.15 Intraoperative (or Remote Location Procedure) Management

No special monitoring is generally required other than ASA standards monitoring routinely employed during any anesthetic procedure. The ECG monitor must detect the pacemaker output in the form of dots or pacing "spikes." In some multi-para monitors, display of pacing "spikes" is optional although pacer output is generally registered by most ECG monitors. It's our responsibility to ensure the display of pacing spikes is "on" in a patient known to have an active pacemaker. In the operation theater where electro surgical units (ESU) are commonly used, the "spikes" are a source of nuisance as their discharge is also picked up by the ECG monitors as pacer output. Sometimes noise filtering setting must be changed to bring back the display of pacemaker "spikes," although, devices such as nerve stimulators, MEP etc. can interfere with detection and display of pacemaker outputs.

Additionally, the patient monitor must have the ability to confirm that each myocardial electrical activity is converted to a corresponding mechanical systole, meaning thereby, we need to monitor the volume of blood displaced within the arterial system for each stroke volume generated by the left ventricle. This is best achieved by either a pulse oximetry plethysmography or a continuous arterial waveform display. Other monitored parameters such as temperature, ABG (acid-base status) may influence or dictate an increase in the pacemaker rate in a pacing dependent patient to meet the increased oxygen demand. Mechanical systole can also be evaluated by a pulmonary-artery catheter (PAC), esophageal Doppler monitor or a trassesophageal echocardiography (TEE) monitor. They can be effectively utilized to evaluate pacing rate and its relationship with the prevailing cardiac output. With respect to anesthetic agents, only isoflurane and sevoflurane is known to prolong the QT interval while halothane appears to decrease it.

As far as ESU use is concerned, monopolar electrocautery has the maximum influence on a pacemaker function—from EMI to device failure. Bipolar ESUs are relatively safer although patients with unipolar electrode configurations are more sensitive to EMI than those with bipolar configurations. "Coagulation" mode of ESU is more likely to cause pacemaker malfunction than the "cutting" mode of ESU. To safeguard the best interest of our patients, a magnet placed over older generations of pacemakers might turn on asynchronous VVI pacing, but newer pulse generators are relatively immune to such effects. If monopolar ESUs have to be used, then the "cautery plate" (current return pad) should be attached to the patient in such a fashion that ESU current path does not traverse the pulse generator unit. For, breast and auxiliary surgeries, the "plate" might be attached to the ipsilateral arm and for head-neck surgeries, the "plate" is best placed under the shoulder contra-lateral to the implanted CRMD. Procedures with special concerns for the implanted CRMDs are dealt in Box 20.6. MRI is a known limitation for CRMDs and in general, MRI is contraindicated in patients with pacemakers and ICDs. The Medtronic corp.

Has launched a new pulse generator and lead system called "Enrhythm MRI sure scan" with special program modes and leads for MRI scanning. It is already used in several European countries the results of which are awaited.

20.16 Pacemaker Failure

In general, there are three causes of pacing failure (in order of occurrence): (1) Failure to capture, (2) Lead failure, and (3) pulse generator failure. The capture failure happens due to a defect at the myocardial level (i.e., the myocytes do not depolarize despite a definite output from the pulse generator) and this remains the most intriguing and difficult problem to tackle. Myocardial conditions that leads to "no-capture" include (but not limited to) myocardial acidosis, electrolyte abnormalities, myocardial ischemia/infarction, supra-therapeutic levels of antiarrythmic, and cardio-selective pharmacologic agents. Also, in general sympathomimetic drugs lower pacing thresholds. During temporary pacing (e.g., transthoracic/transcutaneous pacing, transesophageal), the pulse generator might inhibit internal pacer output at extraneous voltages that will not lead to myocardial capture.

Although, generator and lead failures are rare, often time the reusable pacing cables malfunction after a certain number of use and it goes unrecognized until the time of initiation of temporary pacing (personal experience). The reason behind this may be multi-user and interchangeable nature of the similar looking leads in a workflow. Another common problem with leads are that they are attached to the bare metal wire-needle assembly in the sterile fields by the assistant surgeon often oblivious of the contacts between the two wires producing an "electrical arc" leading to pacing failure. Finally, the modern generators are electronic devices with dual power backup systems and they rarely shut down abruptly because of power failure or battery depletion.

20.17 Post-anesthesia Pacer Evaluation

Any permanent pacing device that was reprogrammed before or during surgery must be interrogated and programmed back appropriately. For, other devices, most manufacturers recommend their interrogation to check remaining battery life (as most surgeries use ESU) and to ensure proper functioning. The weight of evidences is so suggestive that ACC in 2007 published guidelines recommending a post-procedure check of every individual with a pacemaker.

20.18 Implantable Cardioverter-Defibrillators

Implantable Cardioverter-Defibrillators or ICD are one of the major bio-medical engineering breakthroughs of the late twentieth century. These devices prevent death from malignant VT's and they definitely remain superior to anti-arrhythmic drug therapy. Since the first ICD was implanted, a significant number of technical advances have taken place including miniaturization. Also, battery technology improvements have led to pacing capabilities with these devices so much so that current generation ICDs can be easily confused with a pectoral pacemaker. Like pacemakers, ICDS also have a generic code for identification of lead placement and their function. The most comprehensive form of identification is the utilization of "label form" which involves expansion of the fourth position into generic pacemaker code. The position 1 describes shock chamber, II describes antitachycardia pacing chamber and position IV detects antitachycardia pacing chamber as O = none, A = atrium, V = ventricle and D = dual i.e. both atria and ventricle. Position III is for tachycardia detection (E = electrogram; H = hemodynamics) whereas position IV describes programmability (O = none and R = rate modulation).

ICD's measure R-R intervals in each cardiac cycle and categorize HR as either too fast (a short

R-R interval), too slow (a long R-R interval), or normal. If a device detects sufficient number of short R-R interval within a period of time (a programmable feature), the ICD will begin an antitachycardia protocol. The internal computer will decide whether to go for antitachycardia pacing or shock depending on the presentation or programming. The newer devices are programmed to reconfirm VT or VF before discharging to prevent inappropriate shock delivery (ISD). Some ICD initiates antitachycardia pacing while it prepares for shock by charging the capacitor. In an ICD, once a shock is delivered, antitachycardia pacing is not possible any further.

ISD occurs in up to 40% ICD patients for rhythm other than VT/VF. Despite technical advancements, ISDs are still feasible in AF with fast ventricular rate and SVTs. Dual-chamber ICD technology may reduce incidence of ISD in such scenarios along with the following programming available in current ICDs:

Onset criteria:

Generally, onset of SVT has progressively shortening R-R intervals while onset of VT is abrupt.

QRS width criteria:

In general, QRS width in VT is wide (>120 ms), whereas the QRS width in SVT is narrow (<110 ms).

Stability Criteria:

The R-R interval in VT is relatively constant while it is relatively variable in AF with rapid ventricular response. [Artificial intelligence (AI) enabled recognition of morphology and chamber of origin based analytics assisted with comparison of stored templates].

An ICD with an anti-bradycardia algorithm relies on too long a R-R interval sufficient to trigger pacing response.

20.19 Indication of an ICD

Originally, ICDs were implanted in cases of hemodynamically significant VT or VF only. The newer indications with sudden cardiac death (SCD) includes:

Long QT syndrome.

Brugada syndrome (RBBB with ST-elevation in leads $V_1 - V_3$).

Arrhythmogenic RV dysplasia.

Hypertrophic cardiomyopathy in young (primary prevention of SCD).

Any post-MI patient with EF <30% (with a QRS >120 ms).

Any cardiomyopathy (with EF <35%).

20.20 Pre-anaesthetic Assessment of Patients with ICDs

In general, all patients with ICD should be subjected to "reprogramming" so as to disable the anti-tachycardia function preoperatively. However, this may be unnecessary in settings where no EMI is being used and no guidewire insertion is being contemplated.

20.21 Intraoperative Management

Currently, no special monitoring is required for a patient with ICD because of the device per se, but most of them will have severely depressed ventricular function, dilated chambers, and severe valvular regurgitations. ECG monitoring and the facility to cardiovert/defibrillate must be available when an ICD is disabled. The choice of anesthetics will depend on the prevailing hemodynamics and physiologic derangements. However, caution should be exercised during the placement of CVC in any patient with an ICD. Inadvertent shock (30 J) was delivered in a patient because of noise created by the guided wire hitting the ventricular shock coil. The latter is designed to serve as a heart rate sensor which malfunctioned and failed to deliver a shock subsequently when it was actually indicated.

20.22 Post-procedure ICD Evaluation

The device should be re-evaluated and re-enabled if it was disabled prior to the procedure. All events that were recorded in the device intraoperatively must be erased because the next interrogator in the future might not know about the EMI encountered by the patient during the procedure and may misinterpreted them as arrhythmia events. Death has been reported because of failure to reactivate anti-tachycardia in an ICD patient after a routine "cath-lab" procedure.

20.23 Transcutaneous Pacing

Transcutaneous Pacing (TCP) is a temporary means of pacing a patient's heart during an emergency and stabilize the patient until a more permanent means of pacing is available. It is accomplished by delivering electrical impulses across patient's chest wall, stimulating the heart to contract. The most common indication for TCP is symptomatic bradycardia, most commonly resulting from acute MI, sinus node dysfunction, and complete heart block. During TCP, adhesivc pads are placed on the patient's chest either in antero-lateral (AL) or anterior-posterior (AP) positions. The AP position is preferred because it minimizes transthoracic electrical impedance by sandwiching the heart between the two pads. Current is applied until electrical capture [characterized by a wide QRS complex (since the SA node-AV node conducting pathway is bypassed) with tall, broad T-waves on the EKG] occurs (Fig. 20.8).

20.23.1 Indications

1. Hemodynamically significant (hypotension, chest pain, pulmonary edema, altered mental

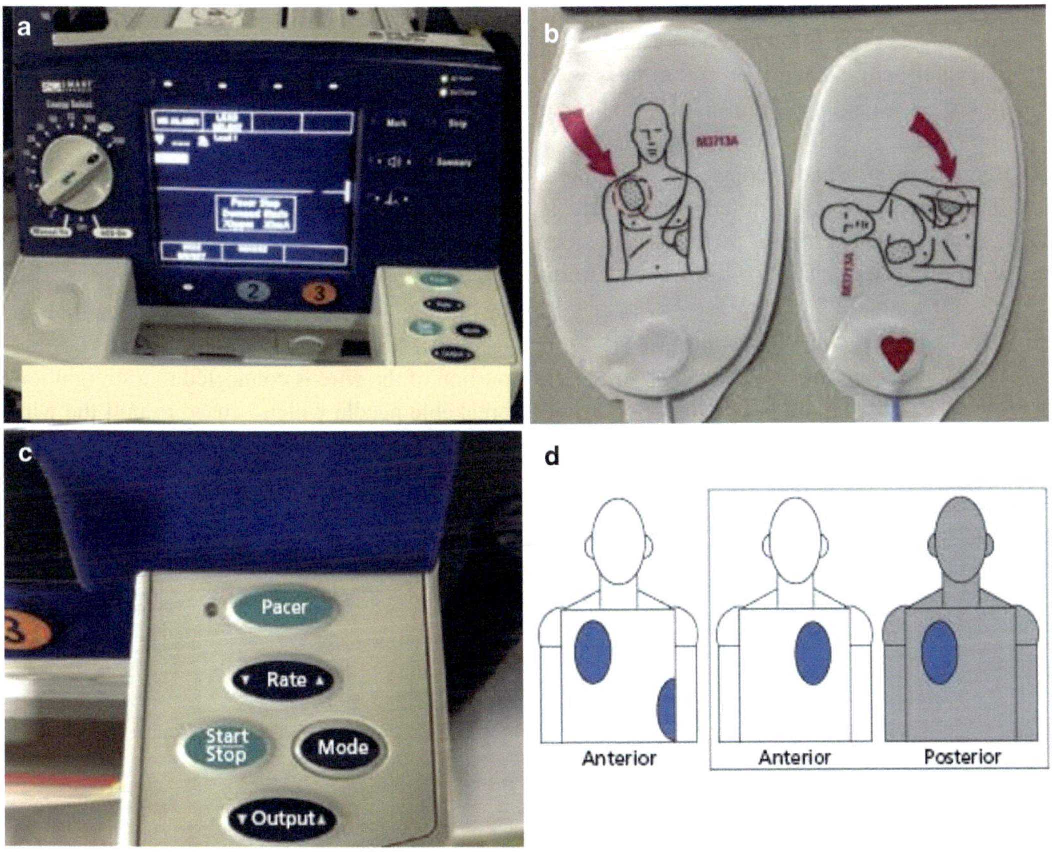

Fig. 20.8 Transcutaneous pacing (TCP). (**a**) Defibrillator with Pacing mode, (**b**) pads used for TCP, (**c**) buttons to change the rate, mode and output TCP, (**d**) placement of pads for TCP

status) bradydysrhythmias unresponsive to atropine, asystole (more likely to be successful when initiated early after a witnessed cardiac arrest. However, unwitnessed cardiac arrest seldom responds to transcutaneous pacing), failed intrinsic pacemaker.

2. When considering institution of transcutaneous pacing, always think about alternate causes for acute dysrrhythmia, e.g., trauma, hypoxia, drug overdose, electrolyte imbalances, and hypothermia.

20.23.2 Technique

1. Ideal pacer pad placement "sandwiches" the heart between the pacing pads and mimics the heart's normal electrical axis. Optimal placement for pads varies by manufacturer, but is generally anterior-posterior or anterior-lateral, with the former being most common. If there is too much hair on the pad placement site, shaving or epilation is warranted so as to minimize electrical impedance.
2. Begin at 30 mA and increase by increments of 10 until capture is noted. Target rate is generally 60–80 bpm. Strongly consider sedation, as TCP can be quite uncomfortable.
3. Most patients cannot tolerate currents of 50 mA and higher without sedation.
4. Often 50–100 mA are required. Ideal current is 1.25× what was required for capture.
5. It is safe to touch patients (e.g., to perform CPR) during pacing.

20.23.3 Pitfalls

1. Skeletal muscle contraction occurs at current levels as low as 10 mA, and does NOT suggest electrical or mechanical capture.
2. Most common reason for not obtaining capture is not adequately increasing the current. Current should be increased as much as necessary for electrical capture.
3. Undersensing is when a pacemaker fails to detect intrinsic activity, and therefore delivers a pace pulse.
4. Oversensing is inappropriate inhibition of the pacemaker due to detection of signals other than R waves (e.g., muscle artifact).
5. Pacing thresholds may change without warning and capture can readily be lost.

20.24 Epicardial Pacing

Epicardial pacing wires (or pacing leads) are fixed onto the epicardium with sutures during or after cardiac surgery which are attached to an external pacemaker (pulse generator box) in turn using a pacing cable (Fig. 20.9).

The epicardial wires are tiny thin stainless steel cables, insulated along most of their length, which comes out through the patient's skin. Inside, they tend to be fixed to the epicardial surface with some resorbable sutures. The "outside" portion of the wire is connected to a straight long breakable needle which is used to pull the wires out through the skin. The wires are finally plugged into a pulse generator using separate pacing cables for atrial and ventricular pacing.

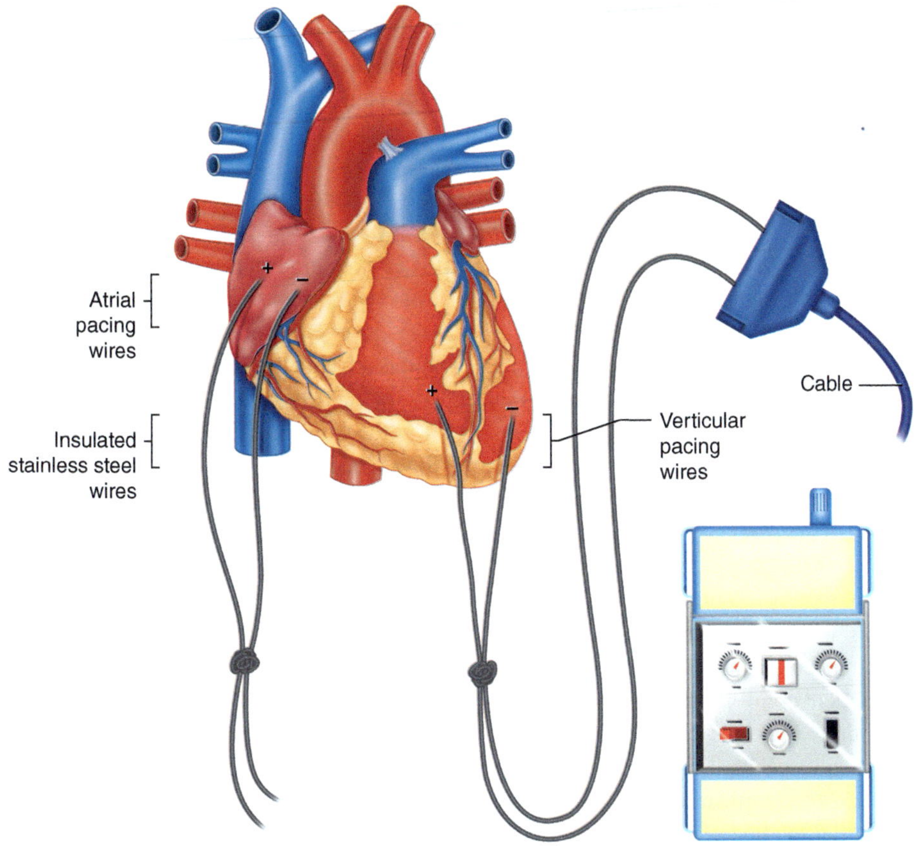

Fig. 20.9 Epicardial lead placement for dual chamber or AV-sequential pacing

20.25 Transvenous Pacing

Temporary transvenous pacing (TVP) is a life-saving procedure which is mainly indicated in patients with symptomatic bradyarrhythmias as well as in patients with specific tachyarrhythmias (i.e., overdrive pacing). Transvenous pacing having bipolar circuit which has both the electrode inside the heart, with the heart muscle and intraventricular blood completing the circuit. Typically, these electrodes are only about 8 mm apart, which reduces the impedance considerably. A unipolar circuit on the other hand relies on a large amount of tissue and body fluid to complete the circuit, and therefore has a much higher impedance.

20.26 Indications

20.26.1 Therapeutic

1. Symptomatic bradyarrhythmias unresponsive to pharmacologic therapy (e.g., systolic blood pressure <80 mmHg, change in mental status, angina, pulmonary edema), including sick sinus syndrome, atrial fibrillation with a slow ventricular response rate.
2. Overdrive pacing may be used to terminate arrhythmias (e.g., sustained supraventricular or ventricular tachycardia).
3. Bradycardia with ventricular escape rhythm unresponsive to pharmacologic therapy.

20.26.2 Prophylactic (in Setting of Acute Myocardial Infarction)

1. Symptomatic sinus node dysfunction or Mobitz type I second-degree AV heart block that is not responsive to atropine therapy.
2. Second-degree Mobitz type II, third-degree, or complete AV heart block.
3. Newly acquired bundle branch block with first-degree AV block.
4. Bilateral or alternating bundle branch blocks.
5. An old right bundle branch block with first-degree AV block and a new fascicular block.

20.26.3 Requirements

1. Transvenous pacing requires central venous access. This method has several advantages over the transcutaneous method, such as enhanced patient comfort and stability of pacing wires but it cannot be initiated as rapidly as transcutaneous pacing (Fig. 20.10).
2. In emergency situations, transcutaneous pacing is the initial method of choice and can be followed by transvenous pacing to pace for a longer period of the time, allowing evaluation of the requirements for permanent pacing.
3. The requirements for transvenous pacing are a central venous access kit, a pacing lead, a temporary external transvenous pacing generator (single-chamber or dual-chamber) and external defibrillator.
4. Fluoroscopy is commonly used for intracardiac lead placement. If fluoroscopy is not available, ECG guidance or echocardiography may be used instead.

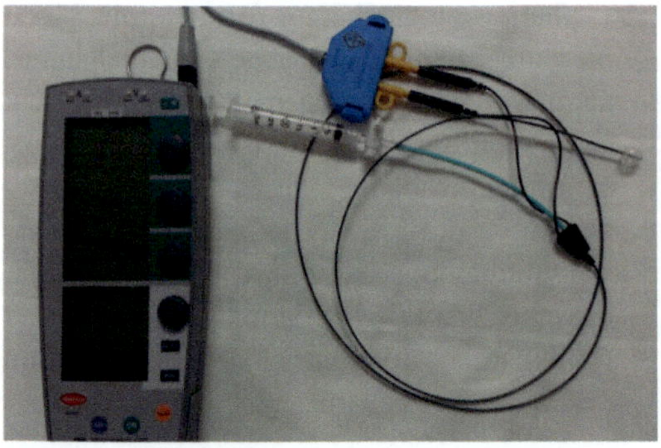

Fig. 20.10 Transvenous pacing

20.27 Procedure

1. After obtaining venous access and placing a transvenous sheath, the balloon-tipped catheter is inserted through the sheath into the vein and is advanced 20 cm (the catheter has markers for each 10 cm).
2. It is then inflated to be advanced with blood flow. The distal electrodes of the catheter are connected to the V_1 lead of the ECG device to record a unipolar ECG. This allows sensing of atrial and ventricular ECGs as the lead enters these chambers.
3. Alternatively, the lead can be paced at maximum output during the insertion, and detection of atrial or ventricular capture will guide the operator as to chamber location.
4. The catheter is advanced through the vein until it reaches the right *atrium* (RA). When the catheter enters the RA, atrial waves are recorded that confirm the catheter position in the RA; or, if the lead is paced at maximum output, then atrial position of the lead is confirmed by atrial capture on a surface ECG or monitor.
5. Advancing further, when the catheter passes the *tricuspid valve* and enters the *right ventricle* (RV) and the catheter is in contact with the RV *endocardium*, the ventricular signal is very large (usually >4 mV) and produces ST segment elevation as an indication of an injury current. From the morphology of the paced QRS on the surface ECG, one can determine the catheter position within the RV.
6. In an emergency, the highest output should be tried first; output should then be gradually reduced until the capture is lost and the pacing threshold is determined.
7. If the situation is not an emergency, the rate is set 10–20 beats/min above the intrinsic heart rate and the output is initially set low and then gradually increased until capture occurs. The ideal capture threshold is less than 1 mA.

8. The lead and sheath are secured to the skin with suture and a transparent dressing applied. The patient is re-evaluated daily, including checking for infection, threshold testing, and evaluation of the paced surface ECG.

Glossary

Asynchronous pacing A type of pacing (VOO, AOO, DOO) in which the pacemaker paces but does not sense. This results in properly timed output pulses that are delivered, regardless of any intrinsic activity going on. Asynchronous pacing modes are rarely used except in specific test or limited situations.

AV-delay Atrio-ventricular delay is the interval a dual-chamber system between atrial event detection (or initiation) and ventricular output.

BPG British pacing group.

Bi-polar Any pacing lead which has two electrodes on the distal end of the lead or any pulse generator which can accommodate such leads.

Capture The occurrence of cardiac depolarization in response to an output pulse.

Chronaxie The point on the strength–duration curve where twice the rheobase voltage value meets the curve; this is generally the innermost portion of the curve of the strength–duration graph. The chronaxie is generally considered a reliable safety margin.

Co-axial lead A type of bipolar lead in which one conductor was wrapped around another conductor.

Dual-chamber pacemaker A pacemaker which senses and paces in both the right atrium and right ventricle of the heart. A dual-chamber pacemaker has two leads (one for the atrium, one for the ventricle).

Escape interval In pacemaker timing cycles, the time from one sensed or paced event to the next sensed or paced event in that same chamber.

Hysteresis A programmable parameter in most pacemakers that establishes the rate at which the pacemaker will be inhibited, when that particular rate differs from the programmed base rate. For example, a pacemaker can be programmed to a base rate of 70 and a hysteresis rate of 60. That means the pacemaker would be inhibited as long as the patient's intrinsic rate was 60 beats a minute or greater. However, when the pacemaker started to pace, it would pace at 70 ppm.

Impedance In pacing, anything that opposes the normal flow of current.

Maximum tracking rate (MTR or max track) The "speed limit" on the pacemaker, the rate over which it will not allow the ventricles to be paced in response to sensed atrial activity.

Mode switching A special feature of many dual chamber pacemakers which allows the device to change modes in the presence of rapid, intrinsic atrial activity. Essentially, mode switching "turns off" the atrial channel of a dual-chamber pacemaker during periods of very high-rate, intrinsic atrial activity. Sometimes called automatic mode switching (AMS).

Multisite pacing Device-based therapy which involves pacing and sensing both the right and left atria (multisite atrial pacing) or the right and left ventricles (sometimes called biventricular pacing).

Myopotential Muscle noise which is sometimes picked up by the pacemaker's sense amplifiers and inappropriately interpreted as cardiac activity.

Output pulse The electrical energy generated by the pacemaker and delivered to the heart. This output pulse is defined by pulse amplitude (voltage) and pulse duration (length of time, measured in milliseconds).

Overdrive suppression The quality of cardiac cells which allows only one electrical impulse to travel on a pathway at any given time; this means that the first impulse to enter the pathway (from the SA node, for example) takes control of the heart and suppresses other electrical impulses which might occur later. Overdrive suppression can be physiological (for example, the SA node is the healthy heart's dominant pacemaker because it suppresses escape rhythms) or a pacemaker algorithm (atrial pacing can overdrive the atrium).

Oversensing A common sensing problem in pacing in which the pacemaker senses signals inappropriately. This causes the pacemaker to "see" intrinsic events that may not be there and to withhold pacing inappropriately. Oversensing typically leads to underpacing and shows up on the ECG in the form of long pauses.

Pacing threshold The minimum amount of energy required to reliably capture (cause depolarization of) the heart. Sometimes called stimulation threshold or capture threshold.

Rate response A feature in modern pulse generators (PGR) that allow them to respond to metabolic needs by utilising a biosensor, e.g., an activity or minute ventilation sensor. It is also better known as rate modulation or adaptation.

Rate responsive AV delay (RRAVD) A timing cycle in dual-chamber pacemakers, that automatically shortens the AV-delay in response to higher atrial rates. This feature is often used with rate-responsive pacing systems. RRAVD can also be useful for patients with high intrinsic atrial rate.

Re-entry circuit An aberrant conduction pathway in the heart which creates an endless loop for electrical impulses and results in tachycardia.

Refractory period A defined period of time (usually measured in milliseconds) during which the heart will not contract. A refractory period may be physiological or it may be part of a pacemaker timing cycle. This is further subdivided into absolute refractory period, when a contraction is impossible, and a relative refractory period, when there is limited response.

Rheobase On the strength–duration curve, the point at which the curve flattens. In setting output parameters, some voltage settings can be made to capture the heart if they are of sufficiently long duration. However, there is a point at which extending the pulse duration becomes moot; for example, for many patients, pacing the heart at a 0.25 V will not capture the heart, even if the pulse duration was a second long. The point at which extending the pulse duration no longer matters is the rheobase.

Sensitivity A programmable parameter which regulates the filter of the pacemaker. Increasing the millivolt setting decreases sensitivity, while the opposite is true for increasing sensitivity.

Spike or Pacing spike A common slang for the typical artefact produced by the pacemaker's output pulse.

Threshold potential The point at which fast sodium channels in cardiac electrical cells open, allowing a sudden influx of positive sodium ions into the cell and causing myocardial cells to depolarize and contract.

Unipolar Any pacing lead which have only one electrode at the distal end of the lead or any PGR which can accept such leads. For such PGRs, the pacer can itself act as an electrode.

Suggested Reading

1. Ideker RE, Chattipakorn N, Gray RA. Defibrillation mechanisms: the parable of the blind man and the elephant. J Cardiovasc Electrophysiol. 2000;11:1008–13. [511–089-939].
2. Badrinath SS, Bhaskaran S, Sundararaj I, et al. Mortality and morbidity associated with ophthalmic surgery. Ophthalmic Surg Lasers. 1995;26:535.
3. Bernstein AD, Irwin ME, Parsonnet V, et al. Report of the NASPE policy conference on antibradycardia pacemaker follow-up: effectiveness, needs and resources. North American Society of Pacing and Electro-physiology. Pacing Clin Electrophysiol. 1994;17(11 Pt 1):1714.
4. Fleisher LA, Beckman JA, Brown KA, et al. ACC/AHA 2007 guidelines on perioperative cardiovascular evaluation and care for noncardiac surgery. A report of the American College of Cardiology/American Heart Association Task Force for practice guidelines. Circulation. 2007;116:e418–500.
5. Rozner MA. Implantable cardiac pulse generator: pace-makers and cardioverter-defibrillators. In: Miller RD, Fleisher L, Johns R, et al., editors. Anesthesia. 6th ed. New York: Churchill Livingstone; 2004.
6. Hayes DL, Strathmore NF. Electromagnetic interference with implantable with implantable devices. In: Ellenbogen KA, Kay GN, Wilkoff BL, editors. Clinical cardiac pacing and defibrillation. 2nd ed. Philadelphia: WB Saunders; 2000. p. 939.
7. Michaloudis D, Fraidakis O, Lefaki T, et al. Anaesthesia and QT interval in humans: effects of halothane and isoflurane in premedicated children. Eur J Anaesthesiol. 1998;15:623.
8. Gregoratos G, Cheitlin MD, Conill A, Epstein AE, Fellows C, Ferguson TB Jr, Freedman RA, Hlatky MA, Naccarelli GV, Saksena S, Schlant RC, Silka MJ. ACC/AHA guidelines for implantation of cardiac pacemakers and antiarrhythmia devices: executive

summary—a report of the American College of Cardiology/American Heart Association Task Force on Practice Guidelines (Committee on Pacemaker Implantation). Circulation. 1998;97(13):1325–35. https://doi.org/10.1161/01.cir.97.13.1325. PMID: 9570207. Mychaskiw G, Eichhorn JH. Interaction of an implanted pacemaker with a transesophageal atrial pacemaker: report of a case. J Clin Anesth. 1999;11:669.

9. Trankina MF, Black S, Gibby G. Pacemakers: perioperative evaluation, management and complications. Anesthesiology. 2000;93(3A):A-1193. [Abstract].
10. Hintringer F, Schwarzacher S, Eibl G, et al. Inappropriate detection of supraventricular arrhythmias by implantable dual chamber defibrillators. A comparison of four different algorithms. Pacing Clin Electrophysiol. 2001;24:835.
11. Verma N, Cunningham D, Falk R. Central venous access resulting in selective failure of ICD defibrillation capacity. Pacing Clin Electrophysiol. 2001;24:394.

Ultrasound Evaluation of Trauma Patient

21

Tej Prakash Sinha, Ayush Srivastava, Anisha, and Debendra Kumar Tripathy

Key Points

- Ultrasound can be used to quickly evaluate the presence of free fluid, such as blood or ascites, in the abdomen or thorax.
- The extended focused assessment with sonography for trauma (eFAST) exam is a commonly used protocol for the initial evaluation of trauma patients.
- Ultrasound is a non-invasive and readily available imaging modality that can be performed at the bedside, making it a valuable tool in the evaluation of trauma patients.
- It is important to remember that ultrasound has limitations and should be used in conjunction with other clinical information and imaging modalities when necessary.
- Focused cardiac ultrasound (FoCUS) is a bedside ultrasound examination used to assess the function and structure of the heart in real-time, that can be used to evaluate a wide range of cardiac conditions in both the emergency and critical care settings.

21.1 Introduction

Ultrasound is a valuable diagnostic tool for evaluating trauma patients in the emergency room. It can quickly identify any internal injuries or bleeding, such as ruptured organs, internal bleeding, or pneumothorax. Extended FAST (eFAST) exam and Focused cardiac ultrasound (FOCUS) are genera approach to the ultrasound evaluation of a trauma patient. The use of ultrasound in evaluating trauma patients in the emergency room can aid in rapid and accurate diagnosis, leading to timely interventions and improved patient outcomes.

21.2 Extended FAST (eFAST)

The FAST (Focused Assessment with Sonography for Trauma) exam is a rapid ultrasound evaluation of the abdomen and pelvis to assess for the

T. P. Sinha (✉) · A. Srivastava · Anisha
Department of Emergency Medicine, JPNTC, AIIMS, Delhi, India

D. K. Tripathy
Professor and Head, Department of Trauma & Emergency, AIIMS Raipur, Raipur, Chhattisgarh, India
e-mail: debendra.anaes@aiimsrishikesh.edu.in

N. Gupta et al. (eds.), *Techniques in Anesthesia, Intensive Care and Emergency Medicine*,
https://doi.org/10.1007/978-981-96-1202-4_21

presence of free fluid, which may indicate internal bleeding. This exam can quickly identify life-threatening injuries and help guide further diagnostic and therapeutic interventions. The eFAST exam includes a FAST exam, as well as an evaluation of the thorax for the presence of pneumothorax or hemothorax. It can help identify injuries to the chest wall, lungs, and heart.

E-FAST is a non-invasive, rapid, repeatable exam and can be performed bedside. It has largely replaced diagnostic peritoneal lavage. Numerous studies have demonstrated sensitivities between 85% and 96% and specificities exceeding 98% [1]. The use of FAST in the initial assessment of abdominal trauma is solely to document the presence of free fluid in intraperitoneal, pericardial, or pleural space. Tough eFAST examination has become standard of care (Box 21.1), it is important to remember that absence of free fluid does not exclude serious intraabdominal or thoracic injury.

Box 21.1 Indication, Contraindication and Cautions of eFAST Scan

- Indications:
  - Blunt or penetrating abdominal or thoracic trauma.
  - Undifferentiated shock as part of RUSH protocol.
- Contraindications:
  - There is no absolute contraindication for E FAST. Though the exam should be commenced only after stabilization of airway and breathing and should not hamper any resuscitative efforts being carried out.
- Cautions:
  - E-FAST is an operator dependent procedure.
  - A very early scan can be false negative as sufficient blood may not have collected that can be detected, similar a late scan may also be false negative in cases where the blood clots to give a similar echogenicity as the tissue.

21.2.1 Techniques and Views

The patient should be in supine position with arms abducted slightly or above the head, though this may vary depending on the patient's conscious level and the presence of any upper extremity injury. The examiner examines the patient by standing to the patients right so that the right hand of the examiner can be used to manipulate the probe position.

The eFAST exam is performed by using a curvilinear or phased array probe in an abdominal preset. The curvilinear probe with a low frequency (1–5 MHz) is the preferred probe to perform the entire examination to avoid delays. However, the linear probe is ideal for examining the lung sliding. The examination is carried out in abdominal preset, that is the probe marker points towards the right in transverse views and towards the head in case of sagittal views (Fig. 21.1).

21.2.1.1 Right Upper Quadrant (ROU) View

It is advisable to begin the examination by examining the Right Upper Quadrant. The RUQ view is the most likely to detect free fluid with an overall sensitivity of 66%. Place the probe over the right mid-axillary line near the lower ribs, with the probe perpendicular to the line of the ribs (Fig. 21.1). Probe marker pointing towards the head. Try to visualize the liver, may have to move the probe cephalad or caudally to do so. Once the liver is seen, turn the probe oblique to maximize the window between the ribs. From here the probe now can be rocked up or down to look for the Morrison's pouch and the hepato-diaphragmatic area (Fig. 21.1). It is important to remember to scan the caudal edge of the left liver lobe as recent retrospective evidence suggests it has the highest sensitivity, exceeding 93%.

Also scan the right hemithorax by sliding the probe cranially above the diaphragm. The presence of the hyperechoic vertebral bodies, or "spine sign," aids in identifying pleural fluid. Sensitivities and specificities of ultrasound for the detection of hemothorax are 92–100%. Ask the patient to take a deep breath, if possible, particularly if the rib shadow obscure the area of interest.

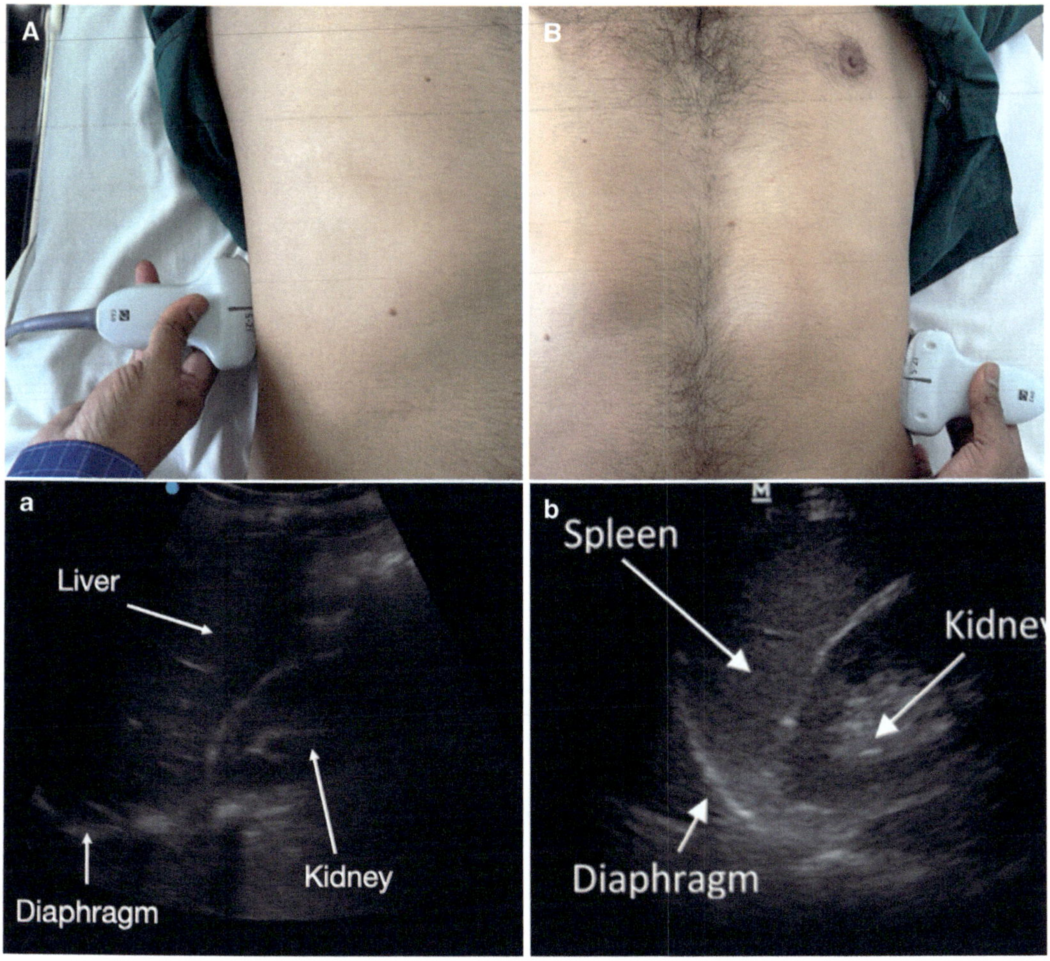

Fig. 21.1 eFAST scan: right upper quadrant (RUQ) and left upper quadrant (LUQ) view. (**A**) Curvilinear probe placement for right upper quadrant (RUQ) view, (**a**) corresponding ultrasound image, (**B**) Curvilinear probe placement left upper quadrant (LUQ) view, (**b**) corresponding ultrasound image

21.2.1.2 Left Upper Quadrant (LOU) View

It is important to remember here, that the spleen is much smaller and much more superior than the liver. Therefore, to visualize the spleen, it may be required to move the probe more posteriorly and superiorly. Again, after finding the window, oblique the probe and rock it to find the lienorenal interface, the sub phrenic area and the left lower hemithorax to rule out any free fluid (Fig. 21.1).

21.2.1.3 Pelvis: Sagittal and Transverse View

Place the probe in the midline just above the pelvis and tilt it down 45° into the pelvis. The view obtained should demonstrate a coronal section of the bladder and pelvic organs. Obtain the transverse view by rotating the probe 90° from the sagittal position while maintaining contact with abdominal wall. Angle the probe into the pelvis. If there is urine in the bladder, it can be visualized as a dark black shadow contained in an oval

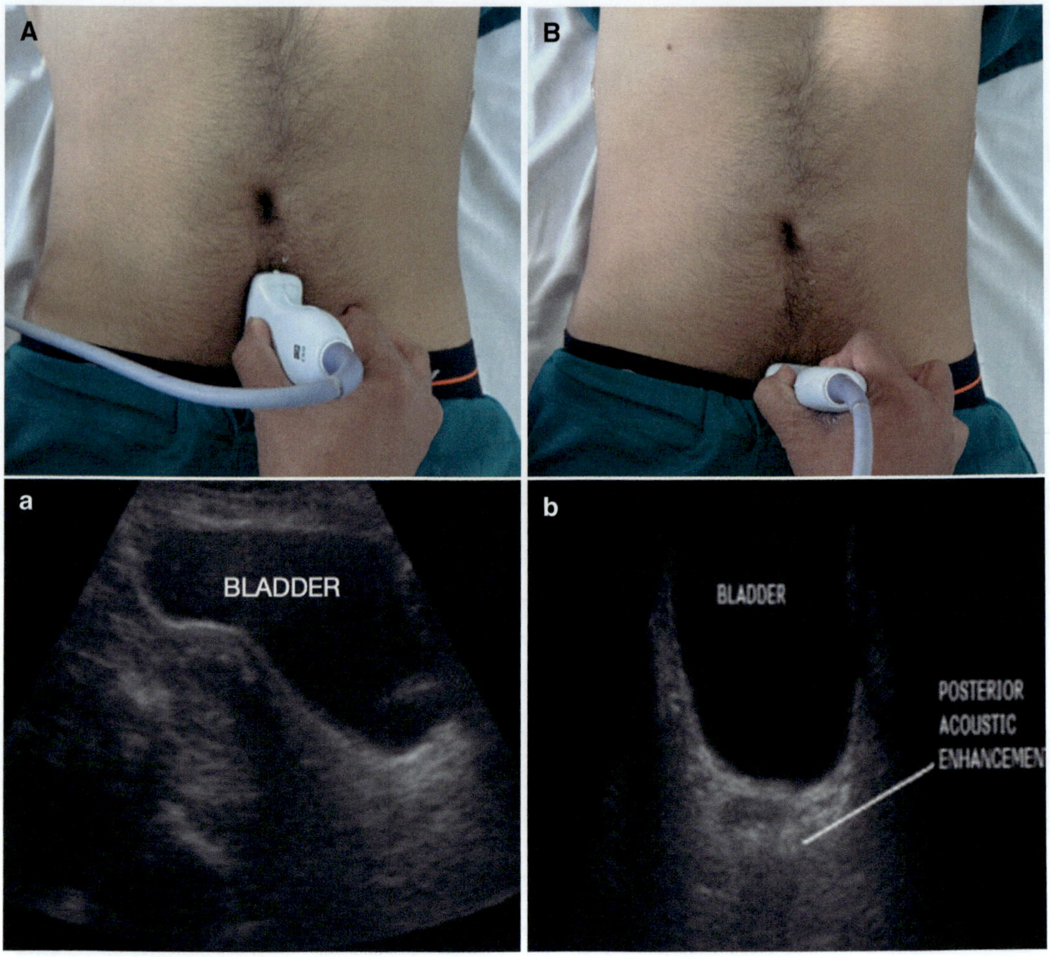

Fig. 21.2 eFAST scan: pelvis (sagittal and transverse view). (**A**) Curvilinear probe placement for sagittal view of pelvis, (**a**) corresponding ultrasound image, (**B**) Curvilinear probe placement for transverse view of pelvis, (**b**) corresponding ultrasound image

shape. If the bladder is empty, what will be visualized is just a bunch of echoes. Sweep the probe for areas of irregular dark black free fluid outside of the bladder (Fig. 21.2).

21.2.1.4 SUBXIPHOID View

For the sub-xiphoid, place the probe flat over the epigastrium, just under the xiphoid process. Push the probe downwards angling it a bit towards the heart. Sweep the probe from left to the right till the cardiac pulsation is visualized. The view obtained utilizes the liver as the acoustic window and should demonstrate four chambers of the heart. Look for the presence of any pericardial effusion. A cardiac tamponade is when the right ventricle collapses during the diastole under the pressure of the effusion.

A subxiphoid view may be a difficult view to obtain especially in obese patients, and in such situation parasternal long axis view or an apical view may be tried. Ultrasound can detect as little as 20 cc of pericardial fluid (Fig. 21.3).

21.2.1.5 THORAX View

Multiple studies have shown ultrasound to be more sensitive than supine chest radiograph for detection of pneumothorax. The probe is placed over the right anterior chest wall at the mid cla-

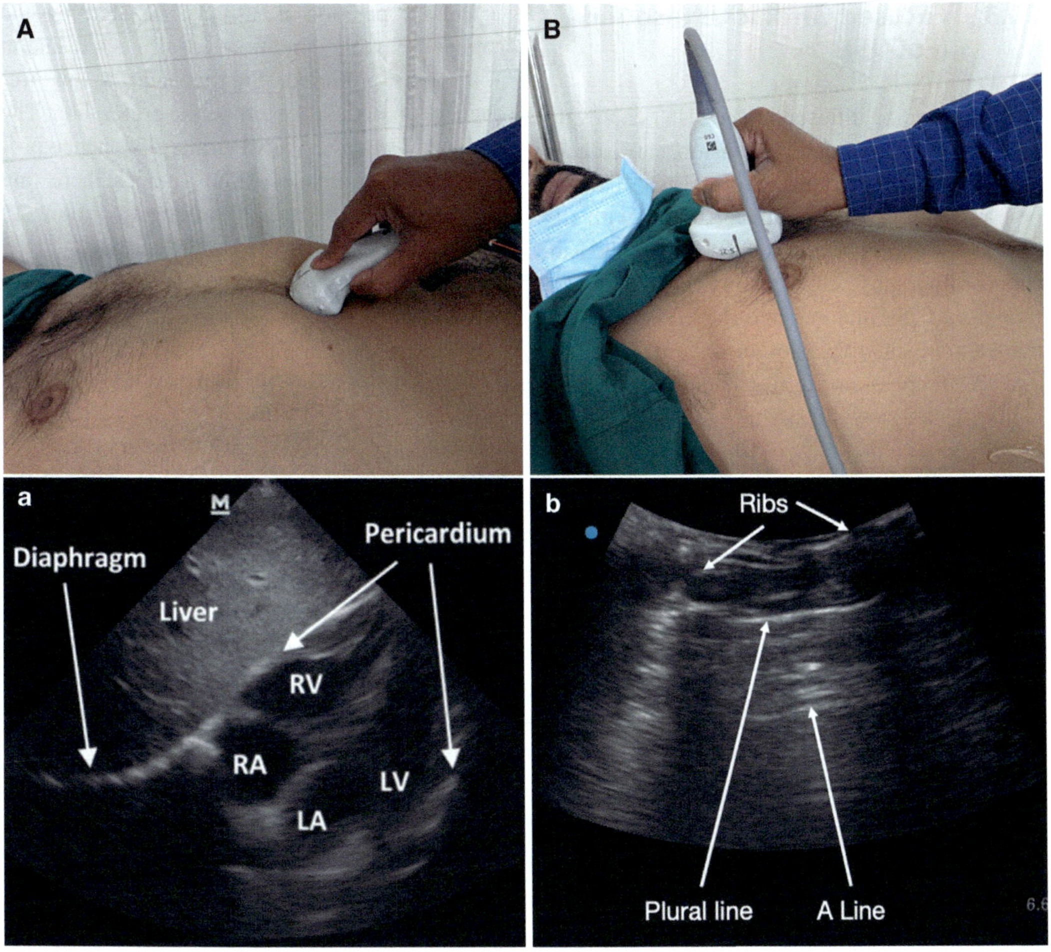

Fig. 21.3 Subxiphoid and thorax view. (**A**) Curvilinear probe placement for subxiphoid cardiac scan, (**a**) corresponding ultrasound image, (**B**) Curvilinear probe placement for thorax scan, (**b**) corresponding ultrasound image

vicular line at the third and fifth intercostal space (Fig. 21.3). Aim is to visualize the pleura between the two rib shadows, and to appreciate the sliding of the pleura to rule out pneumothorax. Pleural line is a bright horizontal echogenic line running just under the ribs. The sliding can be seen as a shimmering or marching of the surface along the plane. The presence of lung sliding excludes pneumothorax. Lung sliding can be graphically depicted on the M-Mode. A normal lung will depict a "sandy beach" appearance, whereas pneumothorax is represented as "Bar code" sign. "Lung Point" is the point where an incomplete pneumothorax ends, depicted by the presence of lung sliding on one side and absence on other.

The probe is slowly moved downwards from zone 1 to 2 and then laterally to zone 3 without lifting the probe from the patient's chest wall and observing the pleural sliding all throughout. The same maneuver is carried over the left side. Absence of lung sliding may be seen in other conditions as well.

1. Chronic obstructive pulmonary disease bleb.
2. Consolidated pneumonia.
3. Atelectasis.
4. Tracheal intubation.

21.3 Focused Cardiac Ultrasound (FoCUS)

Focused cardiac ultrasound (FoCUS) can evaluate the heart for pericardial effusion, cardiac tamponade, and wall motion abnormalities. This can be especially useful in trauma patients with suspected cardiac injury. By performing a bedside echocardiography, the treating physician can incorporate his findings into the clinical assessment and treatment plan of the patient. Time is of essence in commencing resuscitation and establishing a diagnosis in a shocked, arrested of a breathless patient.

The FoCUS exam typically includes a systematic evaluation of the four cardiac chambers, the pericardium, and the aorta. The left ventricle is evaluated for wall motion abnormalities, which may indicate acute myocardial infarction or cardiomyopathy. The right ventricle is evaluated for enlargement, which may indicate pulmonary embolism or chronic pulmonary hypertension. The pericardium is evaluated for the presence of fluid, which may indicate pericardial effusion or cardiac tamponade. The aorta is evaluated for aneurysm or dissection.

The aim of performing a FoCUS examination is to rapidly assess.

- Left and right ventricular (LV and RV, respectively) pump function.
- Pericardial effusion.
- Septal dynamics.
- Valvular morphology and
- Fluid responsiveness.

21.3.1 Techniques and Views

A FoCUS examination does not require the execution of all the views of a comprehensive standard echocardiographic examination. A limited number of views, such as subcostal long axis, subcostal inferior vena cava (IVC), parasternal long axis, parasternal midpapillary short axis, and apical four chamber view can suffice.

Patient position is usually dictated by the patient's clinical condition. Ideally a left lateral position is preferred. Small footprint low frequency phased array probe is preferable. The probe can sit easily between the ribs, hence providing better images. The images here are acquired in the cardiac mode. Important to remember that the marker in the cardiac mode is on the right side of the screen (Figs. 21.4, 21.5 and 21.6).

21.3.1.1 Parasternal Long Axis (PLAX) View

To obtain the PLAX view, place the probe over the anterior chest just left to the sternum at the second intercostal space with the probe marker pointing towards the right shoulder. Slide the probe down along the left sternal border until the desired image comes into view. Usually, the image can be obtained in the third or fourth intercostal space. Occasionally it may be difficult to obtain a view in this plane, placing the patient in the left lateral decubitus position may help enhance the image.

In the image obtained, at the top of the screen we see the right ventricle, and deeper to it lies the left ventricle. We have the interventricular septum in between. To the right of the left ventricle lies the left atrium with the mitral valves in between. We can also visualize the aortic valves and the aortic outflow tract (Fig. 21.4). What is not visualized in a PLAX view is the apex of the heart.

It is also important to identify the descending aorta in the PLAX view as it can help differentiate between a pericardial effusion from a pleural effusion. Pericardial effusion is usually within the pericardium and anterior to the descending aorta, whereas pleural effusion will be posterior to both the descending aorta and the pericardium.

PLAX is good for estimating the ejection fraction. Eyeballing the ejection fraction by looking at the squeeze of the heart and looking at how close the anterior mitral leaflet gets to the ventricular septum can give a good idea of the left

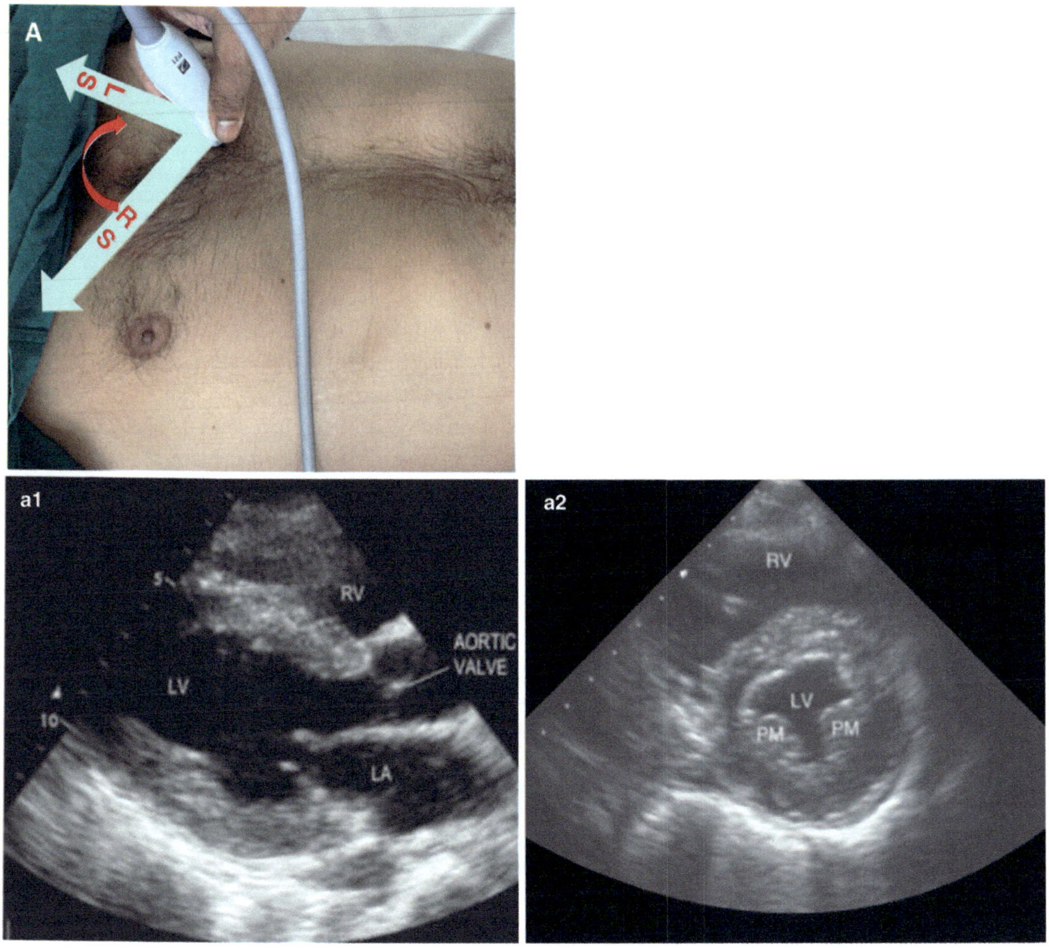

Fig. 21.4 FoCUS: parasternal long axis (PLAX) and short axis (PSAX) view. (**A**) Cardiac probe placed with marker pointing towards right shoulder for PLAX view and then rotated towards left shoulder for PSAX view, (**a1**) PLAX ultrasound image, (**a2**) PSAX ultrasound image

ventricular contractions. The quantification of the ejection fraction can be done by using E point septal separation or EPSS. After obtaining a PLAX view, throw down a M mode spike at the tip of the anterior mitral valve leaflet.

We can assess whether a pericardial effusion is causing a tamponade in this view, by looking at RV collapse during diastole. This corresponds to the time when the mitral valve is open. Diagnosis of tamponade is made when we have a diastolic collapse of right ventricle due to pericardial effusion, with signs of hypo-perfusion like hypotension, tachycardia, and shortness of breath.

21.3.1.2 Parasternal Short Axis (PSAX) View

Once the parasternal long axis view is obtained, rotate the probe 90° to obtain the parasternal short axis view. The probe marker now orients to the patients left shoulder. The transducer beam is now perpendicular to the long axis of the patient's heart. The probe now can be angulated towards the base or the Apex to obtain short axis views at different levels (Fig. 21.4b). Important here is to obtain view at the mid ventricular, or at the level of the papillary muscle group. The left ventricle here appears as a circular muscle ring contracting

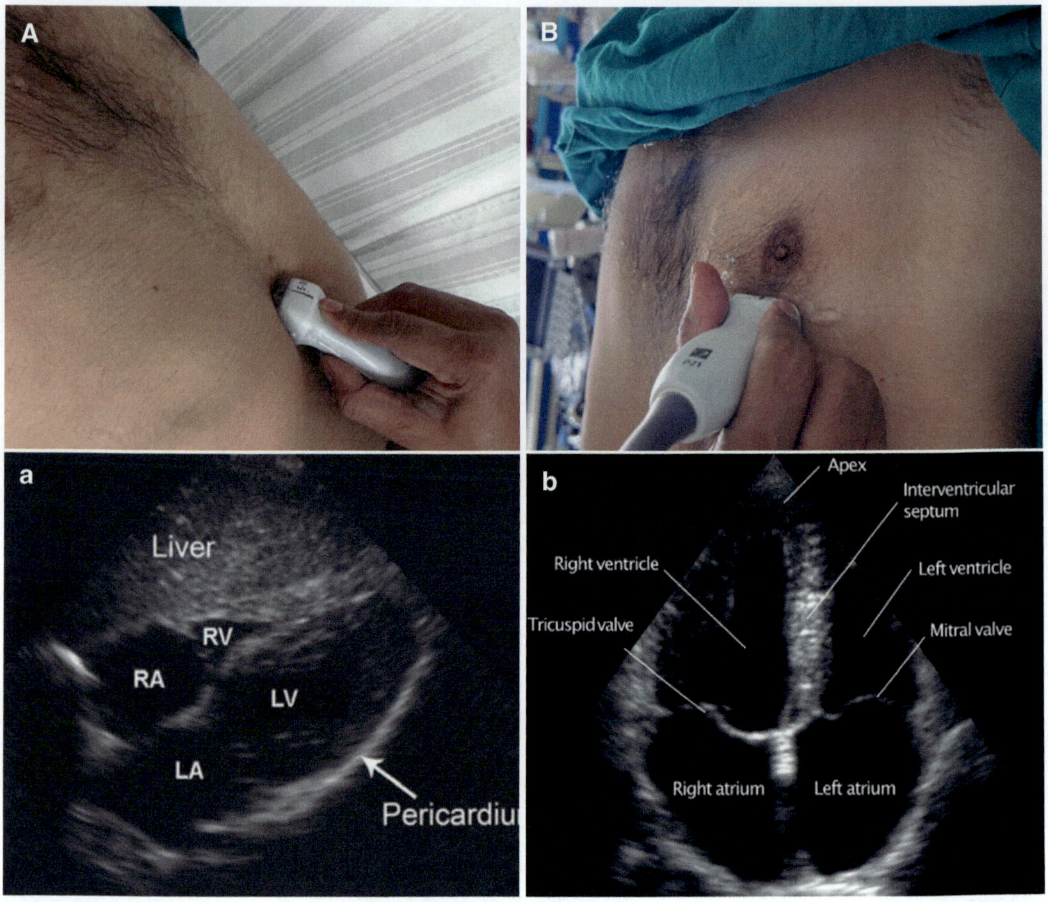

Fig. 21.5 FoCUS: subcostal and apical four chamber view. (**A**) Cardiac probe placement for subcostal four chamber view, (**a**) corresponding ultrasound image, (**B**) cardiac probe placement for apical four chamber view, (**b**) corresponding ultrasound image

towards a hollow center. The ejection fraction again is determined by eyeballing the squeeze of the circular muscle ring and the uniformity of the contraction.

Views can also be obtained at the level of the mitral (fish mouth view) and aortic valve (Mercedes Benz sign). Right ventricular strain in the parasternal short axis view at the level of the mid ventricular, can be determined by observing an enlarged RV and septal bowing (the D sign).

21.3.1.3 Apical Four Chamber View

Apical four view is obtained by placing the probe over the Apex of the heart. The position of the apex can vary from patient to patient. In a patient with COPD, the Apex lies more vertically downwards than laterally. Usually, a good place to start would be by placing the probe at the fifth intercostal space just under the nipple, with the probe marker pointing out towards the left axilla (Fig. 21.5b).

Alternate method is to first palpate the apex, and then to place the probe over that point. Once the apex has been located and a view of the left and right ventricular chambers is on the screen, it is important to place the septum vertical on the screen which can be done by rocking the probe to the right or left. Then by tilting the probe up or down a good view of all four chambers can be obtained. By a general rule, the LV takes up about 2/3 of the screen and the RV 1/3 of the screen. In

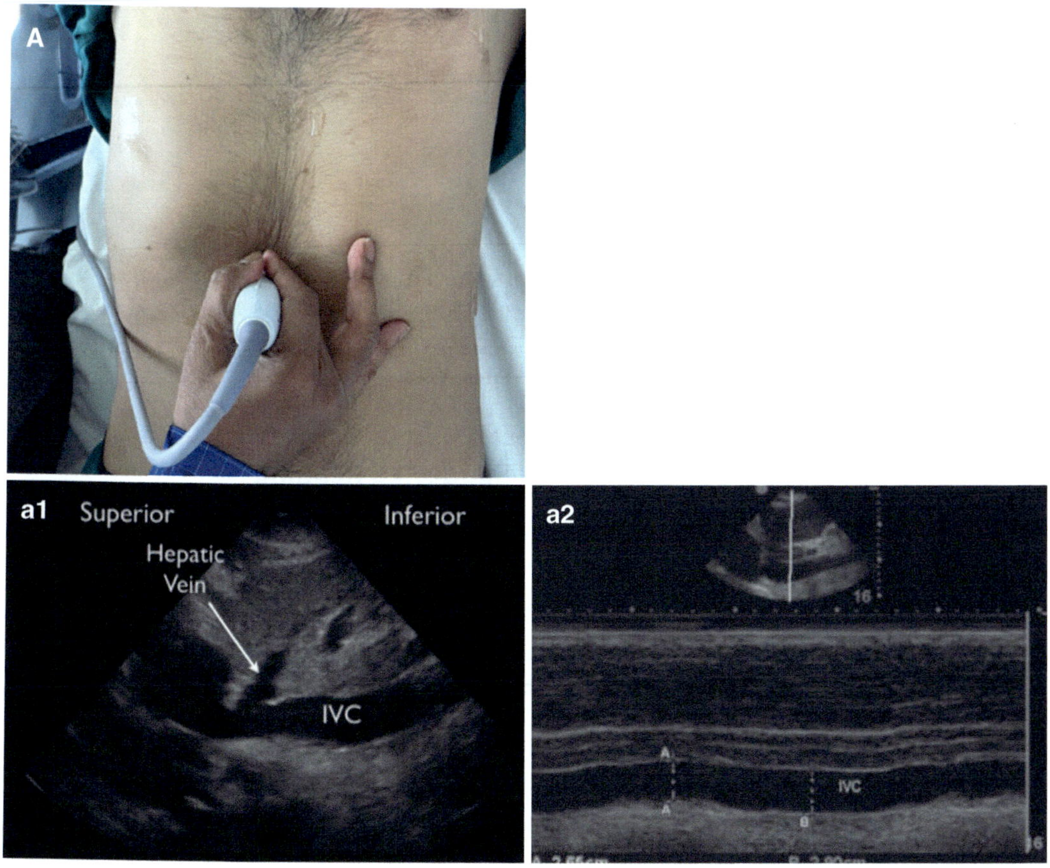

Fig. 21.6 FoCUS: inferior vena cava view. (**A**) Cardiac probe placed with marker pointing cephalad for IVC assessment, (**a1**) Ultrasound image of sagittal view, (**a2**) M-mode image for IVC variation measurements

case of a PE or pulmonary hypertension, the RV will be greater than the LV.

21.3.1.4 Subcostal View

Place the probe flat on the sub-xiphoid region. Here we can ask the patient to bend the knees, if possible, to relax the abdominal muscles. Indicator of the cardiac probe should be pointing to the left side of the patient, unlike in the FAST examination (Fig. 21.5a). Assume an overhand grip on the probe and press it down. Using the liver as a acoustic window, sweep the probe from the left to right direction till cardiac impulse is detected. All four chambers of the heart can be visualized in the sub-xiphoid view. The view is particularly useful in detecting pericardial effusion.

21.3.1.5 Inferior Vena Cava (IVC) Evaluation

To get the view of the IVC, we can start with the sub-costal view of the heart. Here we can narrow in to the right atrium and then turn the probe counterclockwise with probe marker cranially. Slightly turn the probe the to the patients right to bring the IVC into view. The IVC can be seen coursing through the liver into the right atrium (Fig. 21.6).

Other way to approach the IVC view is to hold the probe transversely over the epigastrium to identify the aorta sitting over the spine and the IVC next to it. Now after orienting the IVC at the center of the screen, the probe can be turned 90° with the probe marker pointing cranially. It is important to be sure that one is not scanning the

Table 21.1 IVC diameter measurements

Estimate of RA pressure			
Diameter	Collapse	RAP	Range
<2.1 cm	>50%	3	0–5
		8	5–10
>2.1 cm	<50%	15	10–20

wrong tube before initiating the measurements. The aorta and IVC can be differentiated by following features.

- The aorta is a thick-walled pulsating structure, with no respiratory variation. It dives down beneath the right atrium. In case of confusion, a pulse Doppler can be used to differentiate the two.
- The IVC lies to the right of the midline of the patient and to the aorta. The aorta usually lies a bit on the left.
- An important landmark is the hepatic vein which can be seen entering the IVC at an acute angle, just proximal to its entry into the right atrium.

The measurement of the IVC is done usually 1–2 cm proximal to its entry into the right atrium. The measurement is done perpendicular to the axis of the IVC (Table 21.1).

It is important to measure the IVC at its mid axis, as measuring the diameter at any other axis may result in a falsely low value (side walling). To avoid this, it is better to give some time scanning the IVC to first identify the mid axis.

21.4 Conclusion

Ultrasound is a valuable diagnostic tool for evaluating trauma patients in the emergency room. Its use in trauma evaluation is supported by evidence showing its accuracy, speed, and ability to identify life-threatening conditions. It can help guide further diagnostic and therapeutic interventions and improve patient care. Ultrasound evaluation of trauma patients is an essential part of emergency medicine, and its use should be encouraged to enhance the care of trauma patients in the emergency room.

Suggested Reading

1. Pearl WS, Todd KH. Ultrasonography for the initial evaluation of blunt abdominal trauma: a review of prospective trials. Ann Emerg Med. 1996;27(3):353–61.
2. Rozycki GS, Ochsner MG, Feliciano DV, Thomas B, Boulanger BR, Davis FE, Falcone RE, Schmidt JA. Early detection of hemoperitoneum by ultrasound examination of the right upper quadrant: a multicenter study. J Trauma. 1998;45(5):878–83.
3. Lobo V, Hunter-Behrend M, Cullnan E, Higbee R, Phillips C, Williams S, Perera P, Gharahbaghian L. Caudal edge of the liver in the right upper quadrant (RUQ) view is the most sensitive area for free fluid on the FAST exam. West J Emerg Med. 2017;18(2):270–80.
4. Brooks A, Davies B, Smethhurst M, Connolly J. Emergency ultrasound in the acute assessment of haemothorax. Emerg Med J. 2004;21(1):44–6.
5. Whye D, Barish R, Almquist T, Groleau G, Tso E, Browne B. Echocardiographic diagnosis of acute pericardial effusion in penetrating chest trauma. Am J Emerg Med. 1988;6(1):21–3.
6. Soldati G, Testa A, Sher S, et al. Occult traumatic pneumothorax: diagnostic accuracy of lung ultrasonography in the emergency department. Chest. 2008;133:204–11.
7. Sartori S, Tombesi P, Trevisani L, et al. Accuracy of transthoracic sonography in detection of pneumothorax after sonographically guided lung biopsy: prospective comparison with chest radiography. Am J Roentgenol. 2007;188:37–41.
8. Lichtenstein DA, Menu Y. A bedside ultrasound sign ruling out pneumothorax in the critically ill. Lung sliding. Chest. 1995;108:1345–8.
9. Labovitz AJ, Noble VE, Bierig M, Goldstein SA, Jones R, Kort S, Porter TR, Spencer KT, Tayal VS, Wei K. Focused cardiac ultrasound in the emer-

gent setting: a consensus statement of the American Society of Echocardiography and American College of Emergency Physicians. J Am Soc Echocardiogr. 2010;23(12):1225–30.
10. Andrus P, Dean A. Focused cardiac ultrasound. Glob Heart. 2013;8(4):299–303.
11. Cawthorn TR, Nickel C, O'Reilly M, Kafka H, Tam JW, Jackson LC, Sanfilippo AJ, Johri AM. Development and evaluation of methodologies for teaching focused cardiac ultrasound skills to medical students. J Am Soc Echocardiogr. 2014;27(3):302–9.
12. Spencer KT, Kimura BJ, Korcarz CE, Pellikka PA, Rahko PS, Siegel RJ. Focused cardiac ultrasound: recommendations from the American Society of Echocardiography. J Am Soc Echocardiogr. 2013;26(6):567–81.
13. Via G, Hussain A, Wells M, Reardon R, ElBarbary M, Noble VE, Tsung JW, Neskovic AN, Price S, Oren-Grinberg A, Liteplo A. International evidence-based recommendations for focused cardiac ultrasound. J Am Soc Echocardiogr. 2014;27(7):683–e1.
14. Mok KL. Make it SIMPLE: enhanced shock management by focused cardiac ultrasound. J Intensive Care. 2016;4:1–7.

Needle Thoracocentesis

22

Ripon Choudhary, Ridhima Sharma, and Anju Gupta

Key Points

- A recent chest radiograph should be available prior to pleural aspiration.
- Thoracic ultrasound guidance is strongly recommended for all pleural drainage procedures for pleural fluid.
- In a tension pneumothorax is present, upon entering the pleural space, immediately air bubbles will often be noted in the fluid-filled syringe.
- Continual cardiopulmonary compromise, despite NT indicates inadequate decompression or other coexisting condition.
- In a simple pneumothorax, there is no return of air into the syringe spontaneously but occurs only with aspiration.
- The site of needle insertion is either in the triangle of safety or the second intercostal space in the mid-clavicular line.
- Large bore needle aspiration should be avoided to prevent pneumothorax.
- The procedure should be abandoned once no fluid or air aspirated, there exist symptoms of cough, chest discomfort, or 1.5 L of fluid has been withdrawn.

22.1 Introduction

Thoracocentesis or pleural tap (derived from Greek words, thorax and centesis, puncture) is an invasive procedure to remove air or fluid from the pleural cavity for either therapeutic or diagnostic purposes. The procedure was first performed by Morrill Wyman in 1850 and then described by Henry Ingersoll Bowditch in 1852. There exists a potential space between the inner chest wall and lung in the thoracic cavity and it contains a trace of fluid which acts as a lubricant during the expansion and recoiling of the lung. Any significant collection of air, fluid, or blood is pathological and needs to be removed. A hollow needle or cannula is introduced into the thorax to allow the removal of an abnormal collected air or fluid, in order to reinflate the lung. Thoracentesis can be done either supine or a sitting position depending upon the patient clinical condition and comfort.

R. Choudhary
Department of Anesthesia, LNJP and MAMC Delhi, New Delhi, India

R. Sharma
Department of Anesthesia, AIIMS, Nagpur, India

A. Gupta (✉)
Anesthesiology, Pain Medicine, Critical Care, All India Institute of Medical Sciences, New Delhi, Delhi, India

N. Gupta et al. (eds.), *Techniques in Anesthesia, Intensive Care and Emergency Medicine*,
https://doi.org/10.1007/978-981-96-1202-4_22

22.2 Anatomical Considerations

The thin space between the visceral and parietal pleura is the pleural space and it extends inferiorly to the tenth intercostal space (approximately). The intercostal spaces contain veins, arteries, and nerves lying in the costal groove along with the inferior margin of the superior rib along with intercostal muscles, from above downwards. To evade the neuromuscular bundle injury, needle insertion should be done in the interspace just superior to the rib.

Indication and contraindication for needle thoracentesis are described in Tables 22.1 and 22.2.

Table 22.1 Indications of thoracocentesis

Diagnostic	Therapeutic
1. Establish the cause of pleural effusion (PE) with no known etiology, such as:	1. Decompress the lung in tension pneumothorax as per ATLS guidelines
• Atypical features in suspected CHF: • Unilateral effusion, categorically left-sided • Bilateral effusion, of disparate sizes • Normal Cardiac silhouette on chest radiograph • Widened alveolar-arterial oxygen gradient out of proportion of the clinical settings • B-type natriuretic peptide (BNP) levels inconsistent with heart-failure (HF) • Persistent effusion, despite HF therapy	2. Removal of the pleural fluid in patients with parapneumonic effusions, empyema, i.e., pneumonia and an effusion of more than minimal size, recommend therapeutic thoracentesis
2. To determine the nature of pleural effusion, i.e., transudate or exudate	3. Removal of the pleural fluid, in order to evaluate the status of the underlying lung
3. Pulmonary embolism (PE) (with 10 mm thickness on lateral decubitus X-ray or USG) associated with no obvious cause	4. Relieve the symptoms of respiratory distress, secondary to PE, i.e., dyspnea at rest, increased oxygen requirement and when removal up to 1000–1500 mL is indicated
4. Recurrent PE due to infection or for the confirmation of the malignant cell's presence, due to cancer	

Table 22.2 Contraindications of thoracocentesis

Uncooperative patient
Ruptured diaphragm
Adhesions or pleurodesos
Systemic anticoagulation or bleeding diathesis (INR >2)
PT or PTT greater than twice the normal range
Platelet count less than 25,000/mm^3
Skin infection, cellulitis or herpes zoster at the site of needle insertion
Minimal fluid volume and uncertain location by examination
Altered chest wall anatomy
Serum creatinine concentration of more than 6 mg/dL, uremia
Pneumothorax in the patients on mechanical ventilation with additional PEEP
Uncontrolled coughing

22.3 Pitfall

When the patient is discharged from the hospital after a resolved pneumothorax, recommendations should be made for no flying or scuba diving for a minimum of 2 weeks.

Immediate needle decompression is required in Tension Pneumothorax and prompt insertion of a large over-the-needle catheter into the pleural space is the immediate treatment modality. Evidence propounded that a 5-cm over-the-needle catheter will reach the pleural space >50% of the time, whereas an 8-cm over-the-needle catheter will reach the pleural space >90% of the time.

22.4 Commonly Associated Differential Diagnosis

Tension pneumothorax	*Cardiac tamponade*	*Massive hemothorax*
Decreased or absent breath sounds on ipsilateral affected side Hyper resonant on percussion Trachea deviated away Distended neck veins Obstructive shock	Presence of bilateral breath sounds Normal on percussion Trachea not deviated Distended veins (**Kussmaul's sign**) rise in venous pressure with inspiration when breathing spontaneously, Pulsus paradoxus **Becks triad**; hypotension, distended neck veins, distant or muffled heart sounds Right ventricular diastolic collapse	Decreased breath sounds on auscultation Dull on percussion Trachea midline Collapsed veins

22.5 Pathophysiology

TP is a "one-way valve" air leak from the lungs or through the chest wall (flap-valve mechanism preventing the escape of air entering the pleural space). Air is gushed into the pleural space with no means of escape and eventually collapses the affected lung. The mediastinum is shifted towards the opposite side, reducing cardiac output due to decreased venous return causing "Obstructive" shock.

Prompt clinical diagnosis reflecting air under pressure in the affected pleural space is imperative to prevent mortality. Do not delay therapeutic intervention to obtain radiologic confirmation.

22.6 Role of Needle Thoracostomy in Diagnosis and Treatment of Tension Pneumothorax

Tension pneumothorax (TP) is a life-threatening surgical emergency which requires prompt diagnosis and treatment.

22.7 Most Common Causes of Tension Pneumothorax

1. Mechanical positive-pressure ventilation barotrauma
2. Penetrating or blunt chest trauma
3. Internal jugular or subclavian venous catheter insertion
4. Occlusive dressings, secured on four sides after a traumatic defects or the defect, enact as a flap valve mechanism
5. Percutaneous tracheostomy
6. Conversion of simple pneumothorax to tension pneumothorax

22.8 Clinical Manifestations of Tension Pneumothorax

1. Spontaneous breathing patients often exhibit extreme tachycardia and air hunger whereas mechanically ventilated patients develop explicit signs of hemodynamic collapse
2. Chest pain
3. Respiratory distress, tachypnea
4. Tachycardia, hypotension
5. Tracheal deviation away from the side of injury
6. Unilateral absence of breath sounds
7. Elevated hemithorax without respiratory movement
8. Neck vein distension
9. Cyanosis (late manifestation)
10. Contralateral respiratory excursions, hypoxia or increased oxygen requirement

22.9 Site Selection

S. no.	Site	Advantage
1.	4th or 5th intercostal space in anterior axillary or mid-axillary line	Potential site for subsequent thoracostomy tube insertion as definitive treatment of pneumothorax. Latest tenth update of **Advanced Trauma Life Support** (ATLS) guidelines recommended this site for emergency needle thoracostomy for tension pneumothorax
2.	7th, 8th, 9th space, midway between the posterior axillary line and midline (6–10 cm lateral to spine)	Avoids accidental puncture of liver, spleen, descending aorta and diaphragm
3.	Anterior axillary line in second intercostal space (supine position)	Ease of identification, safe margin, low risk of hemorrhage
4.	Posterior approach	The posterior gutter is deep and is where fluid collects in the erect position. Inter-spaces are wider in the back compared to the front

22.10 Patient Position

1. **Sitting Position**: Place the patient in a sitting position on the edge of the bed, a table with a pillow to lean upon is recommended to maximize the patient's comfort. With the arms resting on the bedside table and the head supported (Fig. 22.1).

2. **Supine or Lateral recumbent Position**: In the patients who are not able to make a sitting position. Elevate the bed end 30–45° (Fig. 22.2a), i.e., the patient at the edge of the bed on the affected side with the ipsilateral arm may be resting on the head. The mid-axillary line should be accessible for the insertion of the needle or in a lateral recumbent with the head and chest elevated 30–45° (Fig. 22.2b).

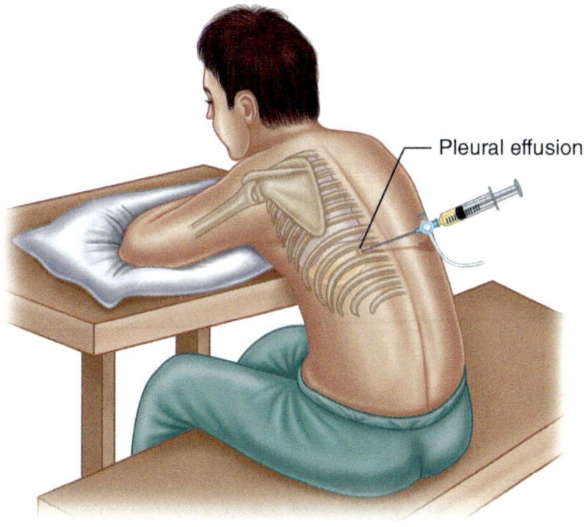

Fig. 22.1 Pleural drainage

22.10.1 Equipment

Povidone iodine or chlorhexidine solution.
Sterile gloves and gown.
12- to-16-gauge catheter over the needle (4.5 cm in length).
5- or 10-mL syringe.

22.10.2 Procedure (Fig. 22.3)

Step 1: The safest and most reliable site for an emergency needle thoracostomy is the second intercostal space in the midclavicular line.

Step 2: After the identification of the correct space, keep the index finger (non-dominant) over the needle insertion site. Apply a 12, 14, or 16-gauge catheter over the needle onto a 5 or 10 mL syringe.

Step3: Insert the catheter-over-the needle perpendicular to the skin and above the superior border of the third rib, thereby avoiding injury to the neurovascular bundle underlying the inferior border of the second rib.

Step4: Few physicians prefer to contact the third rib upper border with the needle tip, walk over it until it goes over the edge, and thereby advance into the pleural space.

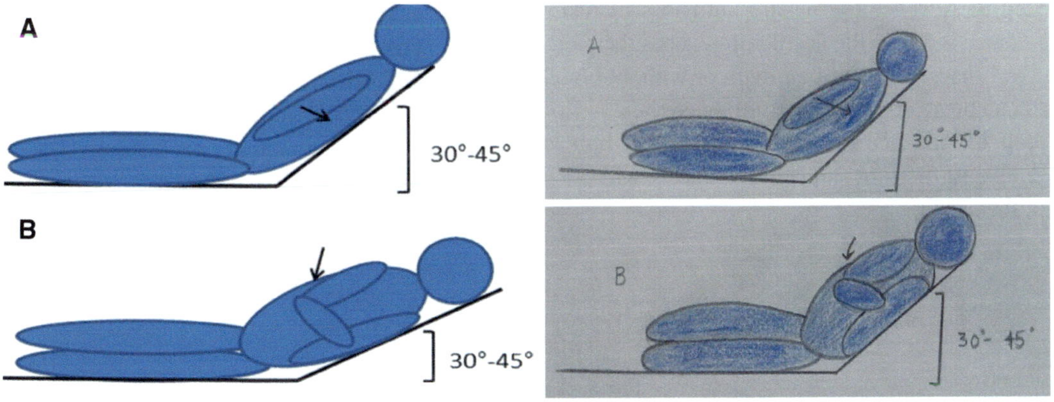

Fig. 22.2 Black arrows indicate the site of procedures. (**a**) Supine position and (**b**) lateral position

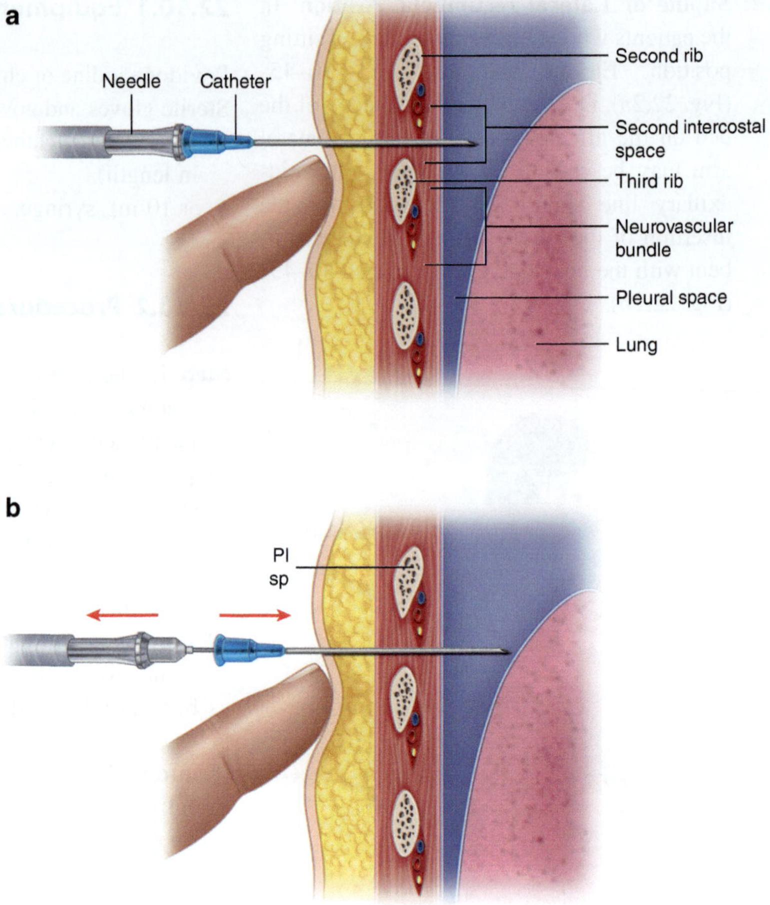

Fig. 22.3 Decompression of a tension pneumothorax with a catheter over the needle. (**a**) The catheter-over—the needle insertion into the pleural cavity. (**b**) The catheter is advanced and the needle is removed

Step 5: Advance the needle until loss of resistance is felt as the needle tip reaches the pleural space. A gush of air, with or without blood can be heard escaping from the syringe.

Step 6: Advance the catheter until the hub is against the skin and simultaneously withdraw the needle.

22.11 Equipment Required for Drainage of Pleural Effusion

The equipment required are listed below (Fig. 22.4).

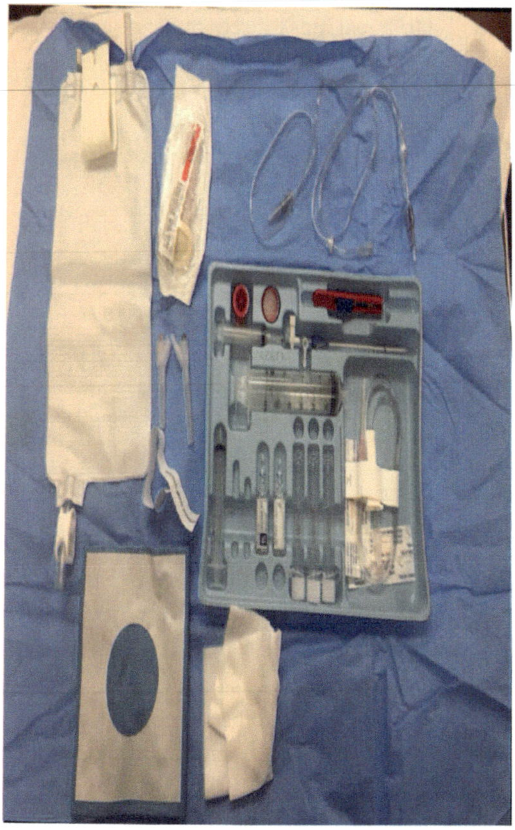

Fig. 22.4 Equipment for needle thoracocentesis

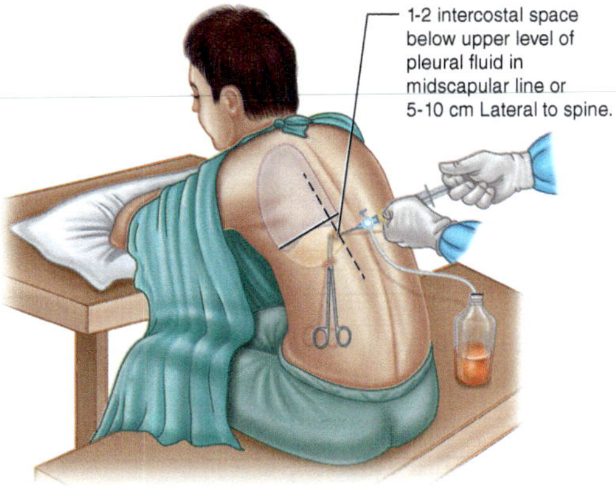

Fig. 22.5 Site of insertion of needle for needle thoracocentesis

22.12 Procedure

Step 1: Position the patient in a sitting or lateral recumbent/supine position, if unable to sit.

Step 2: The needle insertion site should be selected 1–2 intercostal space below the highest level of effusion (Fig. 22.5).

Step 3: Mark the area of needle insertion by a pen or pencil on the skin.

Step 4: Under all aseptic precautions, clean the skin with Povidone iodine or chlorhexidine in a wide area around the site and drape the site with sterile drapes.

Step 5: Give L.A with 1% lidocaine (5 mL syringe with 25 or 27 guage needle) on the skin over the insertion site and then on the superior margin of the rib and the pleura.

Step 6: Insert the needle over the superior margin of the rib to avoid injury to the intercostal nerves and vessels, located near the inferior margin.

Step 7: After the needle insertion, apply negative pressure to the syringe, until a loss of resistance is felt and steady flow of fluid is obtained. This is a pre-eminent step to detect untoward vessel or other structure injury.

Step 8: Note the depth of the needle, once the fluid returns and mark it with a hemostat, as it helps to estimate the approximate depth for the insertion of the thoracentesis needle or angio-catheter.

Step 9: After noting the depth of needle with hemostat, remove the anesthetizing needle. Measure the same depth on the angiocath as the first needle, using a hemostat.

Step 10: After knowing the adequate distance, insert the thoracentesis needle, while exerting steady pressure on patients back with non-dominant hand.

Step 11: Advance needle until it hits the superior aspect of the rib and then continue advancing over the top of the rib. Attach the three-way stopcock and tubing, and aspirate the amount required and thereafter turn the stopcock and evacuate the fluid through the tubing.

Step 12: Remove the necessary amount of pleural fluid (usually 100 mL for diagnostic studies), do not remove more than 1500 mL of fluid at once to avoid increased risk of pleural edema or hypotension.

Step 13: After the removal of the fluid, ask the patient to take a deep breath and hum, then gently remove the needle. This maneuver increases intrathoracic pressure and decrease the plausibility of pneumothorax.

Step 14: Cover the insertion site with a sterile occlusive dressing.

Step 15: A checkbox as shown below should be ticked.

Check-box steps
• Procedure explained to the patient
• Written informed consent obtained
• Patient's identity verified
• Needle insertion site marked
• The verification by all the members of the care team of the patient ensured
• PT, PTI, and INR checked before commencing the procedure
• All aseptic precaution followed during the procedure

22.13 Advantage of Alternative Devices

The main reason for these alternative devices is to outwit the menace of a lung puncture by a sharp needle, which can happen when expanding lung encounters the needle, after the evacuation process.

22.14 Alternative Devices for Thoracentesis

22.14.1 Catheter System (Intracath and EZ Cath)

- In this technique, catheter can be advanced through a needle (Fig. 22.6).

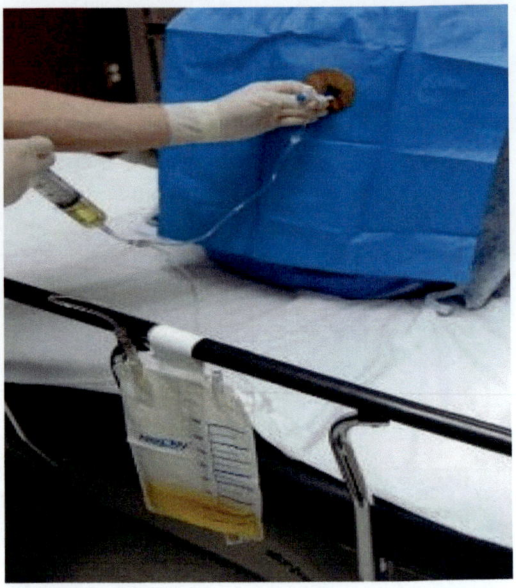

Fig. 22.6 Catheter system for needle thoracocentesis

- The usual size of the needle if 14.
- Insert the needle into the thorax and once the fluid seeps, catheter is steadily advanced into the pleural space and also the catheter should slide without resistance.
- Attach syringe to the catheter and fluid can be drawn for diagnostic purpose.
- In case of resistance slowly withdraw the catheter rather than pulling it back, as it will lead to shearing of catheter. Needle can be reintroduced, and catheter can be advanced, once free flow of pleural fluid is observed.

22.14.2 Modified Husted Needle

- The modified Husted needle is rounded and blunt at the tip.
- The cutting edge is parallel to the shank axis.
- The needle lumen is open eccentrically on the side.
- The blunt tip of the needle helps in reducing the risk of puncture to the lung.

22.15 Complications

Major complications
1. Pneumothorax (11%): Firstly, due to the introduction of air from the outside and is usually asymptomatic. Secondly, accidental puncture of the lung, if asymptomatic, keep the patient under observation and follow with a serial chest X-ray. Generally, the puncture seals spontaneously and if symptomatic, then may require chest tube drainage
2. Hemothorax (0.8%): Accidental injury to an intercostal artery can lead to bleeding, although it is rarely seen
3. Empyema: Strict aseptic precautions can prevent this complication
4. Laceration of the liver, spleen or diaphragm: The lowest recommended level for thoracentesis is between the eighth and ninth ribs, i.e., eighth intercostal space, in order to minimize the injury to the diaphragm
5. Cardiac injury
Minor complications
1. Vaso-vagal syncope
2. Tumour Seeding: High frequency in mesothelioma compared to other tumours patients, although implantation of tumor cells through a thoracentesis needle is a less frequent complication
3. Pain (22%): Reassurance and use of local anesthetic can alleviate the pain, also shoulder pain during the procedure, indicates piercing of the diaphragmatic pleura and low site of insertion
4. Subcutaneous Seroma (0.8%): Collection of fluid under tension can cause, extravasation can occur along the needle track to the subcutaneous tissue
5. Cough (11%)
6. Dry-Tap (13%)
7. Atelectasis
8. Ineffective catheter placement: Most commonly in tension pneumothorax, and needle thoracentesis, with a failure rate of 22–50% in various literature
9. Major vascular injury
10. Persistent or recurrent Pneumothorax: Due to inadequate drainage especially in obese patients or shorter length may be insufficient
11. Iatrogenic Pneumothorax

22.16 Recent Advances

Bedside ultrasound (USG) has become an important imaging modality to identify the exact level of fluid in the chest cavity and identify respiratory variations. USG-guided needle thoracentesis is associated with low complications and failure rate.

USG can be used for the estimation of the required depth of needle insertion from the thoracic wall to fluid volume, pocket and the size of the drainage window for prognostic safety. In cases with a perceived risk of pneumothorax, pre-procedure scanning for the assessment of lung sliding is advocated and can be compared to post-procedure assessment to rule out pneumothorax. The USG-guided site localization should be ideally in the same position as to be assumed during the procedure.

Ultrasound-guided pleural aspiration is associated with a lower failure and complication rate, also the procedure failures or "dry taps" can have further clinically significant complications including visceral injury.

Kohan et al. demonstrated the efficacy of ultrasound-guided pleural aspiration following failed clinical procedures; hence in a failed clinically localized pleural aspiration, image guidance should be performed and further clinical attempts should not be done.

Thoracic ultrasound can be used in the presence of unilateral "white-out" or opaque hemithorax on the chest X-ray. In a prospective study of 50 patients, 9 had no pleural effusion present on thoracic ultrasound, thereby circumventing any inappropriate pleural aspiration and potential procedure-related injury.

In a randomized controlled trial comparing USG-guided pleural aspiration against the blind, there existed a noteworthy higher incidence of dry taps in the presence of small and loculated pleural effusion particularly in the failed clinical guided attempt or in the absence of mediastinum shift.

22.17 Scanning Technique

- The ideal position for scanning is considered sitting upright and leaning forward.
- High-frequency linear transducer, 7.5–10 MHz is considered optimal and is placed in the sagittal or transverse plane on the patient's back.
- The distance from the transducer to the pleural fluid is observed and noted. The probe is then rotated 180° to visualize the pleural fluid between the ribs to ensure that there is only fluid and there is no lung, diaphragm, liver or spleen underneath, at the site of insertion.
- The lung is perceived as an echogenic structure that moves with respiration.
- Observe the deepest pocket of fluid superficial to the lung and freeze the image for the measurement of the approximate depth of the needle insertion, to approach to the maximum amount of fluid (Fig. 22.7).
- The edge of the bone is echogenic and gives shadowing.
- The area should be marked with a pen and under all aseptic precautions, the procedure should be performed.

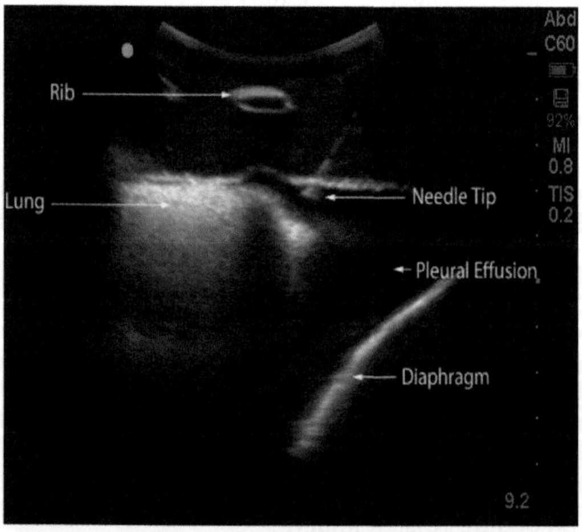

Fig. 22.7 USG-guided thoracentesis

Suggested Reading

1. Krantz BE. Advanced trauma life support for doctors. Chicago, IL: The American College of Surgeons; 1997.
2. Waydhas C, Sauerland S. Pre-hospital pleural decompression and chest tube placement after blunt trauma: a systematic review. Resuscitation. 2007;72(1):11–25.
3. Netto FA, Shulman H, Rizoli SB, Tremblay LN, Brenneman F, Tien H. Are needle decompressions for tension pneumothoraces being performed appropriately for appropriate indications? Am J Emerg Med. 2008;26(5):597–602.
4. Barton ED, Epperson M, Hoyt DB, Fortlage D, Rosen P. Prehospital needle aspiration and tube thoracostomy in trauma victims: a six-year experience with aeromedical crews. J Emerg Med. 1995;13(2):155–63.
5. McPherson J, Feigin D, Bellamy R. Prevalence of tension pneumothorax in fatally wounded combat casualties. J Trauma. 2006;60:573–8.
6. Leigh-Smith S, Harris T. Tension pneumothorax—time for a re-think? Emerg Med J. 2005;22:8–16.
7. American College of Surgeons. Advanced trauma life support ATLS student course manual. The ninth edition, vol. 119. Chicago, IL: American College of Surgeons; 2012.
8. Kwiatt M, Tarbox A, Seamon MJ, Swaroop M, Cipolla J, Allen C, et al. Thoracostomy tubes: a comprehensive review of complications and related topics. Int J Crit Illn Inj Sci. 2014;4:143–55.
9. Evans DC, Stawicki SP, Davido HT, Eiferman D. Obesity in trauma patients: correlations of body mass index with outcomes, injury patterns, and complications. Am Surg. 2011;77:1003–8.
10. Barnes TW, Morgenthaler TI, Olsen EJ, Hesley GK, Decker PA, Ryu JH. Sonographically guided thoracentesis and rate of pneumothorax. J Clin Ultrasound. 2005;33(9):442–6.
11. Jones PW, Moyers JP, Rogers JT, Rodriguez RM, Lee YC, Light RW. Ultrasound-guided thoracentesis: is it a safer method? Chest. 2003;123:418–23.
12. Koh DM, Burke S, Davies N, Padley SP. Transthoracic US of the chest: clinical uses and applications. Radiographics. 2002;22:e1.
13. Roberts JR, Hedges JR. Clinical procedures in emergency medicine and acute care. 5th ed. Amsterdam: Elsevier; 2004. p. 160–74.
14. Introduction to inpatient procedures: a resident-to-resident guide. University of Minnesota internal medicine residency AHCC ambulatory rotation. Second Edition, Revised October 2007.

15. Colice GL, Curtis A, Deslauriers J, et al. Medical and surgical treatment of parapneumonic effusions: an evidence-based guideline. Chest. 2000;118:1158.
16. Riwoe D, Poncia HD. Subclavian artery laceration: a serious complication of needle decompression. Emerg Med Australas. 2011;23:651–3.
17. Wraight WM, Tweedie DJ, Parkin IG. Neurovascular anatomy and variation in the fourth, fifth, and sixth intercostal spaces in the mid-axillary line: a cadaveric study in respect of chest drain insertion. Clin Anat. 2005;18:346–9.
18. Leigh-Smith S, Davies G. Indications for thoracic needle decompression. J Trauma. 2007;63(6):1403–4.
19. Lenaeus MJ, Shepard A, White AA. Routine chest radiographs after uncomplicated thoracentesis. J Hosp Med. 2018;13(11):787–9.
20. Leo F, Makowska M. [Thoracentesis—step by step]. Dtsch Med Wochenschr. 2018;143(16):1186–92.
21. Aelony Y. Thoracentesis without ultrasonic guidance infrequent complications when performed by an experienced pulmonologist. J Bronchol. 2005;12:200e2.
22. Alrajab S, Youssef AM, Akkus NI, Caldito G. Pleural ultrasonography versus chest radiography for the diagnosis of pneumothorax: review of the literature and meta-analysis. Crit Care. 2013;17(5):R208.
23. Elhariri SY, Mohamed H, Burud IAS, Elhariri A. Changing trends in the decompression of tension pneumothorax. J Surg Res. 2019;2:261–6.
24. Clemency BM, Tanski CT, Rosenberg M, et al. Sufficient catheter length for pneumothorax needle decompression: a meta-analysis. Prehosp Disaster Med. 2015;30:249–53.

Intercostal Drainage

23

Ridhima Sharma, Ripon Choudhary, and Anju Gupta

Key Points

- Intercostal drainage is a procedure for removal of air, blood, or fluid collected in the pleural cavity by using a chest drain.
- It is important to counsel the patient and take consent.
- After proper position, it is important to target the safe triangle to minimize the complications.
- One should be aware of potential complication and their management while inserting a chest drain.

23.1 Introduction

Intercostal drainage (chest drain, thoracic catheter) is a procedure done to place a hollow, flexible drainage tube into the chest, for the removal of abnormally collected air, blood, or fluid between the inner and outer lining of the lung. Percutaneous pleural drainage is the third, most common therapeutic procedure after tracheal intubation and vascular catheterization used for the drainage of abnormal collection of air or fluid from the pleural space.

23.2 Historical Background

The concept of chest tube was first illustrated by Hippocrates around 460 BCE, for the treatment of empyema through the insertion of metal-tubes. Playfair was acknowledged as the first physician for the treatment of a child with thoracic empyema and described Water-Seal chest drainage system. In 1910, Robinson added suction to the thoracic drainage by using vacuum air pump. Later on, Lilienthal described the use of a pair of bottles. The 1918 Flu epidemic evolved and perfected the chest tube insertion method and afterwards in the treatment of combat injuries in the world war-II.

23.3 Basic Anatomy and Physiology

The pleural cavity is an air-tight sealed chamber, containing minuscule amount of pleural fluid. The pressure within this space during the breath-

R. Sharma
Department of Anesthesia, AIIMS, Nagpur, India

R. Choudhary
Department of Anaesthesia, LNJP and MAMC Delhi, New Delhi, India

A. Gupta (✉)
Anesthesiology, Pain Medicine, Critical Care, All India Institute of Medical Sciences, New Delhi, Delhi, India

N. Gupta et al. (eds.), *Techniques in Anesthesia, Intensive Care and Emergency Medicine*,
https://doi.org/10.1007/978-981-96-1202-4_23

ing cycle is variable and is sub-atmospheric and decreases during the inspiration.

During the expiration, the intrapleural and intra-pulmonary pressure increases to the level, where they surpass atmospheric pressure, eventually leading the air to flow outside the lungs into the atmospheric surroundings.

Infringement in the pleural integrity creates a severance between the parietal and visceral pleura, thus enabling air or fluid to fill the potential space. The visceral pleura collapses inwards along with the lungs, whereas the parietal pleura recoils along with the chest wall outwards (Fig. 23.1).

23.4 Applied Anatomy

The intercostal spaces contain vein, artery, and nerves along with intercostal muscles, lying in the costal groove along with the inferior margin of the superior rib from above downwards (Fig. 23.2). To evade the neuromuscular bundle injury, chest tube insertion should be done in the interspace just superior to the rib, although insertion very close to the superior margin of the inferior rib may lead to the injury to the intercostal collateral artery.

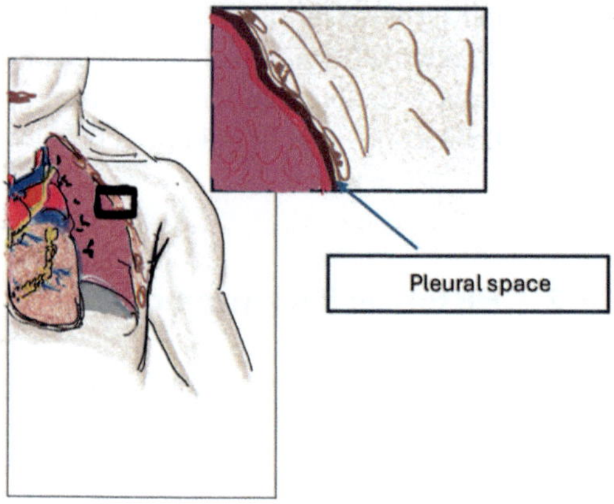

Fig. 23.1 Anatomy of pleural space

Fig. 23.2 Anatomy of intercostal space

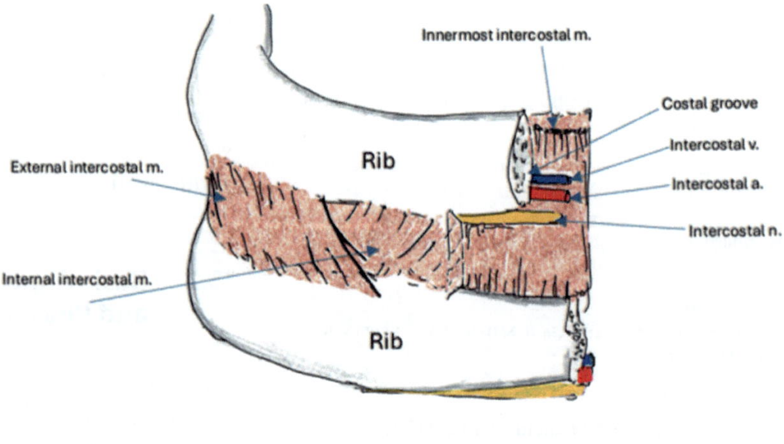

23.5 Indications and Contraindications for ICD Insertion (Table 23.1)

1. Indications
2. Contraindications

   Contraindications are all relative only and the decision depends on the risk versus benefit analysis of the clinical situation (Table 23.2 and Boxes 23.1 and 23.2).

Table 23.1 Indications of ICD insertion

Emergency	Non-emergency
• Pneumothorax – Tension – Spontaneous – Iatrogenic • Hemothorax • Hemopneumothorax • Chylothorax • Bronchopleural fistula • Esophageal rupture, along with gastric leak into pleural space • Penetrating chest trauma • Massive transudative or exudative effusion	• Malignant pleural effusion • Pleurodesis • Empyema • Pleural effusion recurrence • Postoperatively (coronary bypass, thoracotomy, lobectomy) • May be required in the mechanically ventilated patient • Parapneumonic effusions • Therapy-related management

Table 23.2 Contraindications

Contraindications for the chest tube insertion (relative)
• Uncontrolled coagulopathies • Severe thrombocytopenia • Pleural symphysis • Pulmonary/thoracic adhesion • Loculated pleural emphysema or effusion • Pulmonary bullae • Recurrent pulmonary infections • Cardiac patients with more than moderate left ventricular function with small to medium sized pulmonary effusion • Skin infection over the site of skin infection

Box 23.1 Checklist for Patient Preparation

- Clinically evaluate for the need of chest-tube insertion.
- Do chest X-ray, ultrasound or CT scan before insertion of the chest tube and discuss with the radiologist, if required.
- Prior to chest tube insertion, it is wise to avert lung bulla, as it may imitate pneumothorax.
- Explain procedure to the patient or relatives.
- Detailed information about the risk, benefits and complications should be informed.
- Obtain written informed consent.
- The site of the insertion to be marked and verified on the chest X-ray by at least two members involved in the procedure to prevent wrong side insertion.
- Give mild sedation in apprehensive patients.
- Secure intravenous line before the procedure for fluid or medication.
- Apply minimum essential monitoring including saturation, heart rate, blood pressure and electrocardiogram.

Box 23.2 Checklist for ICD Insertion

Insertion Site

The site of chest tube insertion depends upon the indication and location of the abnormality (Table 23.3 and Fig. 23.3). Fluid collects in the dependent part of the chest cavity and air collects in the non-dependent part. In the presence of loculated pleural effusion or empyema, ultrasound-guided needle aspiration to affirm the exact site of insertion of the chest tube is advisable.

Table 23.3 Sites of ICD insertion

Pneumothorax (air)	Tube is inserted above the second intercostal space (anteriorly near the apex of the lung)
Fluids	Tube placed at the 5th or 6th intercostal space (posteriorly near the base of the lung)
Cardiac surgery	Mediastinal tubes to drain fluid around the heart
Hemothorax or both air and blood	Insertion at the base of the lung as well as at the apex

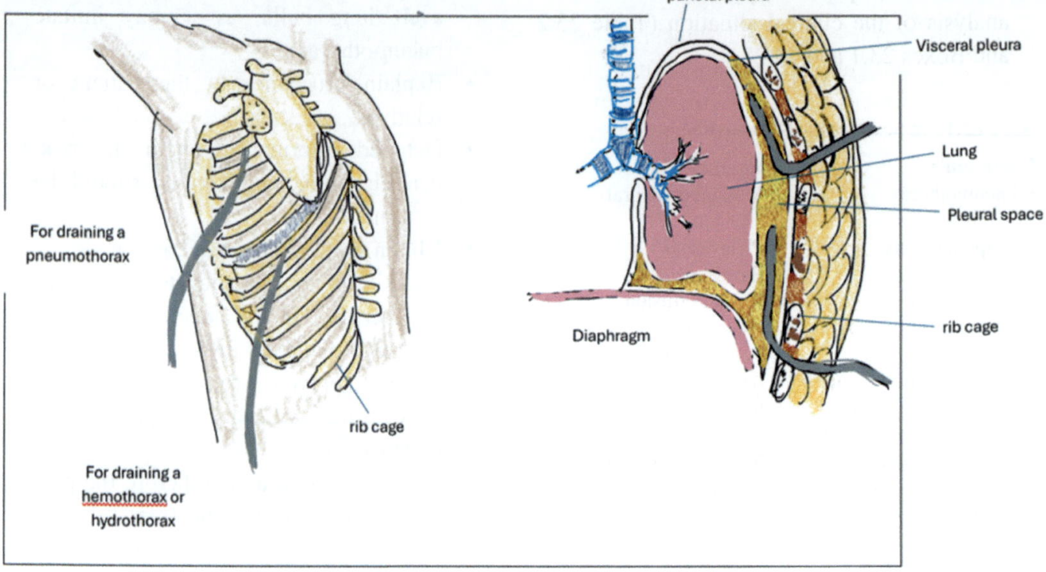

Fig. 23.3 Site of chest tube drainage

23.6 Clinical and Biochemical Assessment Prior to Insertion

- Risk of hemorrhage to be assessed prior to chest tube insertion.
- Routine investigation of the prothrombin time and platelet count are recommended only in patients with existing risk factors.
- Meticulous radiological assessment is required for the differential diagnosis between bullous disease and pneumothorax.
- It is vital to differentiate between the presence of a collapse and pleural effusion particularly in chest X-ray exhibiting a unilateral "Whiteout" picture.
- Lung adherent to the chest wall throughout the hemithorax is a contraindication for the intercostal drain insertion.
- Post pneumonectomy drainage should only be made after the consultation with a Cardiothoracic surgeon.

23.7 Patient Position

The patient is positioned flat generally depending upon the insertion site and content (air or fluid). In order to elevate the body, a small wedge is placed under the shoulder blades, also it gives easy access to the clinician with a wedge placed under the shoulder blades. The arm of the affected lung side is kept away; mostly, it's placed over the patient's head and secured. Excessive adipose tissue may also be needed to be secured out of the way as well.

The British Thoracic Society advocates the use of the "**safe triangle**," an area bordered by

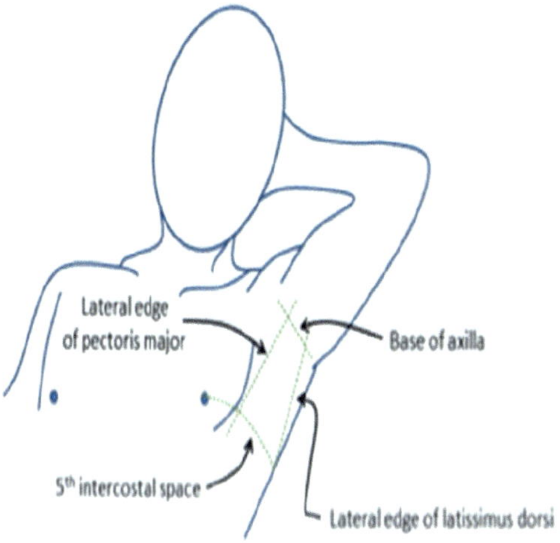

Fig. 23.4 Safe triangle

the anterior border of the latissimus dorsi, the lateral border of the pectoralis major, a line superior to the horizontal level of the nipple, with its apex towards the axillae, the area corresponding to the fifth or sixth space in the midaxillary line (Fig. 23.4).

23.8 Size Selection

There remains constant wrangle about the optimum size of drainage catheter as there exist no large randomized trials, comparing small and large bore tubes. The most appropriate tube size according to weight and age has been shown in the figure.

23.8.1 Selection of Drain Size

- Small bore drains (more comfortable) are recommended more than large bore tubes although there exists no evidence-based therapeutic benefit.

For the monitoring of ongoing further blood loss in acute hemothorax, large bore drains are recommended (Table 23.4).

Table 23.4 Tube size according to age and weight

Tube-size (Fr)	Age	Weight (kg)
8–12	Neonate	>5
10–14	0–1 years	5–10
14–20	1–2 years	10–15
20–24	2–5 years	15–20
20–28	5–10 years	20–30
28–40	>10 years	30–50
32–40	Adults	>50

23.9 Conventional Technique for the Insertion of Chest Tube

1. Identify the proper insertion site, depending upon the pathology. Elevate the head end of the bed (30–60°). Keep the arm of the affected side over the patient's head. Improper positioning can cause vital organ perforation or contralateral pneumothorax.
2. Assemble the chest drainage system according to the recommendations. Connect and adjust the suction to a wall suction outlet until small steady bubbles are observed in the water column.
3. Prepare the skin with Chlorhexidine solution or povidone-iodine and drape the site with sterile sheet.
4. Raise the skin wheel with 25 G needle with L.A (1% solution of Lidocaine with Epinephrine) prior to insertion, e.g., Lignocaine (upto 3 mg/kg). Mild sedation is required in un-cooperated patients.
5. Blunt dissection is advocated for tissues and muscle dissection in the pleural cavity and have become universal (Fig. 23.5). Give 2–3 cm transverse incision through the skin and subcutaneous tissue overlying the interspace. After reaching the superior margin of the rib, close and turn the clamp (Kelly) and push towards the parietal pleura with steady and firm pressure. Open, close and finally withdraw the clamp. Also, prevent the tip of the clamp from penetrating the lung.

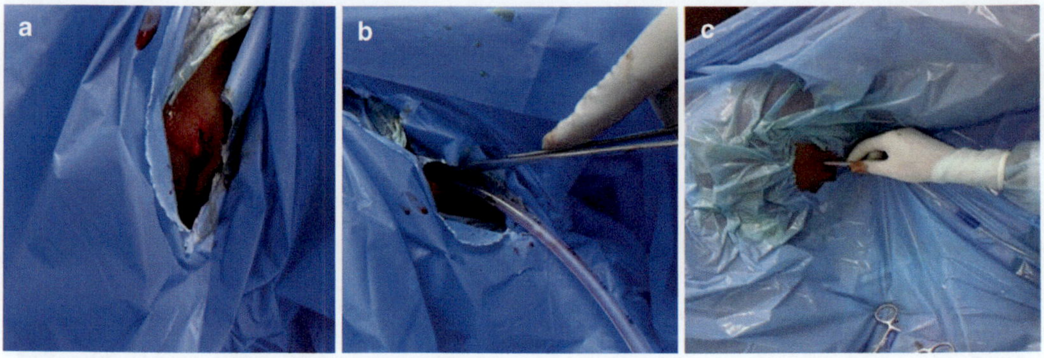

Fig. 23.5 Chest tube insertion technique. (**a**) Stab incision; (**b**) dilatation and insertion of chest tube; and (**c**) chest tube secured in place

6. Insert an index finger to confirm the pleural space, to forbid inadvertent entry into the lung. Also look for any masses or adhesion.
7. Hold the chest tube tip protruding beyond the clamp and advance into the pleural space, guided via finger. Keep the tip direction posteriorly for the drainage of fluid and superiorly for the release of pneumothorax.
8. The proximal hole of the chest tube to be inserted at least 2 cm beyond the rib margin. Finally attach the tube to the pre-assembled suction drainage system.
9. Confirmation of the correct location: Presence of condensation along with the respiration within the tube or drainage of fluid, bubbles at the water-seal level and movement of the water column with respiration confirms the correct placement.
10. 1–0 or 2–0 silk or other non-absorbent suture are used to suture the tube in place. The sutures (two) are tied to provide an airtight seal and pull the soft tissues snugly. First suture is tied across the incision and thereafter both suture ends are winded around the tube and ends will be cut. Place the second suture in a purse-string or mattress suture around the tube at the incision site close to skin. Tie surgeons knot to close the skin around the tube. Wind the loose end and put bow knot around the tube and this knot is later on, after the tube removal is used to close the wound.

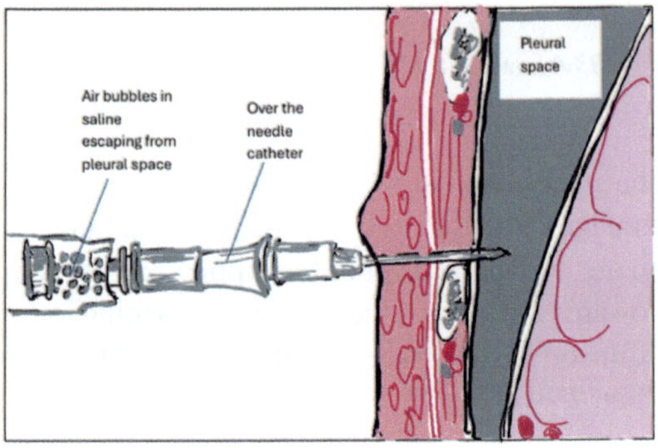

Fig. 23.6 Needle thoracostomy technique

11. Padding should be done to close the wound. Avoid excessive padding and tapes to dress the site which can restrict chest movement.
12. Clinical assessment and chest X-ray should be done for confirmation of the diagnosis. Consider removal once there is less than 100 mL of fluid is drained in 24 h for more than 24 h.

23.9.1 Steps Involved in Chest Tube Insertion

23.9.1.1 Catheter Thoracostomy: Seldinger Method

1. Needle and syringes are used to localize the position of insertion (air/fluid) (Fig. 23.6)
2. Guide wire passed down the hub of the needle, then remove needle and enlarge tract using a dilator

3. Small tube passed over the wire, e.g., pneumonia, effusion, loculated empyema

23.9.1.2 Essential Equipment

- Large or small-bore kit as applicable
- Sterile gown and gloves
- Skin antiseptic solution (e.g., Povidine-iodine or 2% chlorhexidine)
- Sterile drapes
- Gauze swabs
- Syringes and needles (19–25 gauge in adults)
- Local anaesthetic (e.g., lignocaine 1%)
- Scalpel and blade
- Suture kit
- Suture (non-absorbable/1.0–2.0 silk or prolene)
- Instrument for blunt dissection if required (curved clamp)
- Guide wire and dilators for Seldinger technique
- Chest tube

23.10 Chest Drainage System (CDS)

After the chest tube insertion, an integrated CDS is attached. There exist commonly four typed of CDS is attached. There exist four types of CDS

- One-way Heimlich valve
- Three container system
- Digital or electronic CDS
- Simple vacuum bottles

23.10.1 Heimlich Valve

Simple device.

Contains Rubber flutter valve.

Occulted during inspiration (negative intrapleural and intra-tube pressure) thus preventing ingress of air in the pleural cavity.

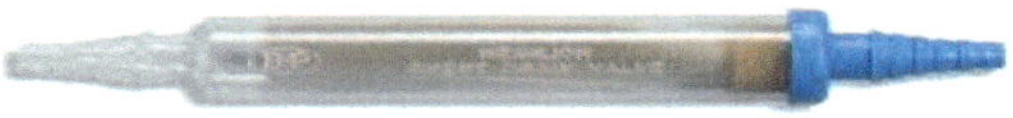

Fig. 23.7 Heimlich valve

Open during expiration (Positive pleural pressure), preventing egress of air of fluid from the pleural space (Fig. 23.7).

Used for pneumothorax, persistent air leaks, tension pneumothorax.

Commercially 8 F catheter coupled with one-way self-contained valve and vent is there.

Allows mobility of the patient.

23.10.2 Three Compartment Chest Drainage System

Most commonly chest drainage system.

Deknatel introduced the first integrated disposable chest drainage unit based on the three-bottle system.

Contains interconnected collecting chamber, water seal and suction control (Fig. 23.8c).

Fluid or air drain into the collecting chamber.

Water seal chamber (usually 2 cm mark to be filled) prevent air from being sucked during inspiration into the pleural space.

Suction chamber may be wet column or dry valve regulator.

Suction mechanism allows suction to adjust for upto -40 cmH_2O (dry), -25 cmH_2O (water).

Mostly, initial pre-set level is -20 cmH_2O.

Connect the drain to the vacuum and gradually increase the suction until gentle bubbling is observed in the suction-control chamber.

Always monitor water levels add sterile water when required.

Bubbling indicate proper functioning.

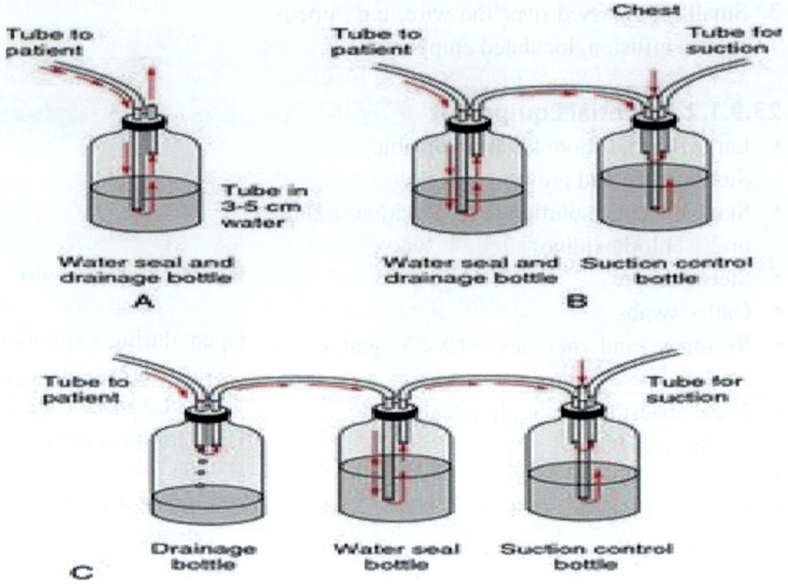

Fig. 23.8 Under water seal drainage system. (**a**) water seal and drainage bottle; (**b**) water seal and drainage bottle with suction control bottle; and (**c**) Drainage bottle with water seal and suction control

23.10.3 Digital Drainage Systems (DDS)

- DDS (Medela, Redax, Thopaz, Dentrex) are used after thoracic surgery and pneumothorax
- Reduced inter-observer variability in air-leak assessment
- Provide continuous digital intra-pleural pressure, fluid drainage and air-leak recording
- Predetermined intrathoracic pressure (usually −8 cmH_2O) is maintained and intervene only to attain the desired value
- Provide ambulation to the patient
- Allows early chest tube removal and shorten the hospital stay also patient can be discharged with these devices in place also, if needed

23.10.4 Vacuum Bottles

- Pleural fluid in the IPC is drained by connecting the exterior one-way valve to a vacuum bottle
- It has 1 L capacity provided by the manufacture or Redon vacuum bottle (disposable); 200, 400, and 600 mL
- In the Aspira catheter, manual pump is connected to the catheter and a collection bag in line
- The patient squeezes the pump to initiate the vacuum effect and the fluid is drained into the collection bag
- Avoid removal of more than 1.5 L in first session
- There exist no data to guide optimal drainage frequency
- Usually varies from once daily to 2–3 times weekly

23.10.5 Wet Suction Control

- The suction control chamber is filled with sterile fluid to the desired height.
- Short suction tubing is connected to a suction source.
- Suction tubing is adjusted to produce bubbling in the suction chamber.
- Increasing suction at the suction source will escalate the airflow through the system, having nominal effect on the chest cavity.
- Excessive source suction will produce loud bubbling disturbing the patient and expediting evaporation of water from the suction control chamber thereby decreasing the suction as the water level lowers.

23.10.6 Dry Suction Control

- Higher suction pressure can be achieved
- Easy set-up

- Self-compensatory regulator instead of a column of water
- Suction can be set at −10, −15, −20, −30, or −40 cm of water
- There is a pre-set −20 cm of water when its opened

23.10.7 Drawback

- Does not provide patient assessment information equivalent to traditional water seal.
- Water level changes indicative of pressure changes in the chest are not there in the dry suction.
- For the detection of adequate air leak, a separate air leak monitor has to be filled with water.

23.11 Potential Sites of Tube Malposition

- Anterior position of the chest tube will cause injury to the muscles and breast tissue.
- More posterior position is uncomfortable and has a high risk of drain leakage.
- Too low chest tube placement has high probability of abdominal placement.
- Inferior placement of the chest tube can perforate the diaphragm and even damage the internal abdominal organs.
- The pathological conditions that elevate the diaphragm including obesity, advanced pregnancy, ascites (massive) and intraabdominal tumours may also perforate the diaphragm.
- The lateral tube insertion in thse fifth, sixth, or seventh intercostal space will enter near the oblique fissure in the chest and if centrally directed can enter the fissure hence both the fissures and the parenchyma are thus potential locus of tube malposition.

23.12 Removal of the Chest Drain

The chest tube should be removed, while the patient is performing Valsalva's maneuver or during expiration (brisk fine movement) and the assistant ties the prior placed closure suture. In pneumothorax, the drain should not be removed until bubbling has ceased.

Clamping of the drain before the removal is generally not required.

23.13 Complications of Chest Tube Insertion (Box 23.3)

Box 23.3 Complications of ICD

Procedure-related lung parenchyma injury	
Complication	Diaphragm injury
	Cardiac or great vessel injury
	Injury to an abdominal organ (stomach, liver, bowel)
	Esophageal injury
	Bronchopleural fistula
	Procedure tract metastases (mesothelioma)
Malposition complication	Tube dislodgment, kinking, occlusion
	Sub-diaphragmatic placement
	Persistent air-leak
	Subcutaneous placement
	Mediastinal placement
	Chest wall tube placement
	Chest drain dislodgement
	Inter-parenchymal placement
	Subcutaneous tube placement
	Chest wall arteriovenous fistula
	Fissural tube placement
Sepsis	Empyema
	Necrotizing chest wall infection
Neuropathic	Horner syndrome
	Phrenic nerve injury
	Intercostal vessel laceration (hemothorax)
	Thoracic duct injury
Shock	Cardiogenic shock from chest tube compression of the right ventricle
	Arrhythmias
Others	Re-expansion pulmonary edema
	Retained catheter fragment
	Recurrent pneumothorax
	Open or tension pneumothorax
	Subcutaneous emphysema

23.14 Role of USG Insertion in ICD Insertion

Chest tubes have been observed to be malpositioned in 20% of cases with expanding figure observed at teaching hospital and in emergency insertion. The American College of Surgeon's advocate chest radiographs (CXR) as the initial choice of imaging followed by gold standard computed tomography (CT).

However, both techniques are expensive, expose the patient to radiations and repositioning causes additional risk and pain. Nowadays, ultrasound (US) has become an important imaging modality in the ICU and emergency departments. Bedside visualization of the pleura by USG is existing part of the eFAST examination· There is no exposure to radiation, requires no shifting and less tube malpositioning is seen.

In order to have high quality images, transducer choice should be optimized. High-frequency linear transducer is used for the best evaluation of the lung, pleural line and delineation of superficial structures. Low frequency transducer helps in the evaluation of deeper thoracic and intra-abdominal structures. For eFAST scan, both high frequency probes are used to evaluate for pneumothorax, low frequency to evaluate intraperitoneal fluid and hemothorax

1. Visualization of the puncture site: The best puncture site is where there is clear visualization of each structures (diaphragm, pleura, organs) and there exist maximum distance between visceral and parietal pleura.
2. Pleural effusion (*V*) is determined by Balik equation *V*(mL)= 20 × Separation (mm).

   Separation = Maximum vertical distance between parietal and visceral pleura in the end of expiration at lung base in supine position with 10–15 elevation.
3. Visualization of the intercostal vessels: Helps in preventing vessel injury. Keep the colour Doppler box on the bottom edge of the rib.
4. Identification for the optimal site for the puncture: Use a low frequency (3.5–5 MHz) ultrasound transducer (convex or phased array probe) to identify the best puncture site.
5. Ultrasound-guided puncture: To minimize the risk of neurovascular bundle injury the transducer to follow the needle trajectory and advanced slowly, at upper edge of the rib at appropriate intercostal space under visualization. For direct needle guidance, the correct position of the needle tip is visualized in real-time and constantly monitored.
6. Guidewire insertion and position check: visualized as a hyperechoic linear structure from the insertion point at the skin surface to the hypoechoic effusion. Vertical rotation of the probe allows visualization of the guidewire over the intercostal space.
7. Ultrasound confirmation. At the end of the procedure, it is mandatory to perform a complete bilateral lung ultrasound scan to exclude any potential trauma or complication.

Suggested Reading

1. Hippocrates (Potter P, trans.). Hippocrates, vol. VI. Cambridge, MA: Harvard University Press; 1988. p. 39–43.
2. Playfair GE. Case of empyema treated by aspiration and subsequently by drainage: recovery. Br Med J. 1875;1:45.
3. Robinson S. Acute thoracic empyema. Avoidance of chronic empyema. Rib trephining for suction drainage. Boston Med Surg J. 1910;163:561–70.
4. Lilienthal H. Thoracic surgery. Philadelphia: Saunders; 1926. vol. I, p. 24, 52–6; vol. II, p. 156–7.
5. Miller KS, Sahn SA. Chest tubes. Indications, technique, management and complications. Chest. 1987;91(2):258–64.
6. Domke MN. Get a positive outcome from negative pressure. In: Nursing made incredibly easy, vol. 8(1). Philadelphia: Wolters Kluwer; 2010. p. 20–9.
7. Durai R, Hoque H, Davies TW. Managing a chest tube and drainage system. AORN J. 2010;91(2):275–83.
8. Azoulay E. Pleural effusions in the intensive care unit. Curr Opin Pulm Med. 2003;9(4):291–7.
9. Kane CJ, York NL, Minton LA. Chest tubes in the critically ill patient. Dimens Crit Care Nurs. 2013;32(3):111–7.
10. English JC, Leslie KO. Pathology of the pleura. Clin Chest Med. 2006;27(2):157–80.
11. Coughlin AM, Parchinsky C. Go with the flow of chest tube therapy. Nursing. 2006;36(3):36–41.
12. Rosenberg ER. Ultrasound in the assessment of pleural densities. Chest. 1983;84:283–5.

13. Bauman M, Handley C. Chest-tube care: the more you know, the easier it gets. Am Nurse Today. 2011;6(9):27–32.
14. Bosman A, De Jong MB, Debeij J, Van den Broek PJ, Schipper IB. Systematic review and meta-analysis of antibiotic prophylaxis to prevent infections from chest drains in blunt and penetrating thoracic injuries. Br J Surg. 2012;99(4):506–13.
15. Da Rocha RP, Vengjer A, Blanco A, de Carvalho PT, Mongon ML, Fernandes GJ. Size of the collateral intercostal artery in adults: anatomical considerations in relation to thoracocentesis and thoracoscopy. Surg Radiol Anat. 2002;24(1):23–6.
16. Ellis H. The applied anatomy of chest drain insertion. Br J Hosp Med. 2007;68(3):M44–5.
17. Webb WR, LaBerge JM. Radiographic recognition of chest tube malposition in the major fissure. Chest. 1984;85(1):81–3.
18. Tomlinson MA, Treasure T. Insertion of a chest drain: how to do it. Br J Hosp Med. 1997;58:248–52.
19. Laws D, Neville E, Duffy J, Pleural Diseases Group, Standards of Care Committee, British Thoracic Society. BTS guidelines for the insertion of a chest drain. Thorax. 2003;58 Suppl 2:ii53–9.
20. Kiefer T. Chest drains in clinical practice. Cham: Springer; 2017.
21. Gogakos A, Barbetakis N, Lazaridis G, Papaiwannou A, Karavergou A, Lampaki S, et al. Heimlich valve and pneumothorax. Ann Transl Med. 2015;3:54.
22. George RS, Papagiannopoulos K. Advances in chest drain management in thoracic disease. J Thorac Dis. 2016;8(Suppl 1):S55–64.
23. Mullon JJ, Burkart KM, Silvestri G, Hogarth DK, Almeida F, Berkowitz D, et al. Interventional pulmonology fellowship accreditation standards: executive summary of the Multisociety Interventional Pulmonology Fellowship Accreditation Committee. Chest. 2017;151:1114–21.
24. Arai H, Tajiri M, Kameda Y, Shiino K, Ando K, Okudela K, et al. Evaluation of a digital drainage system (Thopaz) in over 250 cases at a single site: a retrospective case-control study. Clin Respir J. 2018;12(4):1454–9.
25. Gillen J, Lau C. Permanent indwelling catheters in the management of pleural effusions. Thorac Surg Clin. 2013;23:63–71.
26. Dugan KC, Laxmanan B, Murgu S, Hogarth DK. Management of persistent air leaks. Chest. 2017;152:417–23.
27. Kool DR, Blickman JG. Advanced trauma life support. ABCDE from a radiological point of view. Emerg Radiol. 2007;14:135–41.
28. Chun R, Kirkpatrick AW, Sirois M, et al. Where's the tube? Evaluation of hand-held ultrasound in confirming endotracheal tube placement. Prehosp Disaster Med. 2004;19:366–9.
29. Lichtenstein D, Meziere G, Biderman P, et al. The "lung point": an ultrasound sign specific to pneumothorax. Intensive Care Med. 2000; 26:1434–40.
30. Stone MB, Secko MA. Bedside ultrasound diagnosis of pulmonary contusion. Pediatr Emerg Care. 2009;25:854–5.

24 Spinal Anesthesia

Poonam Motiani and Deepti Agarwal

Key Points

- Spinal anesthesia is a type of neuraxial anesthesia that is used for a variety of lower extremity, lower abdominal, pelvic, and perineal procedures.
- A spinal needle is inserted into the subarachnoid space at the lumbar level to inject an anesthetic solution into cerebrospinal fluid (CSF).
- Spinal anesthesia can be performed in the sitting; lateral decubitus; or, less commonly, prone position.
- Incidence of Post dural puncture headache (PDPH) is lower with smaller gauge (24–27 gauge), pencil point needles and when bevel of cutting needles is kept longitudinal during dural puncture.
- Spinal anesthesia can be performed using a midline or paramedian approach. The midline approach may be easier, while the paramedian approach may be more successful for patients unable to flex the lumbar spine.
- Spinal anesthetic drugs are chosen to achieve the required spinal level and duration of anesthesia.
  - Duration of block is determined by the choice of local anesthetic (LA).
  - Important determinants of the extent of sensory block are the dose and baricity of the anesthetic solution.
  - Adjuvants may be added to LA solutions to alter baricity, improve the quality, or extend the duration of spinal block.
  - After spinal anesthesia, the patient must be monitored as for GA, (Continuous ECG, HR, NIBP, SpO_2, $EtCO_2$). The level of block should be assessed prior to the start of the surgical procedure.

24.1 Background

Spinal anesthesia (SA) or subarachnoid block (SAB) is an integral part of anesthesia practice. In 1898, August Bier, with his assistant, performed spinal anesthesia in six patients using intrathecal cocaine. Even more than a century later, SA continues to be an indispensable anesthetic technique.

Spinal anesthesia provides profound and reversible autonomic, sensory and motor block-

P. Motiani (✉)
Paediatric Anaesthesia, Post Graduate Institute of Child Health, Noida, Uttar Pradesh, India

D. Agarwal
Anaesthesiology and Critical Care, U.C.M.S & GTBH, New Delhi, India

N. Gupta et al. (eds.), *Techniques in Anesthesia, Intensive Care and Emergency Medicine*,
https://doi.org/10.1007/978-981-96-1202-4_24

ade below a spinal dermatome following deposition of a small quantity of local anesthetic in the subarachnoid space, usually sufficient for surgeries on lower limb and lower abdomen. When properly conducted in carefully selected patients, it offers an excellent safety profile. Royal College of Anaesthetists analyzing 324,950 spinal anesthetics reported the incidence of harm (symptoms persisting for more than 6 months) to be 2.6 per 100,000 cases and incidence of paraplegia or death as 2.1 per 100,000 cases, incidence being lower with spinal than with an epidural or CSE block.

24.2 Indications

Spinal anesthesia is usually indicated for infra-umblical surgeries (Table 24.1). Upper abdominal surgeries maybe conducted, under SA, with caution and after weighing the risks-benefits . SA has been particularly useful for cesarean sections as it avoids risk of difficult airway and aspiration.

Table 24.1 Level of spinal anesthesia required for common surgical procedures

Procedure	Dermatomal level
Upper abdominal surgery	T4
Cesarean section	T4
Intestinal, gynecologic, and urologic surgery	T6
Transurethral resection of the prostate	T10
Vaginal delivery of a fetus and hip surgery	T10
Thigh surgery and lower leg amputations	L1
Foot and ankle surgery	L2
Perineal and anal surgery	S2 to S5 (saddle block)

24.3 Contraindications

The absolute and relative contraindications to SA are tabulated (Table 24.2).

Table 24.2 Contraindications of spinal anesthesia

Absolute	Relative
Patient refusal	Coagulopathy (pre-existing or drug induced)
Lack of patient cooperation for positioning	Systemic sepsis
Infection at the site of needle insertion	Fixed cardiac output state (severe MS/AS or HOCM)
Severe uncorrected hypovolemia	Pre-existing neurological deficits
Raised intracranial pressure	
Allergy to drug used	

MS = mitral stenosis; AS = aortic stenosis; HOCM = hypertrophic obstructive cardiomyopathy

24.4 Relevant Anatomy

Spinal cord is invested by three membranes: pia mater, a vascular layer closely adhered to the spinal cord and brain. Outside it lies the arachnoid mater, an avascular layer attached to outer dura mater. Space outside dura mater is the epidural space, between dura and arachnoid is subdural space and that between arachnoid and pia mater is subarachnoid space (Fig. 24.1). Contents of the subarachnoid space include CSF, spinal nerves, and blood vessels. The dural sac of spinal cord extends till S2 vertebral level. The Conus medullaris, terminal end of spinal cord, may lie at the lower border of L1 (in most) or at L2, so it is considered safe to perform a spinal block below L3.

Five ligaments are responsible for maintaining the stability of spine, and three of them are pierced during SAB, namely the supraspinous ligament which joins the tip of the spinous process of each vertebra, the interspinous ligament which joins the adjacent spinous processes and ligamentum flavum which lies just outside the epidural space (Fig. 24.2). Ligamentum flavum, made of right and left ligaments has variable thickness, ranging from 3.65 ± 1.16 to 3.84 ± 1.12 mm in adults (L4–L5 level). The line joining the uppermost border of iliac crests, the intercristal line, passes through the spinous process of L4 vertebra or through the L4–L5 interspace. Mean distance from skin to subarachnoid space is 4.37 ± 0.31 cm.

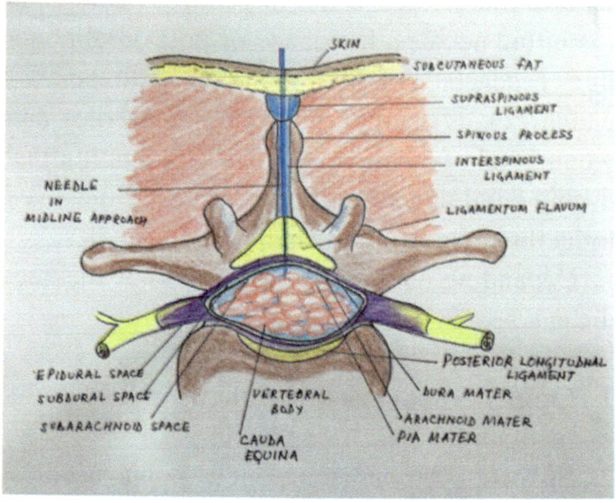

Fig. 24.1 Transverse view at the level L4. Relations of dura mater and contents

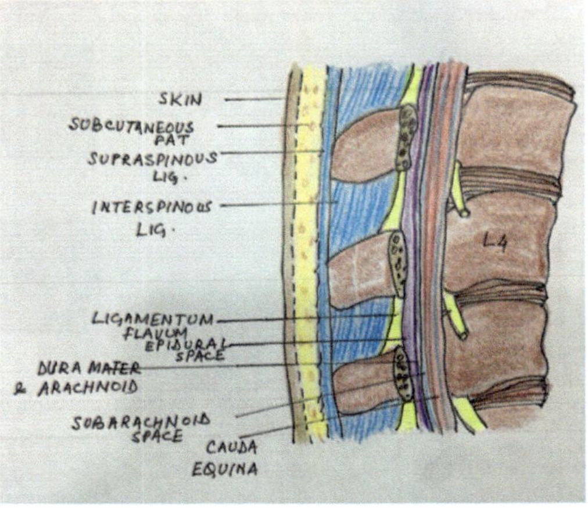

Fig. 24.2 Sagittal view of vertebral anatomy at L4

24.5 Sonoanatomy

On ultrasonography, posterior bony lumbar vertebra cast a dense acoustic shadow and vertebral canal is visualized only through soft tissue acoustic window through either interlaminar or interspinous processes. Using a low-frequency (2–5 MHz), curved-array probe the two most important views to approach vertebral canal are:

Parasagittal oblique view—Probe in slight parasagital plane overlying the articular surface is tilted to direct the beam latero-medially until the humped pattern of articular surface changes to sawtooth pattern of lamina. The gap between the teeth is the interlaminar space and gives soft tissue window for vertebral canal (Fig. 24.3).

Transverse interlaminar view—Probe is placed in midline and moved in cephalad or caudad directions with slight cephalad tilt to make the beam enter the acoustic window between the spinous process (Fig. 24.3).

Ultrasound in spinal anesthesia is particularly a useful adjunct in difficult back scenarios.

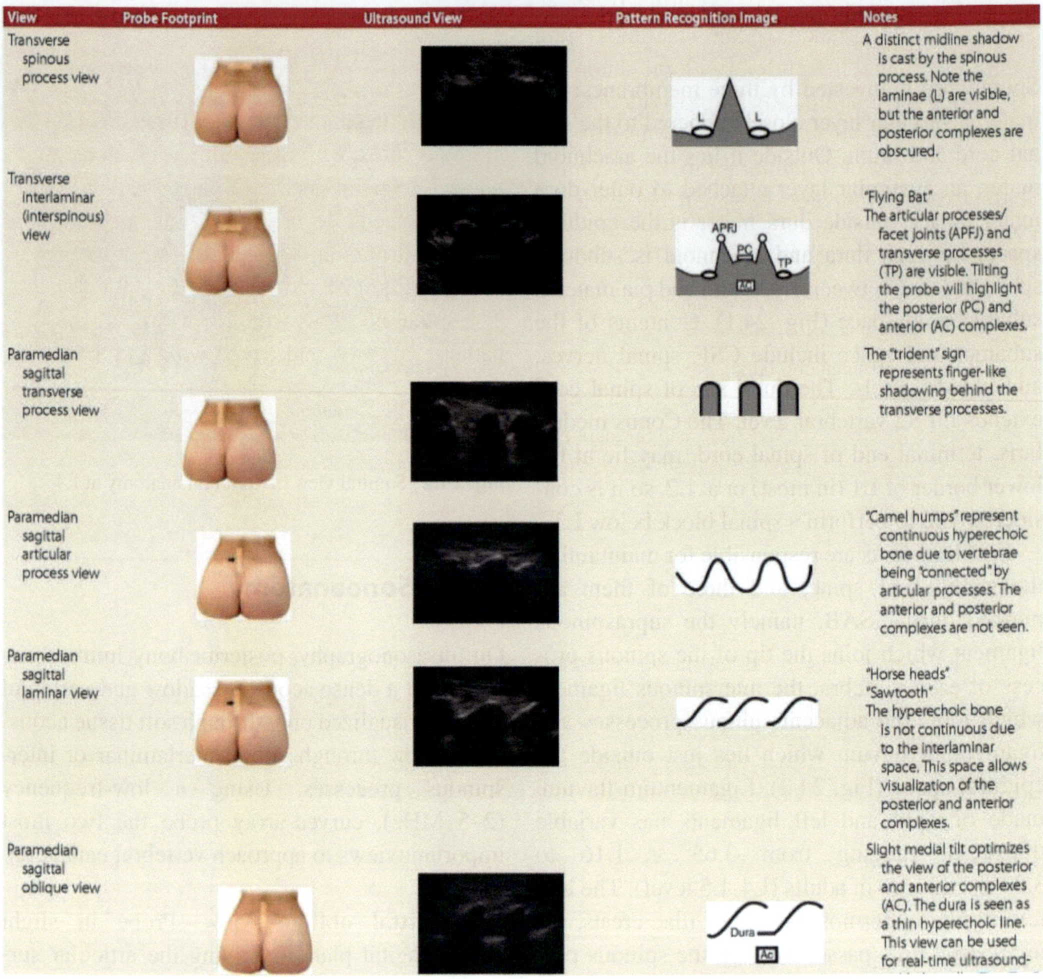

Fig. 24.3 Sonoanatomy of the lumber spine. (Reproduced with permission from Nysora)

24.6 Technique of Subarachnoid Block

24.6.1 Equipment

These include a disposable or sterile tray, sterile gauges, drapes, sponge holding forceps and a small container for skin disinfectant (Fig. 24.4), usually 5–10% povidone iodine or 2–4% chlorhexidine solution in alcohol. The spinal drug should be chosen based on the duration and type of surgery; an adjuvant may be added.

Disposable, single use, styletted spinal needles are commonly used. Pencil point needles give a better tactile sensation of structures but require more force while inserting as compared to cutting needles. Incidence of post dural puncture headache (PDPH) is lower with smaller gauge (24–27 gauge), pencil point needles and when bevel of cutting needles is kept longitudinal during dural puncture. Introducers are often used to facilitate insertion of small gauge needles.

Depending on type of tip (Fig. 24.5) the needle can be:

1. **Quincke-Babcock**—Needle with sharp point, medium length, cutting bevel.
2. **Sprotte**—Atraumatic pencil point needles, noncutting bevel, solid tip and an opening for drug.

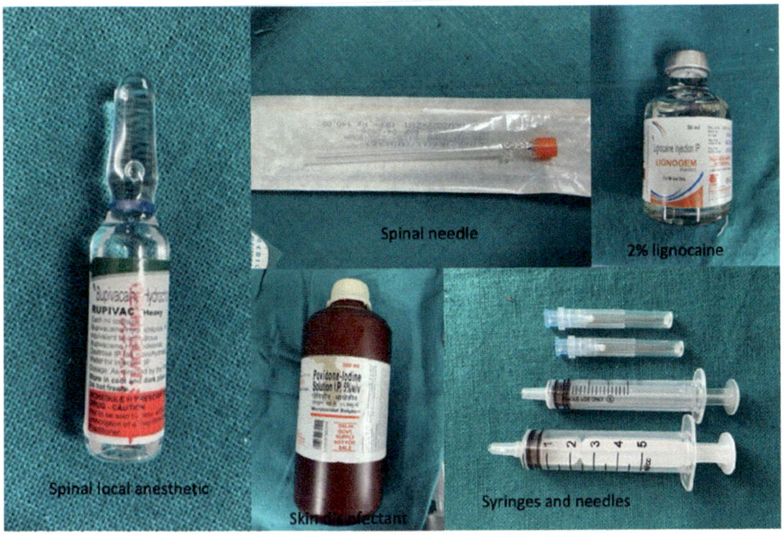

Fig. 24.4 Equipment required for spinal anesthesia

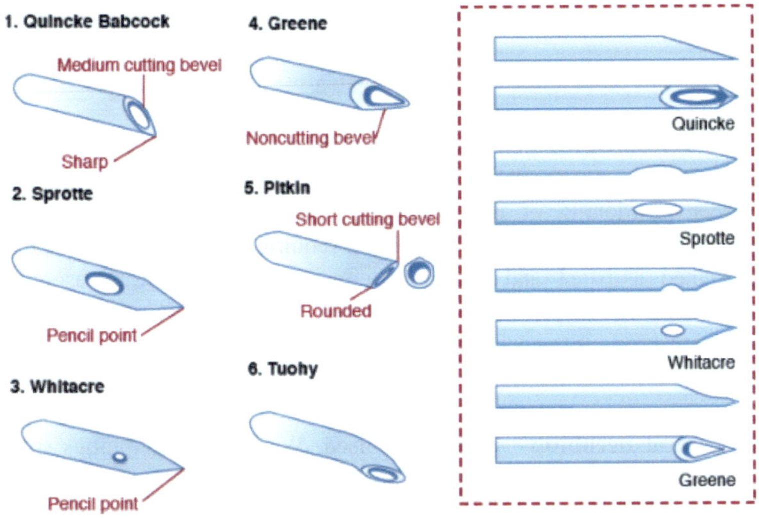

Fig. 24.5 Types of spinal needles

3. **Whitacre**—Pencil point needles with a non-cutting bevel, solid tip and an opening for drug located 2–4 mm proximal to the tip.
4. **Greene**—Needle with rounded point and rounded noncutting bevel.
5. **Pitkin needle**—Needle with rounded point, short length bevel.
6. **Tuohy**—Blunt tip, curved needle, used for catheter insertion.

24.6.2 Minimum Mandatory Monitoring

It is imperative to establish continuous ECG, non-invasive blood pressure, pulse oximetry monitoring, ensuring an intravenous line and resuscitation equipment prior to institution of the block.

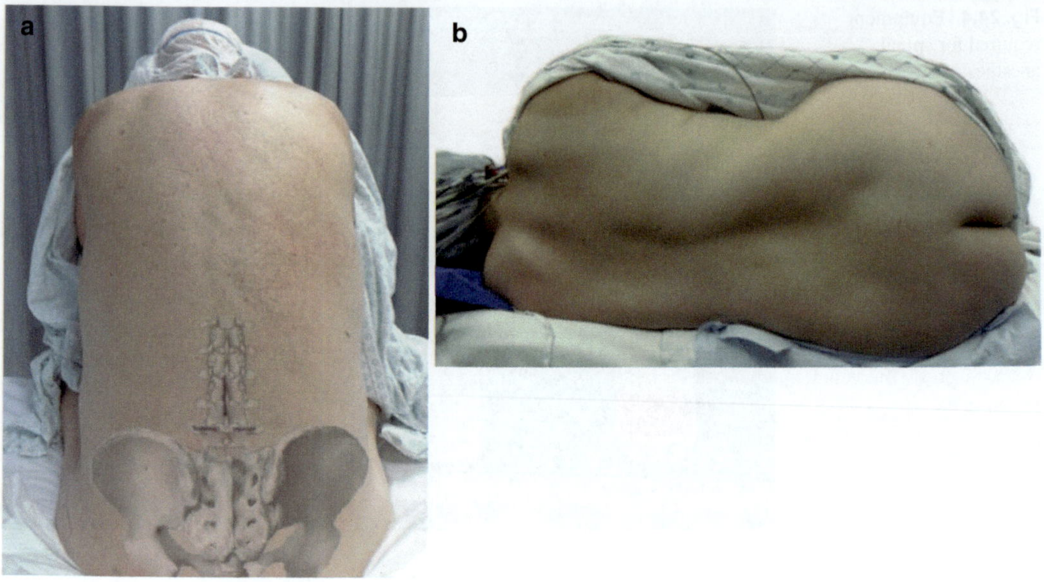

Fig. 24.6 (**a**) Patient in sitting position. (**b**) Patient in lateral decubitus position. (Reproduced from Nysora with permission)

24.6.3 Positioning: Lateral or Sitting

Proper positioning of the patient, of utmost importance for successful performance, requires a trained assistant and patient's cooperation. Depending on nature of surgery and patient factors, can be performed in one of the following positions.

1. **Lateral decubitus**—Commonly used. With the patient lying on his side, the back is positioned parallel to edge of the operating table and knees and hips are flexed to the abdomen and neck flexed (Fig. 24.6b).
2. **Sitting position**—Used when difficult to palpate the lumbar spinous processes. With the patient sitting, legs supported on a stool, a pillow is kept on the lap t and the patient made to flex on it while pushing the lumbar spine backward. Also used for saddle blocks (Fig. 24.6a).
3. **Prone position**—Commonly used for procedures on perineum or rectum, where the operative position of patient is prone. Hypobaric local anesthetic may be used.

24.6.4 Procedure (Midline Approach)

1. ***Prepare the back of patient***—After instituting monitoring and positioning the patient, using an aseptic technique, the back of the patient is prepared using a disinfectant solution, giving adequate time for its action.
2. ***Palpate the lumbar interspinous space***—Thereafter, the back is palpated to identify interspinous spaces and the iliac crests. The intercristal line (Tuffier's Line) is a horizontal line corresponding to the highest points of both the iliac crests and corresponds to L4–L5 interspace.
3. ***Local infiltration h***—The chosen interspace is infiltrated using 2% lignocaine in 2 mL syringe.
4. ***Performing spinal block***—Spinal needle is inserted in the chosen interspace, with a slight cephalic tilt to pierce the skin, subcutaneous fat, supraspinous ligament, interspinous ligament, ligamentum flavum and finally dura mater with arachnoid mater attached to it. A clear pop is felt on passing through the dura. Upon obtaining clear CSF, the syringe (with

spinal drug) is attached to the hub of the spinal needle, using a rotation movement, with the non-dependent hand stabilizing it and drug injected at 0.5 mL/s. If bone is encountered while inserting spinal needle, it should be withdrawn up to the skin and redirected keeping in mind the three-dimensional anatomy of spinal vertebra, after confirming midline and correct patient positioning.

Do's and don't's of spinal anesthesia technique

Do's	Don't's
Position the patient properly keeping in mind patient comfort	Don't inject through an infected area
Follow aseptic precautions strictly	Don't inject if there is blood on aspiration
Perform local infiltration	Don't inject in presence of persistent paresthesia
Inject drugs meant for neuraxial use—read the labels carefully	Continuously monitor ECG, HR, NIBP during procedure
Always be prepared for administering general anesthesia	Don't attempt multiple punctures

24.7 Other Approaches

1. ***Paramedian approach***—In this approach, the spinal needle is inserted 1 cm lateral to the superior border of inferior spinous process, slightly medially angulated (10–15°) to reach ligamentum flavum, and then the dura.
2. ***Taylor approach***—The Taylor, (or lumbosacral approach), a paramedian approach, can be used when other approaches are unsuccessful or cannot be performed. Here, the spinal needle is directed toward the L5–S1 interspace, the largest interspace by inserting it, 1 cm medial and inferior to the posterior superior iliac spine, angulated 45–55° cephalad and medially to reach ligamentum flavum, and then the dura.

24.8 Trouble Shooting a Failed or Partial Spinal Block

- Assess the failure; Inform the surgeon and reassure the patient.
- In case of a partial block, manipulating position of patient, with the use of gravity particularly if a hyperbaric solution has been used, have been used successfully. Sedation and analgesic supplements have also been tried.
- If inadequate/no block, a spinal may be repeated or general anesthesia administered. If the spinal is repeated, due consideration should be given to the interspace and the drug chosen.

Advantages and disadvantages of spinal anesthesia:

Advantages	Disadvantages
Simple and cost-effective technique	Difficult in patients with spinal deformity/previous spinal surgeries
Lower risk of deep vein thrombosis, pulmonary complications and blood transfusion requirements, than GA	Hypotension is the most frequent side effect (due to sympathetic block)
May avoid airway management complications of difficult airway and risk of aspiration	Inadequate block, subdural block, inadvertent high spinal, or total spinal block are known complications
Technique of choice in obstetrics	Inadequate pain relief or discomfort when used alone for intra-abdominal surgeries
Excellent safety profile	May be inadequate for long duration surgeries; may require supplementation with anxiolytics and analgesia

Drugs: **Dose**, **Route**, **Concentration**, **Bolus/Infusion.**

24.9 Local Anesthetics

The choice of local anesthetic is based on potency of the agent, onset and duration of anesthesia, and side effects of the drug. Two distinct groups used are esters and amides (Table 24.3) and provide a duration of action from 45 to 400 min.

Procaine one of the oldest spinal anesthetic, with brief action (<1 h), is used less frequently than lidocaine because of a higher frequency of nausea (unexplained cause) and anesthetic failure rate, and a slower time to recovery; Used as a hyperbaric drug (10%); Dose 50–200 mg.

Lidocaine, often chosen for shorter procedures (<1.5 h); Onset <5 min; Available in two concentrations, 2% and 5%. Transient neurologic symptoms (TNS) have been reported following its use, most frequently after ambulatory procedures with patients in lithotomy or knee arthroscopy positions; No evidence yet, to link these symptoms with subclinical neurologic injury. A Cochrane review of TNS strongly discourages the use of the term, TNS, to avoid linking the clinical symptoms of back and leg pain to neurologic change after the use of lidocaine, which remains unproven.

Long-acting agents for spinal anesthesia include tetracaine, bupivacaine, ropivacaine, and levobupivacaine.

Bupivacaine: Commonly used preparation: 0.5% Heavy; 0.75% Heavy, I 0.5% Isobaric for procedures lasting up to 2–2.5 h.

Ropivacaine, an amide local anesthetic, is 1.8–2 times less potent than bupivacaine and with less effect on the cardiac conduction system.

Levobupivacaine, the isolated (*S*)-enantiomer of bupivacaine, is available for use. However, when used as a spinal anesthetic, where systemic toxicity is minimal, offers little clinical advantage over racemic bupivacaine.

24.10 Spinal Anesthetic Adjuvants

Several classes of medications can be added to the LA solution to improve or change the distribution of the block.

1. **Dextrose**—Lidocaine and bupivacaine are commercially prepared with dextrose in order to make the solutions hyperbaric.
2. **Opioids**—Opioids have been used as intrathecal adjuvants, to improve intraoperative and postoperative analgesia, particularly the discomfort of visceral manipulation during abdominal surgeries (e.g., manipulation of the uterus during cesarean delivery).
   (a) Morphine—A hydrophilic opioid; Dose—75–200 μg; Onset of analgesia: 30–60 min; duration 12–36 h. Common side effects: nausea, vomiting, and pruritus. A less common but serious side effect is delayed respiratory depression (6–18 h after the intrathecal injection).
3. Fentanyl **and** sufentanil—Lipid-soluble opioids; such as fentanyl (10–25 μg) and sufentanil (2.5–10 μg) used as intrathecal adjuvants, improve intraoperative analgesia, and for labor analgesia; provide minimal postoperative analgesia due to short duration of action (4–6 h); not associated with delayed respiratory depression. Pruritus is a common, dose-related side effect.
4. **Alpha adrenergic agonists** (e.g., epinephrine, clonidine)—As intrathecal adjuvants, they increase the density of sensory and motor

Table 24.3 Drug selection for hyperbaric spinal anesthesia

	Dose (mg)		Duration (min)	
Local anesthetic	To T10	To T4	Plain	Epinephrine, 0.2 mg
Lidocaine (5% in 7.5% dextrose)	50–60	75–100	60	75–100
Tetracaine (0.5% in 5% dextrose)	6–8	10–16	70–90	100–150
Bupivacaine (0.75% in 8.5% dextrose)	8–10	12–20	90–120	100–150
Ropivacaine (0.5% in dextrose)	12–18	18-25	80–110	
Levobupivacaine	8–10	12–20	90–120	100–150

block, prolong the duration of action, and may contribute to postoperative analgesia by acting at alpha-adrenergic receptors in the spinal cord.

(a) Epinephrine—Augments the block by direct alpha-adrenergic agonist activity on CNS receptors and by causing vasoconstriction, leading to decreased vascular absorption and subsequent increased neural tissue uptake of the LA; Dose: 100–200 µg.

(b) Clonidine—**Less commonly used; Prolongs the action.**

(c) Phenylephrine—Its mechanism of action and effects are similar to epinephrine. However, has gone into disrepute due to its association with transient neurologic symptoms.

5. **Magnesium**—*N*-methyl-D-aspartate (NMDA) receptor antagonist; modifies nociceptive modulation. Prolongs the duration of spinal anesthesia; limited safety data (i.e., regarding neurotoxicity).

Table 24.4 Factors postulated to alter to spinal anesthetic block height

Patient characteristics
• Age
• Height
• Weight
• Gender
• Intra-abdominal pressure
• Anatomic configuration of the spinal column
Technique of injection
• Site of injection*
• Direction of injection (needle)
• Direction of bevel
• Use of barbotage
• Rate of injection
Characteristics of spinal fluid
• Volume*
• Pressure (cough, strain, Valsalva maneuver)
• Density*
Characteristics of the anesthetic solution
• Density*
• Amount (mass)
• Concentration*
• Temperature
• Volume*
• Vasoconstrictors

24.11 Factors Affecting Block Height

Of more than 20 factors postulated (Table 24.4), only some factors (*) have been documented to influence block height.

24.12 Risks of Spinal Anesthesia: Complications

Complications of spinal blockade are divided into major (rare), moderate (not uncommon), and minor (common) complications (Table 24.5).

Table 24.5 Complications of spinal anesthesia

Minor	Moderate	Major
• Nausea and vomiting • Mild hypotension • Shivering • Itch • Transient mild hearing impairment • Urinary retention	• Failed spinal • Postdural puncture headache (PDPH)	• Direct needle trauma • Infection (abscess, meningitis) • Vertebral canal hematoma • Spinal cord ischemia • Cauda equina syndrome • Arachnoiditis • Peripheral nerve injury • Total spinal anesthesia • Cardiovascular collapse • Death

24.13 Minor Complications of Spinal Anesthesia

1. ***Nausea and Vomiting***:
   (a) Intraoperative nausea and vomiting (IONV) is distressing and may impede surgery. Incidence: Nonobstetric surgery (42%); Higher in parturient (80%).
   (b) Causes: Patient factors—anxiety, decreased lower esophageal sphincter tone, increased gastric pressure, vagal hyperactivity; Surgical factors—exteriorization of the uterus, peritoneal traction; Other causes—systemic opioids, uterotonic drugs, antibiotics, hypotension, intrathecal additives, inadequate block, or high block (higher than T6).
2. ***Hypotension***: Incidence-Variable (15–33%) due to varying definitions of hypotension. Mainly due to blockage of preganglionic sympathetic fibers leading to venodilation and a decrease in preload, others being a fall in afterload, contractility and heart rate. Higher the sympathetic block, more severe is the hypotension. Co-loading with crystalloids, appropriate patient positioning, using minimal dose local anesthetic and appropriate use of vasopressors are some of treatment measures.
3. ***Shivering*** Both neuraxial anesthesia and GA induce shivering strategies suggested to reduce neuraxial shivering include use of a forced air warmer, avoiding cold epidural or intravenous fluids, intrathecal fentanyl 20 μg, intrathecal meperidine 10 mg, or intravenous ondansetron 8 mg. Treatment includes administration of intravenous meperidine 50 mg or intravenous tramadol 0.25–1 mg/kg.
4. ***Itch***: Pruritis, a well-known side effect of opiates, is commoner when administered spinally (46%) than epidurally (8.5%) or through systemic routes. Treatment is naloxone, nalbuphine, ondansetron etc.
5. ***Postoperative Urinary Retention***: Postoperative urinary retention (POUR), after neuraxial block, is due to neural interruption of the micturition reflex (parasympathetic blockade of S2–S4 segments) and bladder overdistention. Patient risk factors include male sex, previous urologic dysfunction; Surgical risk factors include pelvic or prolonged surgery and anesthetic factors are anticholinergic drugs, opioids, and fluid administration (>1000 mL).

24.14 Moderate Complications

1. **Post-dural puncture headache (PDPH)**: a moderately debilitating neurological complication; a common cause for medicolegal claims. Obstetric patients are at higher risk. Multiple punctures, larger needle size, needle type (cutting > separating), lesser body mass index (BMI), female gender, younger age, h/o recurrent headaches, h/o previous PDPH, are all associated with a higher incidence. Use of spinal catheters and timing of ambulation have not been shown to increase the incidence.
   (a) **Major complications of spinal anesthesia** Permanent neurologic disability.

Causes include: ***Direct Needle Trauma***: The elicitation of paresthesias, a risk factor for persistent neurologic injury, indicates that the spinal needle may be adjacent to or penetrating neural tissue; if the latter, injection of local anesthetic into the spinal nerve may result in permanent neurologic damage.

(b) ***Meningitis***: Meningitis, either bacterial or aseptic, can occur after spinal anesthesia. Bacterial meningitis may be caused by contaminated spinal trays and medication, oral flora of the anesthesiologist, and patient infection. In the first half of the twentieth century, most cases of meningitis after spinal anesthesia were aseptic and were traced to chemical contamination and detergents.

(c) ***Vertebral Canal Hematoma***: Rare but devastating complication; Usually occurs in the epidural space, rarely in the subarachnoid space; the source being an injured artery or vein. Spinal hematoma and ischemia carry a poorer prognosis than infective complications. If new or progressive neurologic symptoms develop, an immediate neurosurgery consult should be sought. Magnetic resonance imaging (MRI) spine is confirmatory.

(d) ***Spinal Cord Ischemia***: The anterior spinal cord is more prone to ischemia than the posterior cord, due to its supply by abundant anastomoses. Proposed mechanisms include prolonged hypotension, the addition of vasoconstrictors to local anesthetics, and compression of arterial supply by vertebral canal hematoma.

(e) ***Cauda Equina Syndrome***: Reported with the use of continuous spinal microcatheters. Risk factors include lithotomy position, hyperbaric 5% lidocaine and repeated dosing of LA through continuous spinal catheters.

(f) ***Arachnoiditis***: Causes include infection; myelograms using oil-based dyes; blood in the intrathecal space, neuroirritant or neurolytic substances intrathecally, surgical interventions, intrathecal corticosteroids and trauma.

(g) ***Peripheral Nerve Injury***: The spinal anesthesia induced sensory block, may indirectly result in peripheral nerve injury. Therefore, care must be taken with appropriate positioning, avoidance of tight plaster casts, and observation of distal circulation of limbs rendered insensate by spinal anesthesia.

2. ***Total Spinal Anesthesia*** (TSA): Manifests with respiratory depression, cardiovascular compromise, and loss of consciousness; May be preceded by numbness, paresthesia, or weakness of the upper limb, shortness of breath, nausea or anxiety. It is important to provide cardiorespiratory support and anxiolysis.
3. ***Cardiovascular Collapse***: Cardiovascular collapse, though rare, can occur, after spinal anesthesia.

24.15 Estimating the Risks of the Major Complications of Spinal Anesthesia

The NAP3 study, of the Royal College of Anaesthetist, the best evidence to date on major complications after CNB, the largest prospective audit, with a 100% return rate, reassured us that permanent harm following CNB is rare (incidence of major complications 1 in 24,000–1 in 54,000; Death and paraplegia 1 in 50,000 to 1 in 140,000). Major complications, nonetheless, do happen, and every effort must be made to prevent them. Further, given the catastrophic nature of such complications, ongoing vigilance is of paramount importance. Also, efforts should be made to ameliorate “minor” and “moderate” complications, particularly PDPH.

Clinical Pearls

- **Discharge Readiness**: After spinal anesthesia, patients may be discharged from the recovery room, once the block recedes (at least four dermatomes/spinal level of less than T10), are hemodynamically stable, and comfortable. Outpatients should be able to ambulate without orthostatic changes and void before discharge if, in a high-risk group for urinary retention.

- **Dyspnoea**: Intraoperatively, during high spinal anesthesia, patients occasionally complain of dyspnea. This is not due to decreased inspiratory capacity but due to loss of chest wall sensation, which does not allow patients to experience the reassurance of a deep breath and can be overcome by instructing the patient to raise a hand near the mouth and exhale forcefully. The tactile appreciation of the deep breath provides reassurance.
- **Time efficient**: An important factor for the success of spinal anesthesia in the day-to-day use of anesthesia is that it is time efficient. The patient preparation for surgery can begin almost as soon as the block is administered, with adequate sedation.

24.16 Controversies Regarding Spinal Anesthesia

1. **Regional anesthesia for outpatients**: Earlier it was believed that regional anesthesia was not appropriate for outpatient anesthesia; An increasing number of day-care procedures have challenged this concept. "Walk-in, walk-out" spinals with a low dose lidocaine and opioids for gynecological laparoscopy have created the concept of selective spinal anesthesia. Reintroduction of chloroprocaine may be the solution for bilateral, short acting spinal anesthesia in the future.
2. **Use of neuraxial block in infected or febrile patients**: The decision to perform a regional anesthetic must be made on an individual basis considering the anesthetic alternatives, the benefits, and the risk of CNS infection (which may theoretically occur in any bacteraemic patient). Available data suggest that these patients may safely undergo spinal anesthesia, provided appropriate antibiotic therapy is initiated before dural puncture and the patient has shown a response to therapy, such as a decrease in fever.
3. **Neuraxial anesthesia for immunocompromised patients**:

   Neuraxial analgesia decreases the risk of infection through attenuation of stress response and preservation of immune function. Despite this, spinal anesthesia is not preferred in patients with a neoplasm, immunosuppression after solid organ transplantation, or chronic infection with human immunodeficiency virus (HIV) or herpes simplex virus (HSV) because of the increased risk of infection around or within the spinal canal. The decision to perform a regional anesthetic should be made on a case-to-case basis keeping the risk of CNS infection, hemorrhagic or neurologic complications in mind.
4. **Neuraxial blocks in neurological disorders.**

   The fear of worsening neurologic outcome, local anesthetic toxicity, neural ischemia, and medico legal implications have led many clinicians to completely avoid regional anesthesia in patients with pre-existing central nervous system (CNS) disorders. In a retrospective review, Horlocker et al. analyzed the decision to perform regional anesthesia in these patients and concluded that the risks are not that frequent and CNB should not be an absolute contraindication.
5. **Neuraxial blocks in patients receiving anticoagulants**:

   The safety of neuraxial anesthesia in the anticoagulated patient is based on appropriate timing of needle placement and catheter removal. The decision to perform CNB should be made on an individual basis, weighing the risks with the benefits.

Recommended guidelines for performing spinal procedures in anticoagulated patients:

1. **Warfarin**: Discontinue warfarin 4–5 days before spinal procedure and evaluate INR. INR within the normal range indicates adequate levels of all vitamin K-dependent factors.
2. **Antiplatelet medications**: No contraindications with aspirin or NSAIDs. Thienopyridine derivatives (clopidogrel and ticlopidine) should be discontinued 7 days and 14 days, respectively, prior to procedure. GP IIb/IIIa inhibitors should be discontinued to allow platelet function to recover prior to procedure (8 h for tirofiban and eptifibatide, 24–48 h for abciximab).
3. **Thrombolytics/fibrinolytics**: No data is available to suggest a safe interval between procedure and discontinuation of these medications. Follow fibrinogen level and observe for signs of neural compression.
4. **Low molecular weight Heparin (LMWH)**: LMWH should be withheld for at least 12 h prior or 24 h after a CNB.
5. **Unfractionated SQ heparin**: There are no contraindications to neuraxial procedure if the total daily dose is less than 10,000 units.
6. **Unfractionated IV heparin**: Spinal puncture should be delayed 24 h after last dose, after documenting normal aPTT. Heparin may be restarted 1 h following procedure.

Note: NSAIDs = Nonsteroidal anti-inflammatory drugs; GP IIb/IIIa = Platelet glycoprotein receptor IIb/IIIa inhibitors; INR = international normalized ratio; LMWH = low-molecular-weight heparin; aPTT = activated partial thromboplastin time

Suggested Reading

1. Cook TM, Counsell D, Wildsmith JA. Major complications of central neuraxial block: report on the Third National Audit Project of the Royal College of Anaesthetists. Br J Anaesth. 2009;102(2):179–90.
2. Kolte VS, Khambatta S, Ambiye MV. Thickness of the ligamentum flavum: correlation with age and its asymmetry—an magnetic resonance imaging study. Asian Spine J. 2015;9(2):245–53. https://doi.org/10.4184/asj.2015.9.2.245.
3. Hazarika R, Choudhury D, Nath S, Parua S. Estimation of skin to subarachnoid space depth: an observational study. J Clin Diagn Res. 2016;10(10):UC06–9. https://doi.org/10.7860/JCDR/2016/21679.8755.
4. Ghosh SM, Madjdpour C, Chin KJ. Ultrasound-guided lumbar central neuraxial block. BJA Educ. 2016;16(7):213–20.
5. Spinal Anaesthesia. Nysora.com.
6. Miller RD. Miller's anaesthesia. 7th ed. Amsterdam: Elsevier; 2012. ISBN 978-0-443-06959-8.
7. Dahl JB, Jeppesen IS, Jørgensen H, et al. Intraoperative and postoperative analgesic efficacy and adverse effects of intrathecal opioids in patients undergoing cesarean section with spinal anesthesia: a qualitative and quantitative systematic review of randomized controlled trials. Anesthesiology. 1999;91:1919.
8. Liu S, Chiu AA, Carpenter RL, et al. Fentanyl prolongs lidocaine spinal anesthesia without prolonging recovery. Anesth Analg. 1995;80:730.
9. Belzarena SD. Clinical effects of intrathecally administered fentanyl in patients undergoing cesarean section. Anesth Analg. 1992;74:653.
10. Maehara Y, Kusunoki S, Kawamoto M, et al. A prospective multicenter trial to determine the incidence of transient neurologic symptoms after spinal anesthesia with phenylephrine added to 0.5% tetracaine. Hiroshima J Med Sci. 2001;50:47.

Spinal Anesthesia in Pediatric Patients

25

Anju Gupta and Anu Kewlani

Key Points

1. Spinal anesthesia is a safe and useful technique for anesthesia in children.
2. Spinal anesthesia is a useful modality for ex-preterm infants and other children where the risk of general anesthesia can be prohibitive.
3. Hemodynamic changes are infrequent in children particularly below 5 years of age.
4. L4–5/L5–S1 intervertebral spaces should be chosen but Tuffier's line is a reliable landmark.
5. Hyperbaric bupivacaine is the most commonly used local anesthetic agent.
6. Complications are infrequent in this population
7. Ultrasound is a new promising modality especially for young infants.

25.1 Background

August Bier, in 1898, first reported the successful use of spinal anesthesia (SA) in an 11-year-old child for surgery on a thigh tumor. Following this, Bainbridge (1901), Tyrell Gray (1909), Berkowitz and Greene (1950) described SA as an excellent alternative to general anesthesia (GA) in children including thoracic surgeries (lobectomy, pneumonectomy). Spinal anesthesia was an innovative and popular technique in pediatric anesthesia in the first half of 1900, but then its use decreased significantly due to developments in general endotracheal anesthesia along with lack of expertise for SA (fear of adverse effects, lack of patient co-operation).

The new interest in the use of spinal anesthesia rose three decades ago when awake spinal anesthesia was introduced for herniotomies in preterm neonates with a high risk of apnea associated with general anesthesia (GA). However, SA is a feasible technique not only in neonates but also in older children and adolescents.

25.2 Indications

The various surgical and miscellaneous procedures where SA has been used are listed in Table 25.1.

A. Gupta (✉) · A. Kewlani
Anaesthesia, Pain Medicine, Critical Care,
All India Institute of Medical Sciences,
New Delhi, Delhi, India

N. Gupta et al. (eds.), *Techniques in Anesthesia, Intensive Care and Emergency Medicine*,
https://doi.org/10.1007/978-981-96-1202-4_25

Table 25.1 Uses of spinal anesthesia in pediatric patients

1. Premature, ex-premature infants, specifically those undergoing inguinal herniorrhaphy
2. Outside neonatal period (a) General surgeries (rectal biopsy, incision of rectal abscess, colostomy) (b) Urological surgery (orchidopexy, circumcision, urethroplasty, posterior urethral valve fulgurations) (c) Lower limb orthopedic surgery (amputations, closed reduction of hip, club foot repair, arthrogram, muscle biopsy, tendon lengthening) (c) Meningomyelocele repair
3. Patients in whom GA may pose a significant risk (a) Facial dysmorphia, difficult airway (b) Medical diseases-muscular dystrophy, mucopolysaccharidosis, family history of malignant hyperthermia, bronchopulmonary dysplasia (c) Emergency-full stomach with aspiration risk, chest infections
4. In combination with GA (a) Preoperative morphine spinal anesthesia combined with GA for scoliosis surgery-reduced blood loss and better pain control (b) Cardiopulmonary bypass- to blunt the stress response, protects hemodynamic status, decrease opioid requirement, and reduces perioperative morbidity and mortality
5. Miscellaneous Radiotherapy, congenital abnormalities, chronic pain management

25.3 SA in Premature and Ex-premature Infants

SA is mainly used for premature and former premature infants, those undergoing lower abdominal or lower limb surgeries (of duration less than 90 min). These patients often have a history of apnea of prematurity or have associated anomalies such as bronchopulmonary dysplasia, and chronic lung disease and thus have an increased incidence of post operative apnea (45% in <48 weeks post conceptional age). Former premature infants remain at risk for same until after 60 weeks post conceptional age (PCA). General anesthesia increases the risk of apnea, desaturation, and bradycardia in these patients whereas SA has been found safe.

The incidence of postoperative apneas correlates with gestational age at birth, the post-conceptional age at the time of surgery, weight, anemia (hematocrit less than 30%), and history of apneas.

Special considerations for choosing spinal anesthesia for neonates or infant include the following:

- The expertise of the anesthesia provider to perform procedure on neonate/infant.
- The motivation of the surgeon to perform surgery on awake infant under SA.
- The estimated length of surgery should be less than 90 min.

25.4 Contraindications

Contraindications to SA in children are mostly similar to those in adults. Here are the contraindications listed below:

- Coagulation abnormalities
- Systemic sepsis or local infection at the puncture point
- Uncorrected hypovolemia
- Parental refusal or an uncooperative child
- Neurological abnormalities with increased intracranial pressure
- Anatomic abnormalities such as spina bifida, occult spinal dysraphism, and meningomyelocele are relevant in this age group
- Procedures lasting more than 90 min

25.5 Anatomical Differences Between Adults and Children

1. *Delayed ossification and growth of iliac crests*: Tuffier line, which joins anterior superior iliac spinous processes, crosses the spine at L5 or lower in infants. This line passes over L5–S1 interspace in neonates instead of L4–L5 interspace as in adults. The shape of the infants' and children's pelvis is more circular, and the position of the iliac crest is lower than that in adults.
2. *Cartilaginous structure of bones and vertebrae*: Reduced resistance to penetration by sharp needles. So, there is a risk of direct trauma and bacterial contamination of ossification nuclei which can compromise further bone or joint growth. Thin and sharp needles should be avoided; use short and short beveled ones instead. Do not apply excessive force on needle: if resistance is felt, stop trying to insert the needle farther.
3. *Spine and ligaments*: Ligaments are less densely packed. Hence, feel of loss of resistance is less marked. Increased spine flexibility limits normal thoracic kyphosis and facilitates cephalad spread and higher level of sensory block. Laminae are cartilaginous; hence, paramedian approach should be avoided.
4. *Dural Sac and lower termination of spinal canal*: Dural sac terminates at S3 and spinal cord at L3 vertebral levels, at birth. Adult level (S2 and L1 respectively) is reached at around 2nd year of life. Thus, it is important to use a low approach (L4–5 or L5–S1) to avoid direct trauma to spinal cord.
5. *CSF*: Children require higher dose of local anesthetic (LA) drug due to higher total CSF (neonates—10 ml/kg, infants and young children—4 ml/kg, adults—2 ml/kg).
6. *Delayed myelinization of nerve fibers:* Facilitates intraneural penetration of local anesthetics. Onset time is shortened, and diluted local anesthetic is as effective as more concentrated anesthetic in adults.
7. *Meninges*: Highly vascular piamater and high cardiac output lead to rapid re-absorption of LA and shorter duration of block in children.

25.6 Technique

25.6.1 Preparation

- The procedure should be explained to the parents (and child if appropriate), with a description of risks and benefits. Informed consent from parents and assent from older children should be obtained.
- A full blood count including platelet count and coagulation screen (prothrombin time, PT; activated partial thromboplastin time, APTT) may be performed preoperatively where clinically indicated. Blood tests are not usually required for a routine herniotomy.
- The operating room should be warmed. Warm blankets and heaters should be used for neonates and infants to prevent heat loss.
- The room should be quiet and surgical instruments should be covered to minimize patient anxiety for older children.
- The child should be fasted as for GA (4–6 h for milk and 2 h for clear liquid).
- Premedication can be used according to institutional preferences. Usually, older children require some premedication for easy parental separation, IV cannulation, and spinal puncture.
- Topical anesthesia using EMLA (eutectic mixture of local anesthetics) can be applied 60–90 min prior to SA. EMLA cream should not be used preterm (<37 weeks) as there is risk of methemoglobinemia.

25.6.1.1 Equipment Preparation

- All drugs and equipment should be prepared and checked prior to starting.
- Table 25.2 shows the list of equipment needed for performing spinal blocks.

Table 25.2 Equipment required for spinal anesthesia

Disposable or sterile tray with sterile gauges, drapes, sponge holding forceps, and a small container for keeping disinfectant
Skin disinfectant (5–10% povidone iodine or 0.5–2% chlorhexidine solution in alcohol)
A 1ml syringe for loading spinal drug and a 2 ml syringe for local infiltration
Hypodermic needles-2
The spinal local anesthetic drug, adjuvant if required
Spinal needle (sizes and length of needle depending on the child's age)
Lignocaine 1% for skin infiltration

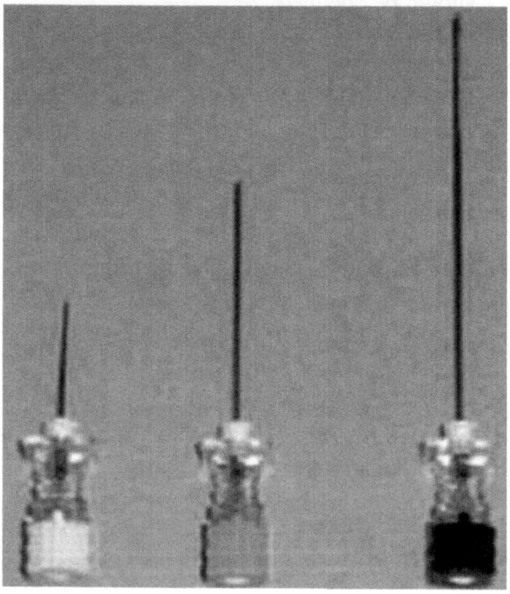

Fig. 25.1 Types of spinal needle

25.6.1.2 Spinal Needle

- Spinal needles used in children range from size 22–25 G with stylets, preferred length 25–50 mm (25–30 mm for infants, 50 mm for small children) (Fig. 25.1).
- A 25 G or 26 G needle with stylet is generally preferred for neonates and infants.
- There are studies in which a 90 mm adult spinal needle has been used for children successfully. However, a shorter pediatric needle is preferred because of the smaller dead space and it allows more precise movement.
- Both needle types (pencil point and cutting type) have a similar success rate.
- Most important feature of the needle to determine the success of the block is the distance separating the tip of the needle from its distal orifice; this distance must be as short as possible to avoid extradural leakage.
- Needle without a stylet should not be used since it can deposit skin tags (epithelial tissue) in the intrathecal space and increase the risk of epidermoid tumors of the neural axis.
- Contradictory to older studies, recent studies have concluded that needle design does affect the incidence of post-dural puncture headache (PDPH) in children. Pencil-point tip needle has a lower incidence of PDPH as compared to the cutting type.

25.6.1.3 Local Anesthetic Drugs and Doses

- The duration of spinal block is shorter in infants than in adults, probably due to the larger volume of CSF. In addition, there is proportionally greater blood flow to the spinal cord with the more rapid uptake of drugs from the subarachnoid space. These phenomena are most pronounced in preterm infants compared to full-term infants.
- Various drug used in SA, doses according to weight and their duration of action is mentioned in Table 25.3. Dosage of LA agents varies inversely with the body weight.
- **Isobaric and hyperbaric bupivacaine (0.5%)**—remain the most popular drug for pediatric SA. Baricity of LA drug is not important because both isobaric and hyperbaric solutions have similar block characteristics in children.
- **Levobupivacaine (0.5%)**—has similar properties to bupivacaine and is required in similar doses. Due to its lower toxicity, its use is preferable in newborns and younger infants or in patients with impaired liver function.
- **Ropivacaine 0.5%**—Duration of motor block is significantly shorter than equipotent doses of bupivacaine.
- Studies have shown 1 mg/kg of isobaric solutions of 0.5% bupivacaine and ropivacaine and

Table 25.3 Recommended doses and approximate duration of LA for SA in infants and children

Type of LA	<5 kg	5–15 kg	>5 kg	Duration range (min)
0.5% bupivacaine/levobupivacaine (hyper/isobaric)	0.5–0.6 mg/kg (0.1–0.12 ml/kg)	0.4 mg/kg (0.08 ml/kg)	0.3 mg/kg (0.06 ml/kg)	30–180 (80)
0.5% isobaric ropivacaine	0.5–1 mg/kg (0.1–0.2 ml/kg)	0.5 mg/kg (0.1 ml/kg)	0.5 mg/kg (0.1 ml/kg)	34–210 (96)
0.5% hyperbaric tetracaine	0.5–0.6 mg/kg (0.1–0.12 ml/kg)	0.4 mg/kg (0.08 ml/kg)	0.3 mg/kg (0.06 ml/kg)	35–240 (90)

1.02 mg/kg of L-bupivacaine have similar potency in infants. However, the safety of such high doses is questionable because of the risk of neurotoxicity.

- **Tetracaine 0.5%**—was a commonly used drug earlier**.** Tetracaine is no longer available in some countries.
- **Isobaric lignocaine 2%**—not used currently because of its shorter duration of action and reports of neurological complications in adults.

25.6.1.4 Spinal Anesthetic Adjuvants

1. **Epinephrine (1 in 100,000)**: Dose 2–3 mcg/kg. Extends the duration of blockade by 30%. Epinephrine has been implicated in several reports of ischemic spinal injury; however, not been proven by any study.
2. **Clonidine**: Dose 1–2 mcg/kg. The addition of clonidine to hyperbaric bupivacaine increases the duration of blockade and analgesia but may cause hypotension, bradycardia, and sedation. A dose of 1 mcg/kg doubles the time of full recovery from blockade as compared to bupivacaine alone, with less incidence of hemodynamic or respiratory depression symptoms. With a dose of 2 mcg/kg, the incidence of adverse effects is higher. Close monitoring of these patients for 24 h is recommended.
3. **Fentanyl**: Dose 0.2–2 mcg/kg. Increases the duration of SA and also prolongs postoperative analgesia without causing hemodynamic and respiratory alterations. It also does not delay discharge from PACU.
4. **Morphine**: A dose of 4–5 mcg/kg provides effective and safe analgesia in a variety of surgical procedures. In Cardiac surgeries, 10 mcg/kg provides hemodynamic stability with 24-h analgesia (patients extubated in OR). In scoliosis surgery (15 mcg/kg) has been reported with decreased blood loss, safe and prolonged analgesia.
5. **Neostigmine:** Dose 0.75 mcg/kg. Causes significant prolongation of the block, with no increase in emesis or delayed recovery.

25.6.1.5 Procedural Sedation

- Regional anesthesia in children is usually performed under sedation. The primary aim of sedation is to achieve anxiolysis in children and to prevent any movement during the procedure. Performing spinal puncture in a struggling, agitated child may cause trauma to delicate neurovascular structures and should be avoided. Ketamine, midazolam, propofol, dexmedetomidine, and inhalational agents like sevoflurane or nitrous oxide are commonly used.
- Children should be monitored closely during sedation.
- Sedation is avoided in preterm and former preterm infants because of the risk of apnea. These infants may be soothened with flavored pacifiers or sugar dip.
- Intraoperative sedation may not be required if SA is successful because de-afferentiation itself produces sedation.
- Loose soft restraints may be applied to prevent the infant from reaching onto the sterile field.
- Some older children who prefer not to be sedated, music or watching a cartoon can be used for distraction.

25.6.2 Position

Proper positioning of the patient is of utmost importance for the successful performance of the spinal block. A trained assistant is required in this regard. In children, spinal anesthesia can be performed in one of the two positions of the patient: lateral decubitus and sitting.

Lateral decubitus position: The patient is positioned at the border of the surgical table and held firmly by an assistant. The patient is curled up and flexed at the hip joint. In neonates and infants, care must be taken to avoid neck flexion because it can cause upper airway obstruction leading to hypoxia (decreases transcutaneous O_2 tension by almost 28 mmHg). The child's neck should be extended, to ensure an open airway. Elevating the head end of the table by 45° while puncture is made in a lateral position in infants, increases the CSF pressure by widening subarachnoid space, thus increasing the success of the block in infants.

Sitting position: Both sitting and lateral positions have been found to be suitable for performing spinal punctures. The child is seated with the back flexed. The assistant is required to firmly maintaining the sitting position. Neck flexion is not necessary because it does not facilitate the performance of the block in small children. Functional /hysterical scoliosis makes puncture more difficult.

The lateral position may be easier than the sitting position for older patients for whom intravenous sedation may be indicated.

25.6.3 Procedure

1. A midline approach is usually recommended over a paramedian approach.
2. The desired dose of spinal local anesthetic should be calculated and prepared in a syringe before dural puncture to ensure that the correct dose is administered.
3. Because the volume of local anesthetic needed is small in neonates, it is important to measure the volume corresponding to the hub of the needle (0.02–0.04 ml) and to count this volume, too, in the total dose of local anesthetic.

(a) **Prepare the back of the patient**: The anesthesiologist performing the block should scrub and don a sterile gown and gloves. After setting up monitoring, intravenous access, and resuscitation equipment, the patient is positioned and the back of the patient is prepared using a disinfectant solution (2% chlorhexidine or povidone-iodine), giving adequate time for its action.

(b) **Palpate the lumbar interspinous space**: Dural puncture is performed in the lumbar area, and because the spinal cord ends at L3 in infants and even lower in some neonates, needle placement should be at L4/5 or L5/S1 interspace. The iliac crest is at the level of the fifth lumbar vertebra in young children, and the position is even lower in neonates, and a puncture at the intercristal level will be below the spinal cord.

(c) **Local infiltration of the site**: After palpating the space, the midline should be infiltrated with 0.1 ml of 1% lignocaine. Care must be taken to avoid deep penetration.

(d) **Performing spinal block**: Spinal needle is inserted in the midline to pierce the skin, subcutaneous fat, supraspinous ligament, interspinous ligament, ligamentum flavum and finally dura mater with arachnoid mater attached to it. Ligaments are less densely packed, hence feel of loss of resistance is less marked.

The needle is advanced slowly, and the stylet is frequently removed to check for the free-flowing return of CSF.

Depth of insertion at L4–L5 varies with age: newborn 10–15 mm, up to 5 years 15–25 mm, 5–8 years 30–40 mm.

The distance between skin and subarachnoid space can be related to height or weight using the formulae:

Distance from the skin to subarachnoid space (cm)	0. 03 × height (cm)
Distance from the skin to subarachnoid space (mm)	[2 × weight (kg)] + 7 (mm)

The subarachnoid space is very narrow (diameter is 6–8 mm in term newborn), so a slight deviation of the midline can result in puncture failure.

The barbotage method is not recommended, as it may result in a higher level of motor blockade and has a potential for the total spinal blockade.

The drug is injected slowly, over 20 s, to avoid the extensive spread of the block.

After the procedure, the child is placed supine. Raising the legs above the trunk (for e.g., while applying cautery) or Trendelenburg position should be avoided to prevent the risk of high or total spinal block. In the case, if there is rapid rise in the level of blockade, the patient can be placed in the reverse Trendelenburg position.

Hematic punctures are more common in infants than in adults, with an incidence of 8–19%. So, it is recommended not to make more than 3 attempts at spinal puncture unless GA is contraindicated.

25.6.3.1 Assessing the Block

Assessing the level of the blockade is difficult in infants and young children, particularly if patients have received sedation or if the block is being performed under general anesthesia. Transcutaneous electrical stimulation has been seen useful in infants to assess the block.

In infants, the sensory block can be assessed by loss of response to cold stimuli (alcohol swab) or pinprick. The level of the block is assessed by observing the ventilation rate and pattern.

In older children, the motor block can be assessed by modified Bromage score and pain by various scales example FLACC in infants, CHEOPS in children 1–7 years of age, and Visual Analogue scale or VAS in older children.

25.7 Complications of Pediatric Spinal Anesthesia

There are few studies to date that have described the complications of SA in neonates and infants. In older children, complications of SA are similar to those seen in adults and are usually minor complications and infrequent.

A few complications are listed below.

1. Cardiorespiratory insufficiency: Hypoxia and hypotension due to SA although rare in children, can be seen in premature or ex premature infants. However, they can be secondary to the flexed neck while the procedure, high spinal blockade, or due to sedation. The incidence of intraoperative bradycardia under SA alone in 1554 infants was noted to be 1.6%.
2. High or total spinal anesthesia (0.6–0.8%): Drug overdose, barbotage, or Trendelenburg position post spinal block can result in high or total spinal anesthesia. Total spinal anesthesia may induce bronchospasm secondary to decreased circulatory catecholamines.
3. Intravascular injection and local anesthetic toxicity: The relative dose of local anesthetic required in neonates/infants is much higher than that needed in older children and adults. Neonatal jaundice may increase the risk of toxicity from amide local anesthetics.
4. Subdural hematoma: Two cases of subdural hematoma have been reported in infants following SA. Both were treated conservatively and children were normal at follow-up 2 years after their diagnoses.
5. Post-dural puncture headache (PDPH): It is the most common complication in children with an incidence of 8–25%. Incidence is the same in children of all age groups. Incidence is lower with the thinner needle (4–5% with 25 G or 27 G needle vs 12–15% with 22 G needle). According to recent studies, the incidence is lower with pencil point needles compared to cutting needles (0.4% vs. 5%)

   Symptoms are usually mild to moderate and last for a few days. Along with headaches, children may also have nausea and vomiting and associated symptoms from other cranial nerves, such as blurred vision, vertigo, tinnitus, or diminished hearing. The diagnosis of PDPH is difficult in neonates and infants because of their inability to communicate their symptoms; postural distress may be the only clue. Treatment is mainly conservative. Epidural blood patch with 0.2–0.3 ml/kg blood in severe cases or if symptoms persist for more than 1 week.
6. Backache (5–10%): is a minor common complaint, relieved with mild analgesics. As such backache is a frequent postoperative complication, and the type of anesthesia (regional or general anesthesia) does not affect its incidence.

Thus, the association of spinal anesthesia with increased risk of backache is not known yet.

7. Transient neurological symptoms (3–4%): Often start as pain and dysesthesia in the gluteal region radiating to lower limbs. It is usually subclinical neurotoxicity due to local anesthetic. Symptoms are mild.
8. Meningitis: Aseptic or septic meningitis after SA is a rare complication, only a few case reports are available. Lumbar puncture is advised in patients who develop a fever after spinal block for diagnosis.

25.8 Recent Updates

Ultrasound: Ultrasound guidance for the pediatric spinal block is an attractive modality since it is easy to perform in children <6 months of age since the posterior arch of the vertebra is not yet ossified and provides a perfect acoustic window. The lumbosacral part of the spinal canal with the conus medullaris and the cauda equina are especially beautifully depicted with a high-resolution linear array probe. It can be used either as a pre-scan to determine the depth of dura and midline or for real-time guidance. A recent Cochrane review on the use of ultrasound for neuraxial block in children determined that ultrasound guidance is particularly advantageous in young children as it improves the success rate and reduces the time to perform the procedure [1]. However, additional data are required before definitive conclusions can be made on its practical utility in this population.

Suggested Reading

1. Guay J, Suresh S, Kopp S. The use of ultrasound guidance for perioperative neuraxial and peripheral nerve blocks in children: a Cochrane review. Anesth Analg. 2017;124:948–58.
2. Bier A. Experiment regarding the cocainization of the spinal cord. Zentralbl Chir. 1899;51:361–9.
3. Bainbridge WS. A report of twelve operations on infants and young children during spinal anesthesia. Arch Pediatr. 1901;18:570–4.
4. Gray HT. A study of subarachnoid block in children and infants. Lancet. 1909;2:913–7.
5. Berkowitz S, Greene BA. Spinal anaesthesia in children: report based on 350 patients under 13 years. Anesthesiology. 1951;12:376–87.
6. Abajian JC, Mellish RW, Browne AF, et al. Spinal anesthesia for surgery in the high-risk infant. Anesth Analg. 1984;63:359–62.
7. Brown TC. History of pediatric regional anesthesia. Pediatr Anesth. 2011;22(1):3–9. https://doi.org/10.1111/j.1460-9592.2011.03636.x.
8. Gupta A, Saha U. Spinal anesthesia in children: a review. J Anesthesiol Clin Pharmacol. 2014;30(1):10–8. https://doi.org/10.4103/0970-9185.125687.
9. Williams RK, Adams DC, Aladjem EV, et al. The safety and efficacy of spinal anesthesia for surgery in infants: the Vermont Infant Spinal Registry. Anesth Analg. 2006;102:67–71.
10. Krane EJ, Harberkern CM, Jacobson LE. Postoperative apnea, bradycardia and oxygen desaturation in formerly premature infants: prospective comparison of spinal and general anesthesia. Anesth Analg. 1995;80:7–13.
11. Forkin KT, Nemergut E. Miller anaesthesia 8th edition. Anesthesiology. 2016;124(4):977–8.
12. Geiduschek JM. Pediatrics. In: Brown DL, editor. Regional anaesthesia and analgesia. 1st ed. Philadelphia: WB Saunders Company; 1996. p. 559–62.
13. Dohi S, Seino H. Spinal anesthesia in premature infants: dosage and effects of sympathectomy. Anesthesiology. 1986;65:559–61.
14. Kokki H. Spinal blocks. Paediatr Anaesth. 2012;22:56–64.
15. Hirabayashi Y, Shimizu R, Saitoh K, Fukuda H. Spread of subarachnoid hyperbaric amethocaine in adolescents. Br J Anaesth. 1995;74:41–5.
16. Nickel US, Meyer RR, Brambrink AM. Spinal anesthesia in an extremely low birth weight infant. Paediatr Anaesth. 2005;15:58–62.
17. Puncuh F, Lampugnani E, Kokki H. Use of spinal anesthesia in pediatric patients: a single centre experience with 1132 cases. Pediatr Anesth. 2004;14:564–7.
18. Gupta A, Saha U, Sinha SK, Gupta N. Subarachanoid block (SAB) versus general anaesthesia (GA) in children undergoing surgeries below umbilicus. J Anaesthesiol Clin Pharmacol. 2008;24:425–8.
19. Kokki H, Heikkinen M, Turunen M, Vanamo K, Hendolin H. Needle design does not affect the success rate of spinal anaesthesia or the incidence of postpuncture complications in children. Acta Anaesthesiol Scand. 2000;44:210–3.
20. Kokki H, Turunen M, Heikkinen M, Reinikainen M, Laisalmi M. High success rate and low incidence of headache and neurological symptoms with two spinal needle designs in children. Acta Anaesthesiol Scand. 2005;49:1367–72.
21. Shaywitz BA. Epidermoid spinal cord tumors and previous lumbar punctures. J Pediatr. 1972;80:638–40.

22. Apiliogullari S, Duman A, Gok F, Akillioglu I. Spinal needle design and size affect the incidence of postdural puncture headache in children. Paediatr Anaesth. 2010;20:177–82.
23. Kokki H, Tuovinen K, Hendolin H. Spinal anaesthesia for paediatric day-case surgery: a double-blind, randomized, parallel group, prospective comparison of isobaric and hyperbaric bupivacaine. Br J Anaesth. 1998;81:502–6.
24. Kokki H, Ylönen P, Heikkinen M, Reinikainen M. Levobupivacaine for paediatric spinal anesthesia. Anesth Analg. 2004;98:64–7.
25. Kokki H, Ylönen P, Laisalmi M, Heikkinen M, Reinikainen M. Isobaric ropivacaine 5 mg/ml for spinal anaesthesia in children. Anesth Analg. 2005;100:66–70.
26. Frawley G, Smith KR, Ingelmo P. Relative potencies of bupivacaine, levobupivacaine, and ropivacaine for neonatal spinal anaesthesia. Br J Anaesth. 2009;103:731–8.
27. Goldman LJ. Complications in regional anaesthesia. Paediatr Anaesth. 1995;5:3–9.
28. Rochette A, Raux O, Troncin R, Dadure C, Verdier R, Capdevila X. Clonidine prolongs spinal anesthesia in newborns: a prospective dose ranging study. Anesth Analg. 2004;98:56–9.
29. Duman A, Apiliogullari S, Duman I. Effects of intrathecal fentanyl on quality of spinal anesthesia in children undergoing inguinal hernia repair. Paediatr Anaesth. 2010;20:530–6.
30. Finkel JC, Doyle JM, Conran AM. A comparison of three intrathecal morphine doses during SA in children having open heart surgery. Anesthesiology. 1997;87:A1052.
31. Eschertzhuber S, Hohlrieder M, Keller C, Oswald E, Kuehbacher G, Innerhofer P. Comparison of high- and low-dose intrathecal morphine for spinal fusion in children. Br J Anaesth. 2008;100:538–43.
32. Batra YK, Rajeev S, Panda NB, Lokesh VC, Rao KL. Intrathecal neostigmine with bupivacaine for infants undergoing lower abdominal and urogenital procedures: Dose response. Acta Anesthesiol Scand. 2009;53:470–5.
33. Arthrus OJ, Murray M, Zubier M, Tooley J, Kelsall W. Ultrasongraphic determination of neonatal spinal canal depth. Arch Dis Child Fetal Neonatal Ed. 2008;93:F451–4.
34. Wright TE, Orr RJ, Haberkern CM, Walbergh EJ. Complications during spinal anesthesia in infants: high spinal blockade. Anesthesiology. 1990;73:1290–2.
35. Kachko L, Simhi E, Tzeitlin E, Efrat R, Tarabikin E, Peled E, Metzner I, Katz J. Spinal anesthesia in neonates and infants - a single-center experience of 505 cases. Paediatr Anaesth. 2007 Jul;17(7):647–53.
36. Aouad MT, Moukaddem FH, Akel SR, Kanazi GE. Respiratory failure in a former preterm infant following high spinal anesthesia with bupivacaine and clonidine. Paediatr Anaesth. 2008;18(10):1000–1.
37. McDougall RJ, Barnes R, Danks RA, Ditchfield M. Subdural haematoma following infant spinal anaesthesia. Childs Nerv Syst. 2016;32:579–81.
38. Janssens E, Aerssens P, Alliet P, et al. Postdural puncture headaches in children. A literature review. Eur J Pediatr. 2003;162:117–21.
39. Kokki H, Sakonvaara M, Herrgård E, Onen P. Postdural puncture headache is not an age-related symptom in children: a prospective, open-randomised, parallel group study comparing a 22-gauge Quincke with a 22-gauge Whitacre needle. Paediatr Anaesth. 1999;9:429–34.
40. Oliver A. Dural punctures in children: what should we do? Paediatr Anaesth. 2002;12(6):473–7.
41. Kokki H, Hendolin H. Comparison of 25G and 29G Quincke spinal needles in pediatrics day care surgery. A prospective randomized study of puncture characteristics, success rate and postoperative complaints. Pediatr Anesth. 1996;6:115–9.
42. Kokki H. Spinal anaesthesia in infants and children. Best Pract Res Clin Anaesthesiol. 2000;14:687–707.

26 Epidural Block

Geetanjali Chilkoti

Key Points

- Epidural block is regional anesthesia that involves injecting medication into the epidural space of the spinal cord.
- It is commonly used for analgesia for labor pain and various surgeries.
- Typically, a combination of local anesthetic (such as bupivacaine) and a narcotic (such as fentanyl).
- It can cause temporary side effects like hypotension, headache etc.
- It is important to discuss the risks and benefits of epidural block with patients

26.1 Introduction

Epidural block, also called extradural block, refers to placement of local anesthetics or other drugs in the epidural space at different levels of the vertebral column.

When used in anesthesia, it provides optimal pain relief with less hemodynamic instability compared to general anesthesia (GA). It also reduces the surgical stress response, the time to return of GI function, the incidence of perioperative thromboembolic events, and the risk of cancer recurrence. Lastly, epidural block possibly reduces the overall morbidity and mortality associated with major surgery.

26.2 Anatomy

Epidural surrounds the dura mater with the following boundaries: foramen magnum superiorly, sacrococcygeal membrane inferiorly, posterior longitudinal ligaments anteriorly, and pedicles intervertebral foramina laterally. Posterior boundary is formed by ligamentum flavum, lamina and spinous process of vertebra, interspinous and supraspinous ligaments from inside to the exterior (Fig. 26.1).

Contents of the epidural space include nerve roots, and fat, areolar tissue, lymphatics, and blood vessels. The venous plexus is valve-less and is continuous with the iliac vessels in the pelvis and the azygos system in the abdominal and thoracic body walls.

Ligamentum flavum is the posterior midline fusion of the right and left ligamentum flava. Its thickness may vary which may be presented as the midline gaps as well as it can get calcified with aging; this may lead to difficulty in identifying the entry point for epidural as well as to failure in identifying the epidural space.

G. Chilkoti (✉)
Department of Anesthesiology and Critical Care, UCMS and GTB Hospital, New Delhi, India

N. Gupta et al. (eds.), *Techniques in Anesthesia, Intensive Care and Emergency Medicine*,
https://doi.org/10.1007/978-981-96-1202-4_26

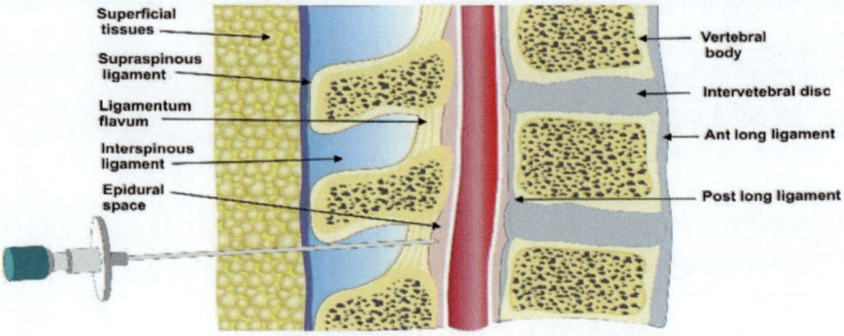

Fig. 26.1 Anatomy of epidural space (original)

Advantages
- Improved perioperative analgesia
- Reduced surgical stress response
- Reduced risk of postoperative complications especially pulmonary complications
- Reduced incidence of perioperative thrombo-embolic events
- Reduces the risk of cancer recurrence

Indications for epidural block

For anesthesia Primary anesthetic technique (single shot/ continuous infusion) or Combined spinal epidural block (CSE) Epidural block integrated along with GA	Perioperative or peripartum pain management Improved perioperative or peripartum pain management
Chronic pain management	Epidural steroids in patients with radicular pain or radiculopathy

Surgical indications for epidural block

Obstetric surgery	Cesarean delivery, labor analgesia
Orthopedic surgery	Hip and knee surgery, open reduction and internal fixation, arthroscopy, arthrotomy and amputation of lower limb bones
Gynecologic surgery	Hysterectomy, pelvic floor procedures, hysteroscopy, dilation& curettage, urinary incontinence procedure, reversal of lap ligation
General surgery	Breast, hepatic, gastric, colonic and anorectal surgery, various genitourinary surgeries
Vascular surgery	Amputation of lower extremity, revascularization procedures
Cardiothoracic surgery	Thoracotomy, esophagectomy, thymectomy, coronary artery bypass grafting (on and off pump) (In cardiothoracic surgery, it is administered along with GA and the risk of epidural hematoma may be higher than other surgeries

Contraindications

Absolute	Relative
• Refusal of the patient • Local infection at the site of administration • Severe bleeding diathesis	• Increased intracranial pressure • Preload dependent states, e.g., significant aortic stenosis, hypertrophic obstructive cardiomyopathy • Other bleeding diathesis, e.g., thrombocytopenia • Right to left shunt and pulmonary HTN • Bacteremia • Previous back surgery, pre-existing neurologic injury, back pain • Placement in anesthetized patients

26.3 Complications

It can be related to the technique, drug, or equipment. Often, more than one factor could be involved.

Procedure-related
- Inadvertent intrathecal or intravascular injection leading to total or high spinal anesthesia

- Pneumocephalus—a rare complication when large amount of air is used for LOR technique for identification of epidural space.
- Subdural injection of local anesthetic
- Epidural hematoma/abscess
- Hypotension
- Nausea, vomiting
- Post-dural puncture headache
- Epidural hematoma
- Epidural abscess/spinal epidural abscess
- Aseptic meningitis
- Osteomyelitis
- Back pain

Drug-related
- Local-anesthetic induced side effects
- LA systemic toxicity
- Allergy to LA
- Transient neurological syndrome
- The adjuvants like opioids, alpha-2 agonists, benzodiazepines etc. may have their own side effects
  - Steroids-related side effects include localized increase in pain, Non-positional headaches resolving within 24 h, facial flushing, anxiety, sleeplessness, fever, high blood sugar, a transient decrease in immunity

Equipment

Epidural needles	It allows easier identification of tissue and for facilitation of passage of the epidural catheter
Loss of resistance syringe	It allows the detection of the change in resistance once the epidural space is reached
Epidural catheters	It is used for continuous epidural anesthesia/analgesia
Spinal needle	For administration of subarachnoid block via epidural needle or in a different space
Hydrophobic filter	Hydrophobic 0.2 micron filter is available for additional safety and control against microbial infection

Epidural needles: Various designs, i.e., Tuohy, Crawford, Weiss, etc. are available; Tuohy being the commonest one (Fig. 26.2). Available in 16 or 18 G and 3.5 inches long (up to 6 inches for obese patients). The Tuohy needle has a curved tip (Huber point) with a blunt bevel designed to allow easier identification of tissue and for facilitation of passage of the epidural catheter. Wings at the junction of the needle shaft is for better controlled holding. The Crawford epidural needle is a Quincke type with an extremely short, and thus a very blunt and flat (approx. 60° with horizontal axis) bevel. Weiss needle is the modification of Tuohy's needle with metal wings attached to the needle hub. Whitacre or Quincke type needle has also been utilized for epidural steroidal injections and the Whitacre needle had been found to have the benefit of reducing the incidence of intravascular injection with and minimum amount of radiation exposure with minimal differences in technical difficulties (Fig. 26.3).

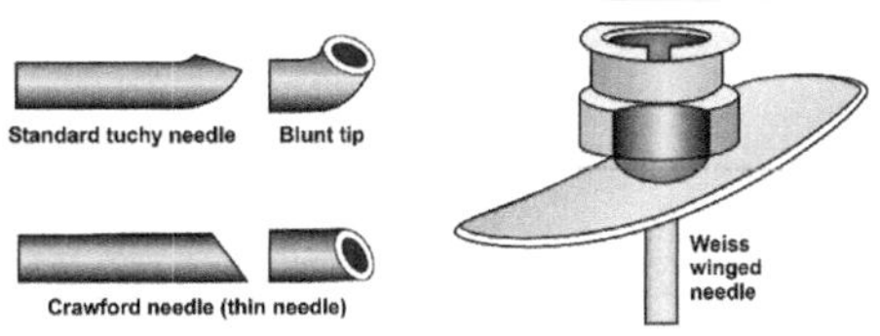

Fig. 26.2 Epidural needles (original)

> TNS is a rare and self-limiting complication with the use of lidocaine in spinal and epidural block and is presented with post-operative symmetrical back pain radiating to the buttocks and legs without any neurological deficit. The cornerstone of treatment is the management of systemic pain by NSAID, amitriptyline, gabapentine and epidural steroids

The suggested image of combined spinal epidural block has been incorporated as Fig. 26.4.

- Loss of resistance syringe: It is either made of plastic or glass. The latter has exceptionally low friction and thus allows the detection of the change in resistance once the epidural

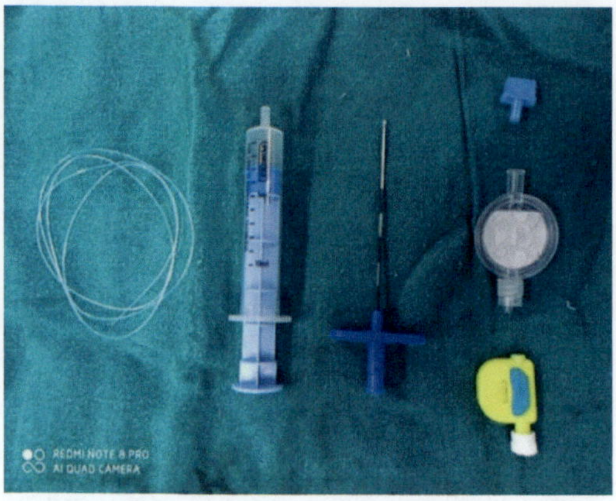

Fig. 26.3 Epidural set

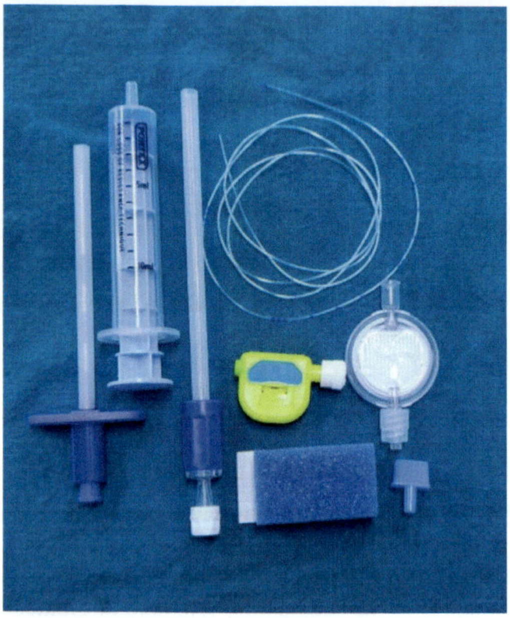

Fig. 26.4 Combined spinal epidural set (original)

space is reached. The loss of resistance can be checked by filling the syringe with air or saline and the choice of either of them has not been found to affect the success at identifying the epidural space.

- Epidural catheters: used for continuous epidural anesthesia/analgesia. The catheter may have a single hole or multiple holes. Very often in these kits, 19 G and 20 G catheters are paired with 16-G and 18-G needles, respectively.
- Epidural set- contains epidural needle and epidural catheter only. In these kits, 16 G or 18 G epidural needle is paired with an epidural catheter (Fig. 26.3).

Techniques:

1. According to location: Lumbar, thoracic, cervical
2. Approach: Midline and lateral
3. Position: Sitting or lateral position
4. Based on identification of epidural space
5. Single shot and continuous techniques

26.4 Procedure

Preprocedural preparation and considerations

- An intravenous access must be instituted for administration of fluid and medication.
- Avoid excessive sedation to have patients' cooperation during the positioning.
- Minimal mandatory monitors as recommended by American Society of Anesthesiologist (ASA) should be applied.
- Few important surface anatomic landmarks for epidural block are the most prominent spinous process (C7), the scapular spine (T3), and the inferior border of the scapula (T7).
- The patient may be positioned either in a sitting or lateral decubitus position.
- Sitting position is technically easier, used more commonly; however, preferred in obese, obstetric or scoliotic patient as it allows better exposure of intervertebral interspaces.
- Lateral decubitus position is preferred because of better tolerated hemodynamic changes, a reduced incidence of unintentional intravascular and dural puncture and easier attainment of unilateral blocks especially in orthopedic procedures. The block is instituted under aseptic precaution following thorough part preparation using Chlorhexidine with alcohol or povidone iodine Care must be taken to keep needles and drugs away from the skin disinfectants as the latter is considered neurotoxic.
- The desired interspace is identified using anatomic surface landmarks and palpation or with

ultrasonography. Compared to the conventional method of palpation of landmarks, US assistance (i.e., preprocedural scanning) results in fewer needle passes/insertions and skin punctures and provides similar pain relief.

> For sonography-guided epidural block, structures are identified using linear array transducer after skin disinfection and application of a sterile transducer sheath and gel. After local anesthesia with 2 ml preservative-free lignocaine (1%), the intervertebral space was visualised longitudinally and an 18-G epidural needle (Tuohy) was inserted and advanced under sonographic guidance into the epidural space of the sacral canal. Two ml of air is injected to check correct needle placement which will appear as hypoechoic zone as judged by real-time sonography.

- Infiltrate the skin and subcutaneous tissue with local anesthetic agent we can avoid using abbreviations too frequently (most commonly 1–2% lignocaine) uniformly we use lignocaine between adjacent spinous processes.
- Following LA, the epidural needle must be advanced along with its stylet with its bevel pointing toward the patient's head.
- Few of the hand positions commonly used during the advancement of the epidural needle are shown in Fig. 26.5a, b.
- The epidural needle is advanced through the skin, subcutaneous tissue, supraspinous, and interspinous ligaments, then the stylet is removed, and the loss of resistance (LOR) syringe (filled up with either saline, air or both) is firmly attached to the hub of the epidural needle.
- Air or saline for LOR can also be included in Controversies section to be created now.
- The air or saline for LOR has been incorporated in Controversies section.

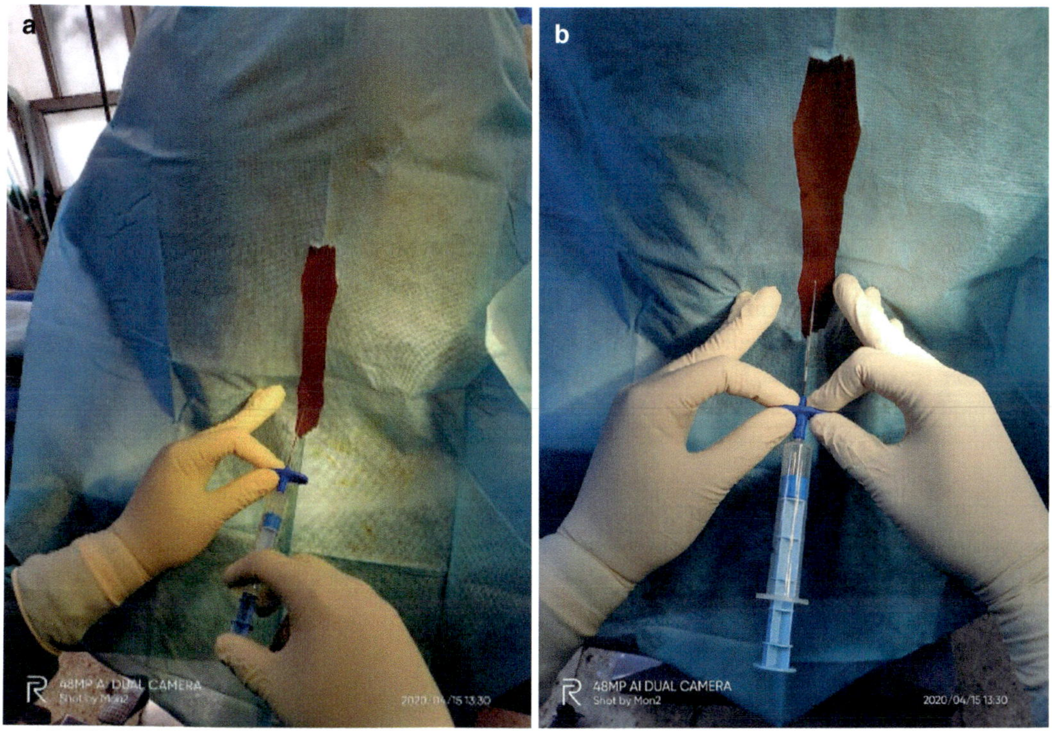

Fig. 26.5 (**a**, **b**) Epidural needle advancement with single hand (**a**) or two hands (**b**)

The needle can be engaged in either of any aforementioned ligaments before initiating epidural blockade using LOR technique. The interspinous ligament feels gritty and ligamentum flavum offers more resistance.

- While applying the pressure to the plunger of LOR syringe, the needle is slowly advanced further. As soon as the ligamentum flavum is pierced, a loss in resistance will be noted; this indicates the epidural space. The rough formula for calculation has been discussed below.

One must inject only the desired quantity during LOR technique especially while using air.
The sub-atmospheric pressure of the epidural space is diminished significantly from cervical to lumbar region, thus confounding various techniques for epidural space identification.

- The needle is fixed in this position and 5–10 ml of saline may be injected to expand the epidural space as it may decrease the risk of inadvertent vascular injury.
- Single-shot epidural technique
  - During single-shot epidural technique, the calculated LA dose may be administered directly through the needle in divided doses over several minutes. However, this technique is used less commonly now-a-days.
- Continuous epidural blockade
  - For continuous epidural blockade, an epidural catheter is inserted into the space. The marking on the epidural needle at the skin is noted. It represents the *depth to epidural space*, i.e., depth from the skin to the epidural space. This depth is subtracted from the total length of the needle (which is commonly 9 cm).
  - The epidural catheter is inserted via the Tuohy's needle until the 15-cm mark on the catheter approaches the hub of the epidural needle.
  - The needle is carefully removed taking care that the catheter doesn't dislodge.
  - To determine where the catheter should be secured at the skin, we can add 4–6 cm to the previously calculated *depth to epidural space*, e.g., if the latter is 8 cm, the catheter should be secured or taped at 12 cm or 13 cm mark at the skin (Fig. 26.6).

The catheter should not be threaded more than 4–6 cm into the epidural space, i.e., secured at around 10–11 cm mark at the skin.

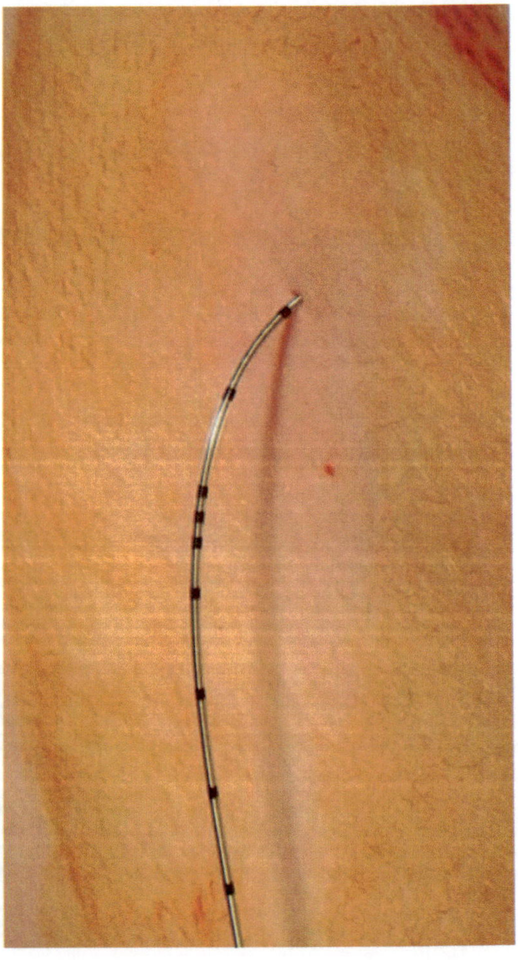

Fig. 26.6 Depicting 13 cm fixation mark on the epidural catheter

- The epidural filter is connected to the distal end of the epidural catheter. Following which, a sterile clear dressing is put.
- It is paramount to communicate with the patient throughout the procedure.

26.5 Test Dose to Rule Out Catheter Mal-placement

- The catheter mal-placement into the subarachnoid, intravascular, or subdural should be ruled out before administration of drug via catheter. The classical test dose combines 3 mL of 1.5% lidocaine with 15 mcg of epinephrine.
- If the catheter is intrathecal, 45 mg of lidocaine should produce a significant motor block; although recent evidences have questioned its reliability.
- If intravascular, the aspiration test would be positive; however, false negative cases may occur. A change in heart rate of 20% or greater or an increase in heart rate of 10–25 beats/min) within one minute suggests that the catheter is intravascular and should be replaced.
- It has been recommended to observe the patient for 5 min before labelling the test dose to be negative.
- Rarely catheter migration may occur after initial confirmation of the correct epidural placement of the catheter; therefore, it is advisable to fractionate the therapeutic dose in a 3–5 ml aliquots so that each bolus dose acts like a test dose.
- Exceptions have been observed in labouring, hypertensive, anesthetized patients, and patients receiving β-adrenergic blocking agents. In labouring patients, the concerns with the test dose are false-positive interpretation due to painful uterine contractions leading to change in HR and epinephrine-induced decrease in uterine blood flow. In hypertensive and pregnancy-induced hypertension, an exaggerated and not so well tolerated increase in BP may occur following the test dose. Under anesthesia, false negative result with test dose may occur due to the interference of inhalational anesthetic agents with epinephrine in the test dose. Similarly, in patient on beta blocker, the heart rate changes may not be reliable.

> During integrated epidural block and GA, the correct catheter placement must be evaluated before administering GA.

26.5.1 Paramedian Approach

- It is different from midline approach as the midline structures like supraspinous and interspinous ligaments are not traversed rather needle penetrates the paraspinous tissue which offers lesser resistance.
- It may be indicated in patients with spine deformities, difficulty in positioning e.g. orthopedic patients, or epidural technique in mid-thoracic regions as the tips of the spinous processes is directed caudally making midline technique difficult.

Steps:

1. Identify the intended interspace and infiltrate LA, one cm lateral and caudal to the inferior aspect of superior spinous process of the desired spinal level.
2. The epidural needle is inserted at around 15-20 degree towards midline with a cephalad tilt. If bone is encountered, the needle is redirected laterally, again with a cephalad tilt.

26.5.2 Taylor Approach

It is a paramedian approach utilizing the large L5-S1 interspace. It may be indicated in patients with ossified ligaments or where there is difficulty in positioning or as a rescue technique where the conventional paramedian approach fails.

Steps:

1. Following identification of the intended interspace, LA is infiltrated one cm medial and one cm caudal to the posterior superior iliac spine.
2. The epidural needle is inserted from this site, 45-55 degree cephalad and medially.
3. If the needle encounters bone, the needle should be walked of the bone resistance of the ligamentum is encountered and entry into the epidural space is achieved.

26.6 Drugs: Dose, Concentration

The duration and the level attained with epidural block are determined primarily by the site of injection, volume and the concentration of the drug used. As a general guideline, the initial loading is determined by the level of injection e.g. 1–2 mL of LA per segment to be blocked in a lumbar epidural, 0.7 mL/segment for a thoracic epidural, and 3 mL/segment for a caudal epidural. For surgical anesthesia, higher concentration (0.5% bupivacaine) and lower concentration (0.125% or 2.5% bupivacaine) for analgesia is administered. For maintenance of anesthesia, either a continuous infusion (4–15 ml/h) or top up dosages (one third or one quarter of the initial loading dose at time intervals depending upon the duration of LA used) are recommended.

Several drugs can be used in different combinations to achieve neuraxial anesthesia:

Local anesthetics: Lidocaine 1% and 2%, bupivacaine 0.25%, 1.5% and 2%, ropivacaine 0.75%, levobupivacaine 0.5%, chloroprocaine 2% and 3%.

Epidural additives: Vasoconstrictors such as epinephrine and phenylephrine are used to decrease the vascular absorption of local anesthetics.

Opioids: fentanyl, morphine, hydromorphone, oxycodone, or sufentanil (augment analgesic effects of the LA).

Alpha-agonists: clonidine and dexmedetomidine prolongs epidural analgesia.

26.7 Maintenance of Analgesia Techniques

It could be intermittent injection of analgesics or continuous epidural infusion or patient-controlled epidural analgesia (PCEA) (Fig. 26.7). Intermittent bolus offers a better area of distribution and less LA consumption; however, provide fluctuation between pain and analgesia.

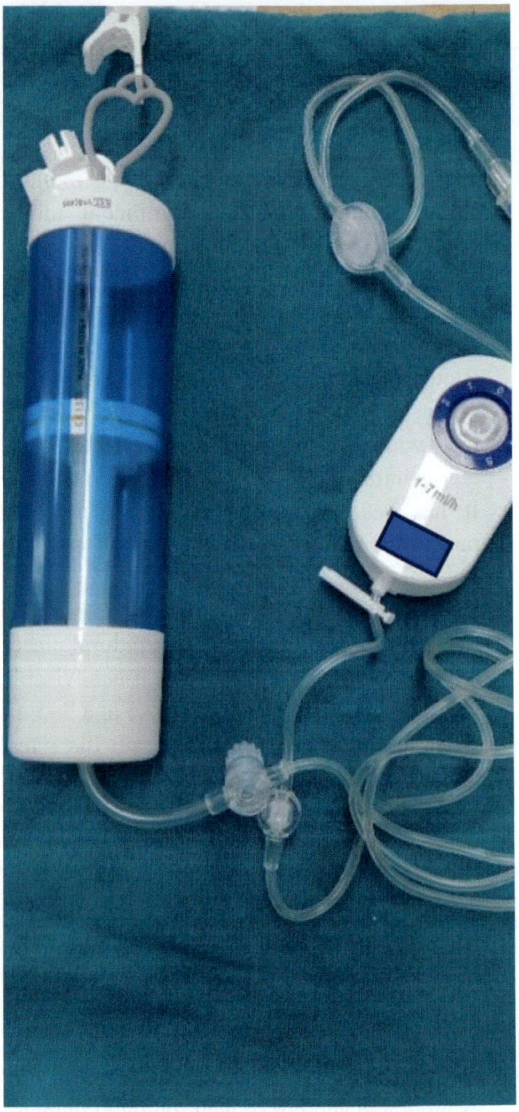

Fig. 26.7 Single dose PCEA infusion pump (original)

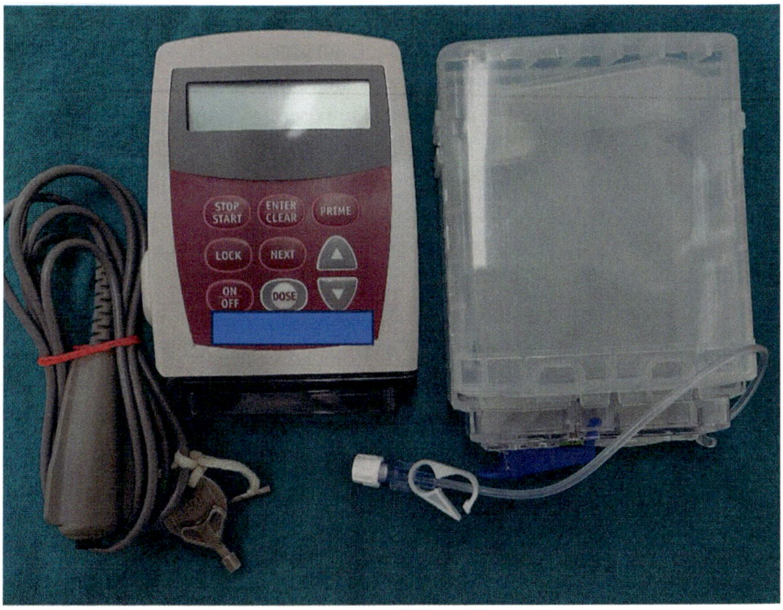

Fig. 26.8 Portable PCEA pump with cassette reservoir (original)

Continuous infusion of local anesthetics and opioids provides stable analgesia. However, it has been associated with increased local anesthesia consumption and, therefore, profound and sustained motor blockade. Patient-controlled epidural analgesia allows the patient to adjust the time of local anesthetic dosing to contractions and modify the intervals as labour progresses. The limitations include elevated cost of the equipment, more training and staff education are involved. On the other hand, PCEA has shown lower total dose usage of bupivacaine and ropivacaine compared to the continuous infusion technique (Fig. 26.8).

26.8 Cervical Epidural Block

- Cervical epidural anesthesia (CEA) is indicated for various surgical and pain procedures involving carotid artery, thyroid, breast, airway, upper limb and other head and neck surgeries, cervical-brachial neuraxial pain conditions etc.
- The commonly utilized positions for cervical epidural block are prone, sitting and lateral decubitus.
- Both midline and paramedian approaches have been utilized with or without fluoroscopic assistance.
- Single-shot injections of drug should be slow; whereas, for continuous techniques, the catheter must not be more than 2–3 cm into the cervical epidural space.

> In the cervical region, C7-T1 interspace is the widest along with largest skin-epidural space and epidural space-dural sac distance than at other cervical levels.
> Discontinuous ligamentum flavum at midline in the cervical region may contribute to false LOR.
> LOR with air is avoided as it can cause pain and pneumocephalus

- There have not been any dogmatic guidelines regarding its indication. The relative benefits or harm of CEA has been evaluated but the evidence is limited and is based on small studies. The clinical use of CEA has no place in routine practice; however, can only be considered in extensive carotid artery surgeries and possible oral-hypopharyngeal cancer surgeries. Its use warrants a strong rationale and must be considered under an expert anesthesiologist.

26.9 Thoracic Epidural Block

- Thoracic epidural anesthesia (TEA) is a commonly used and is known to have analgesic as well as non-analgesic effects such as reduced intraoperative blood loss, attenuated perioperative stress response and enhanced gastrointestinal motility leading to reduced duration of hospital stay [1].
- TEA is commonly used for upper abdominal and thoracic surgery, including gastrectomy, esophagectomy, lobectomy, and descending thoracic aorta procedures. The role of high TEA in cardiac surgery and off-pump coronary artery bypass (OPCAB) surgery is contentious with the higher risk of epidural hematoma.
- TEA, where combined with GA should be administered with patient either lightly sedated or awake before inducing general anesthesia as it warns the anesthetists of the potential neurological damage and early evaluation of the extent of sensory analgesia.
- The surface landmarks may be difficult in obese patients. Counting of the thoracic segment can be done from C7 vertebra for upper TEB or iliac crest for lower TEB. Fluoroscopy or ultrasound can be used to guide placement at a precise segment and verify appropriate catheter position after injection of contrast media.
- The Sitting position with neck and upper back flexion can be preferred. However, lateral decubitus position can be used in critically ill or recovering patient.
- Two approaches exist to the thoracic epidural space—midline or paramedian. The midline approach could be difficult in TEB due to the extreme caudal angulation of the thoracic spinous processes. The difficulty in lower TEB is same as that of lumbar epidural block due to the similar angulation of the spinous process.
- A paramedian approach is preferred in mid and high thoracic regions due to the extreme angulation of the thoracic spinous process. For paramedian approach, one cm lateral to the inferior tip of the spinous process corresponding to the designated vertebra, LA is injected both to the skin and lamina of vertebral body below. The approach of the needle is about 15° to the midline and 60–65° from the coronal plane. The LOR syringe is attached to the epidural needle which is then moved forward till the loss of resistance is attained. The epidural needle is stabilised and the stylet is removed and thread the catheter.
- After low-thoracic epidurals more cranial spread occurs than after high- and mid-thoracic epidurals, this could be attributable to the progressive increase in the width of the epidural space from 1–1.5 mm at C5 (as a result of cervical cord expansion) to 2.5–3 mm at T6 and 5–6 mm at L2. Therefore, insertion of a low thoracic epidural should correspond to the midline of the surgical incision, whereas a high-thoracic epidural should be inserted at a relatively more cranial point in respect to the incision.

26.10 Side effects

- Neurologic complications-including spinal cord injury, especially with upper TEB may arise due to direct nerve trauma by the needle or catheter. However, no study has reported neurological sequelae following TEA till now. Recently, the anatomic explanation for this low incidence was given following MRI thoracic canal studies of 50 patients which confirmed that the cord and the cauda equina touches the dura mater posteriorly in the lumbar region and anteriorly in the thoracic region

- Dural puncture-The incidence is 0.4–1.2% but has not been not found to be related to neurological sequelae.
- Unsuccessful catheter placement, post-operative radicular pain and peripheral nerve lesions.
- Epidural hematoma/abscess.
- Adverse effects related to medications used in TEA include nausea, vomiting, pruritus, hypotension, urinary retention, sedation, and respiratory depression.

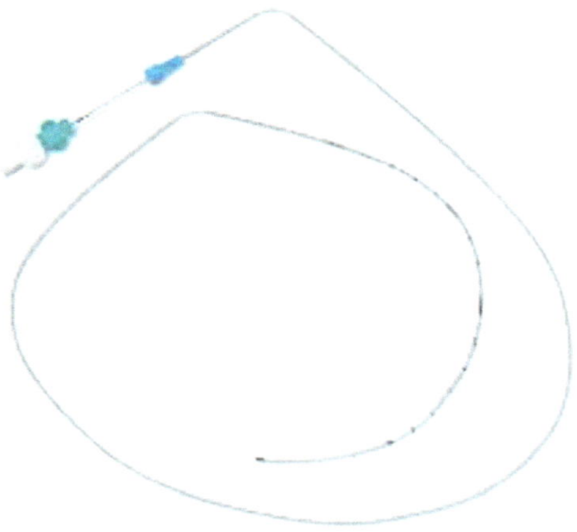

Fig. 26.9 Wire reinforced epidural catheter

26.11 Caudal Anesthesia

It is a variation of epidural anesthesia and administered at sacral level and is useful for interventions under the umbilicus line, e.g., circumcision, herniotomy, and orchiopexy. It shall be discussed in the subsequent chapter.

26.12 Controversies and Recent Advances

- Air vs Saline for LOR technique- When air is used for LOR, it may result in a false LOR as air is compressible and has also been associated with an increased incidence of complications such as pneumoencephalus. PDPH, incomplete or patchy block, venous air embolism or subcutaneous emphysema etc. The use of either air or saline for loss of resistance technique for identification of the epidural space has not been found to be related to difference in the complications rate.
- Wire-reinforced catheter is the recent technological advance in epidural catheter design. The addition of a circumferential stainless-steel coil within a nylon or polyurethane catheter has greater flexibility and thus, decreased incidence of venous cannulation, intrathecal placement, catheter migration (Fig. 26.9).
- The newer but less commonly used modern methods such as epidrum and acoustic devices have also been found to be efficacious as compared to the loss of resistance technique for identification of the epidural space and need further exploration. In the future, new methods of detecting misplaced catheters, such as acoustic signal guidance, nerve stimulation, and ultrasound-guided insertion, may replace the classical test dose method (Fig. 26.10).

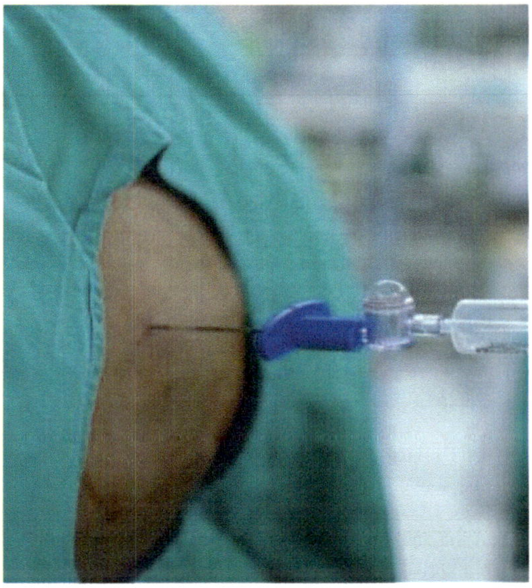

Fig. 26.10 Epidrum device (original)

- Thoracic epidural block in sepsis and critically ill patients has been a relative contraindication for thoracic epidural block. However,

recently, various experimental and few human studies have shown that TEB not only increases the gastrointestinal blood flow in sepsis, thus preventing splanchnic ischemia, it also attenuates ischemia- or infection-related inflammatory responses originating from splanchnic region by other mechanisms.
- Hematoma and abscesses after epidural anesthesia

Epidural anesthesia and thromboprophylaxis: The American Society of Regional Anesthesia and Pain Medicine (ASRA) and the European Society of Anaesthesiology (ESA) have published their consensus statements in this regard with the aim to minimize hemorrhagic complications; however, these recommendations allow variations based on the subjective judgment of the anesthesiologist and the institution protocol.

Suggested Reading

1. Youssef N, Orlov D, Alie T, Chong M, Cheng J, Thabane L, Paul J. What epidural opioid results in the best analgesia outcomes and fewest side effects after surgery? A meta-analysis of randomized controlled trials. Anesth Analg. 2014;119(4):965–77.
2. Popping DM, Zahn PK, Van Aken HK, Dasch B, Boche R, Pogatzki-Zahn EM. Effectiveness and safety of postoperative pain management: a survey of 18 925 consecutive patients between 1998 and 2006 (2nd revision): a database analysis of prospectively raised data. Br J Anaesth. 2008;101:832–40.
3. Rigg JR, Jamrozik K, Myles PS, et al. Epidural anaesthesia and analgesia and outcome of major surgery: a randomised trial. Lancet. 2002;359:1276–82.
4. Wijeysundera DN, Beattie WS, Austin PC, Hux JE, Laupacis A. Epidural anaesthesia and survival after intermediate-to-high risk non-cardiac surgery: a population-based cohort study. Lancet. 2008;372:562–9.
5. Landoni G, Iselle F, Greco M, Zangrillo A, Royse CF. Benefits and risks of epidural analgesia in cardiac surgery. J Cardiothorac Vasc Anesth. 2015;115(1):25–32.
6. Antibas PL, do Nascimento P, Braz LG, Vitor Pereira Doles J, Módolo NS, El Dib R. Air versus saline in the loss of resistance technique for identification of the epidural space. Cochrane Database Syst Rev. 2014;7:CD008938.
7. Agarwal D, Mohta M, Tyagi A, Sethi AK. Subdural block and the anaesthetist. Anaesth Intensive Care. 2010;38(1):20–6.
8. Abbatemarco JR, Rae-Grant AD. Transient neurologic syndromes: a diagnostic approach. Cleve Clin J Med. 2018;85(2):155–63.
9. Li WX, Luo RY, Chen C, et al. Effects of propofol, dexmedetomidine, and midazolam on postoperative cognitive dysfunction in elderly patients: a randomized controlled preliminary trial. Chin Med J. 2019;132(4):437–45.
10. Shirmohammadie M, Ebrahim Soltani A, Arbabi S, Nasseri K. A randomized-controlled, double-blind study to evaluate the efficacy of caudal midazolam, ketamine and neostigmine as adjuvants to bupivacaine on postoperative analgesic in children undergoing lower abdominal surgery. Acta Biomed. 2019;89(4):513–8.
11. Sanwatsarkar S, Kapur S, Saxena D, Yadav G, Khan NN. Comparative study of caudal clonidine and midazolam added to bupivacaine during infra-umbilical surgeries in children. J Anaesthesiol Clin Pharmacol. 2017;33(2):241–7.
12. Zorrilla-Vaca A, Makkar JK. Effectiveness of lateral decubitus position for preventing post-dural puncture headache: a meta-analysis. Pain Physician. 2017;20(4):E521–9.
13. Elgueta MF, Duong S, Finlayson RJ, Tran DQ. Ultrasonography for neuraxial blocks: a review of the evidence. Minerva Anestesiol. 2017;83(5):512–23.
14. Olawin AM, Das J. Spinal anesthesia. In: StatPearls. Treasure Island: StatPearls Publishing; 2019.
15. Gupta S, Raval D, Patel M, Patel N, Shah N. Addition of epidural Clonidine enhances postoperative analgesia: a double-blind study in total knee-replacement surgeries. Anesth Essays Res. 2010;4(2):70–4.
16. Capogna G, Camorcia M, Stirparo S, Farcomeni A. Programmed intermittent epidural bolus versus continuous epidural infusion for labor analgesia: the effects on maternal motor function and labor outcome. A randomized double-blind study in nulliparous women. Anesth Analg. 2011;113(4):826–31.
17. Boutros A, Blary S, Bronchard R, Bonnet F. Comparison of intermittent epidural bolus, continuous epidural infusion and patient controlled-epidural analgesia during labor. Int J Obstet Anesth. 1999;8(4):236–41.
18. van der Vyver M, Halpern S, Joseph G. Patient-controlled epidural analgesia versus continuous infusion for labour analgesia: a meta-analysis. Br J Anaesth. 2002;89(3):459–65.
19. Standl T, Burmeister MA, Ohnesorge H, Wilhelm S, Striepke M, Gottschalk A, Horn EP, Schulte Am Esch J. Patient-controlled epidural analgesia reduces analgesic requirements compared to continuous epidural infusion after major abdominal surgery. Can J Anaesth. 2003;50(3):258–64.

20. Shanthana H, Mendis M, Goel A. Cervical epidural analgesia in current anaesthesia practice: systematic review of its clinical utility and rationale, and technical considerations. Br J Anaesth. 2016;116(2):192–207.
21. Zawar BP, Mehta Y, Juneja R, Arora D, Raizada A, Trehan N. Nonanalgesic benefits of combined thoracic epidural analgesia with general anesthesia in high risk elderly off pump coronary artery bypass patients. Ann Card Anaesth. 2015;18:385–91.
22. McLeod GA, Cumming C. Thoracic epidural anesthesia and analgesia. Contin Educ Anaesth Crit Care Pain. 2004;4(1):16–9.
23. Giebler RM, Scherer RU, Peters J. Incidence of neurologic complications related to thoracic epidural catheterization. Anesthesiology. 1997;86:55–63.
24. Lea˜o DG. Thoracic epidural anesthesia: analysis of 1240 cases. Rev Bras Anestesiol. 1997;47:138–47.
25. Imbelloni LE, Gouveia MA. Low incidence of neurologic complications during thoracic epidurals: anatomic explanation. Am J Neuroradiol. 2010;31(10):E84.
26. Toledano RD, Tsen LC. Epidural catheter design: history, innovations, and clinical implications. Anesthesiology. 2014;121(1):9–17.
27. Carvalho, et al. Commonly-used versus less commonly-used methods in the loss of resistance technique for identification of the epidural space: a systematic review and meta-analysis of randomized controlled trials. J Clin Anesth. 2017;38:41–51.
28. Adolphs J, Schmidt DK, Korsukewitz I, Kamin B, Habazettl H, Schäfer M, et al. Effects of thoracic epidural anaesthesia on intestinal microvascular perfusion in a rodent model of normotensive endotoxaemia. Intensive Care Med. 2004;30:2094–101.
29. Horlocker TT, Wedel DJ, Rowlingson JC, et al. Regional Anesthesia in the patient receiving antithromboticor thrombolytic therapy; American Society of RegionalAnesthesia and Pain Medicine evidence-based guidelines (Third Edition). Reg Anesth Pain Med. 2010;35(1):64–101.
30. Gogarten W, Vandermeulen E, Van Aken H, Kozek S, Llau JV, Samama CM. Regional anaesthesia andantithrombotic agents: recommendations of the European Society of Anaesthesiology. Eur J Anaesthesiol. 2010;27(12):999–1015.
31. Bos EME, Haumann J, de Quelerij M, et al. Haematoma and abscess after neuraxial anaesthesia: a review of 647 cases. Br J Anaesth. 2018;120(4):693–704.

27 Dural Puncture Epidural Analgesia

Vinayak PS

> **Key Points**
> - Dural puncture epidural technique has the potential to fasten onset and improve quality of labor analgesia when compared with conventional epidural technique.
> - Also, DPE has fewer maternal adverse effects compared to CSE.
> - DPE is a valuable addition to the obstetric anesthetists' armamentarium.

The experience of childbirth ranges from agony to ecstasy. It has intense physical, psychological, emotional, developmental, social, cultural, and spiritual components. Pain scores during labor have shown that degree of pain ranges between that of cancer pain and amputation of a digit.

Techniques of labor analgesia are classified as non-pharmacological and pharmacological. Several nonpharmacological methods are described in the literature. Epidural analgesia (EA) is the most commonly employed technique and enjoys widespread reputation for its efficacy and success. Onset of epidural block has a more gradual onset compared to spinal but with the advantage of being more controllable levels of block and continuous infusion through a catheter. Combined spinal epidural (CSE), on the other hand, combines the benefits of both spinal and epidural techniques but it can cause hemodynamic instability, foetal bradycardia, pruritis and other adverse effects due to the intrathecal drugs.

In 1996, Suzuki and colleagues published the first study on the dural puncture epidural (DPE) technique in patients undergoing lower abdominal surgery. This was followed by a series of publications on the novel technique of DPE wherein a dural hole is created prior to epidural injection. DPE is a modification of conventional epidural analgesia that involves the intentional puncture of the dura with a spinal needle through the needle placed in the epidural space, without a medication being injected intrathecally.

27.1 Dural Puncture Epidural Technique

The DPE technique involves first locating the epidural space with the epidural needle and then passing a spinal needle through the shaft of the epidural needle to create a dural puncture with CSF confirmation; however, no medications are directly administered through the spinal needle. The spinal needle is withdrawn, and the epidural catheter inserted and dosed with a conventional

Vinayak PS (✉)
Department of Anaesthesiology, MS Ramaiah Medical College, Bangalore, India

Manipal Hospital, Bangalore, India

N. Gupta et al. (eds.), *Techniques in Anesthesia, Intensive Care and Emergency Medicine*,
https://doi.org/10.1007/978-981-96-1202-4_27

dose (12–20 mL) of dilute local anesthetic (e.g., bupivacaine 0.125%) with or without an opioid (fentanyl 2 μg/mL).

27.2 Mechanism of Action

The translocation of epidural medications through the dural puncture into the subarachnoid space has been postulated as a possible mechanism by which the DPE technique improves analgesia or anesthesia. The mechanism by which DPE produces analgesia has been found to be directly proportional to the size of the needle, volume of epidural drug mixture and injection time. Size of the dural puncture: The gauge of the needle utilized for the dural puncture plays a significant role in the migration of the drug. In a primate model, Bernards et al. suggested that drug movement through the meningeal hole following dural puncture with 18–25 G needles is responsible flux of medication administered by epidural into the subarachnoid space. Recent studies have shown the spinal needle used to create the dural puncture should be larger than 27 G. Faster onset to analgesia and better sensory block characteristics with the DPE technique have been found when 25/26 G needles are used. Volume of the epidural drug mixture: Larger volumes of epidural top-ups have been found to have faster and better bilateral blocks in DPE. Short injection times: Epidural injection over 1–6 min have been found to have a faster onset.

The analgesia produced has been found to be inversely proportional to the intact meningeal surface area exposed to the drug and the intrinsic diffusion capacity of the drug through an intact dura. If a drug readily crosses the spinal meninges, the presence of a physical hole in the dura will minimally impact its transfer to the subarachnoid space. In contrast, a drug with a slow trans meningeal transfer rate will greatly benefit from "dry" dural puncture. This explains why, in Bernards et al.'s study, trans meningeal flux of morphine in a monkey model increased in the presence of 27-G dural holes but translocation of lidocaine was comparable between native specimens and those pierced with a 27-G Whitacre needle. Distance of the dural puncture from the site of epidural drug administration also could have influence on the onset, quality, and duration of analgesia. All published trials have used a needle through needle technique for DPE.

27.3 Advantages and Disadvantages of DPE

Advantages include shorter time for onset of analgesia as suggested by low VAS score at 20 min, reduction in the overall number of epidural top-ups, better sacral analgesia and improved hemodynamic stability compared to CSE or spinal. CSF through the spinal needle in the DPE technique also indicates that the epidural needle is properly placed in the epidural space. Unlike the CSE, epidural is immediately activated in DPE. When used for labor analgesia, DPE produces more rapid onset and better quality of block with reduced unilateral block.

DPE has few disadvantages as well. First, lux through a 25 G dural puncture may be limited only to a limited period of time after the puncture depending on the volume or epidural pressure generated with epidural medication bolus. Second, dural puncture with small (i.e., 26- or 27-G) spinal needles seems to confer either minimal benefits or improved analgesic quality and lower pain scores in the first 10 min whereas dural puncture with 25-G spinal needles has been reported to provide higher success.

Further studies are required to refine the technique (drug concentration, volume, effect on labor, etc. (Table 27.1).

Table 27.1 Comparison of standard neuraxial analgesia techniques versus DPE technique

	Epidural	CSE	DPE
Block characteristics			
Onset of analgesia	Slowest	Fastest	Intermediate
Spread of analgesia	Average	Very good	Good
Block symmetry	Lower	Higher	Higher
Block quality	Average	Excellent	Very good
Failed block	Higher risk	Lower risk with CSF return	Lower risk with CSF return
Catheter testing	Immediate	Delayed	Immediate
Catheter adjustment/replacement rate	Higher	Lower	Lower
Incidence of adverse events			
PDPH	No difference	No difference	No difference
Motor block	Higher	Lower	Lower
Maternal hypotension	Low	High	Low
Pruritis	Low	High	Low
Need for top-ups	Early	Intermediate	Intermediate
Uterine tachysystole	Low	High	Low
Fetal bradycardia	Low	High	Low
Emergency LSCS due to fetal Bradycardia	No difference	No difference	No difference

CSE combined spinal epidural, *DPE* dural puncture epidural, *PDPH* postdural puncture headache

Suggested Reading

1. Suresh M. Shnider and Levinson's anesthesia for obstetrics. Philadelphia: Lippincott Williams & Wilkins; 2013. p. 882.
2. Gunaydin B, Erel S. How neuraxial labor analgesia differs by approach: dural puncture epidural as a novel option. J Anesth. 2019;33(1):125–30.
3. Heesen M, Rijs K, Rossaint R, Klimek M. Dural puncture epidural versus conventional epidural block for labor analgesia: a systematic review of randomized controlled trials. Int J Obstet Anesth. 2019;40:24–31.
4. Chau A, Tsen LC. Update on modalities and techniques for labor epidural analgesia and anesthesia. Adv Anesth. 2018;36(1):139–62.
5. Bernards CM, Kopacz DJ, Michel MZ. Effect of needle puncture on morphine and lidocaine flux through the spinal meninges of the monkey in vitro. Implications for combined spinal-epidural anesthesia. Anesthesiology. 1994;80(4):853–8.
6. Wilson SH, Wolf BJ, Bingham K, Scotland QS, Fox JM, Woltz EM, et al. Labor analgesia onset with dural puncture epidural versus traditional epidural using a 26-Gauge Whitacre needle and 0.125% bupivacaine bolus: a randomized clinical trial. Anesth Analg. 2018;126(2):545–51.
7. Layera S, Bravo D, Aliste J, Tran DQ. A systematic review of DURAL puncture epidural analgesia for labor. J Clin Anesth. 2019;53:5–10.

28 Nasogastric and Orogastric Tube Insertion

Sachin Kumar, Anju Gupta, and Nishkarsh Gupta

28.1 Background

Nasogastric (NG) or orogastric (OG) tubes as their name suggest are small tubes that are placed either through the nose or the mouth and their tip end in stomach. Dr. Abraham Louis Levin first described their use in 1921. Nasogastric tube is also known as Ryle's tube in Commonwealth countries, after John Alfred Ryle. NG/OG tubes may be used for feedings, medication administration, treatment of drug overdose, or removal of contents from the stomach via aspiration, suction, or gravity drainage.

28.2 Relevant Anatomy

The nares are the anterior opening of the nose. Nasopharynx is situated 5–7 cm posterior to nares. Nasopharynx then continues with oropharynx. The length of the pharynx from the base of the skull to the start of the esophagus is 12–14 cm. Total length of the esophagus starting from upper esophageal sphincter to the stomach is 25 cm. Stomach is 25 cm long though it's length can vary being a distensible structure. Thus, an approximately 55 cm of the tube length is inserted in adult patient if one aims at inserting it till middle of stomach from nares.

S. Kumar · A. Gupta (✉)
Anesthesiology, Pain Medicine, Critical Care, All India Institute of Medical Sciences, New Delhi, Delhi, India

N. Gupta
Department Onco-Anesthesiology and Palliative Medicine at DRBRAIRCH, All India Institute of Medical Sciences, New Delhi, Delhi, India

28.3 Types of NG Tubes

- Levine tube: It is a single lumen nasogastric/orogastric tube. It is usually made of plastic with several drainage holes near the gastric end of the tube. This is more appropriate for administration of medication/nutrition.
- Salem sump tube: It is a two-lumen nasogastric/orogastric tube. The large lumen allows for easy suction of gastric contents, decompression, irrigation, and medication delivery. The smaller lumen allows atmospheric air to enter in to stomach and create pressure balance once the stomach contents are aspirated so that gastric mucosa does not adhere to suction eyelets.
- Moss tube: It is a triple-lumen nasogastric tube. The first lumen is used to inflate gastric balloon to occlude the cardioesophageal junction. The second lumen is an esophageal aspiration port and third is used for duodenal feeding.

N. Gupta et al. (eds.), *Techniques in Anesthesia, Intensive Care and Emergency Medicine*,
https://doi.org/10.1007/978-981-96-1202-4_28

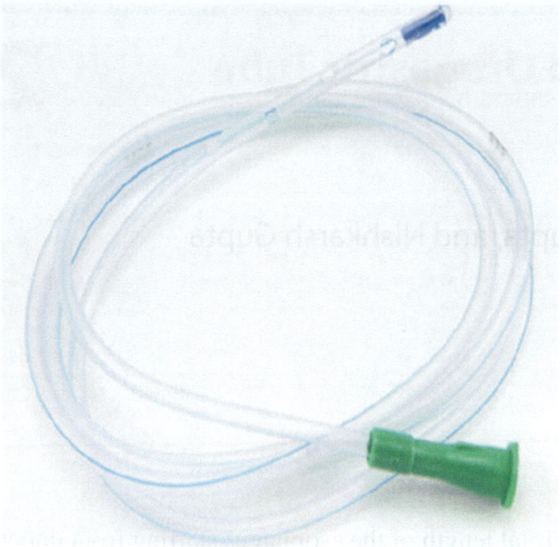

Levine tube

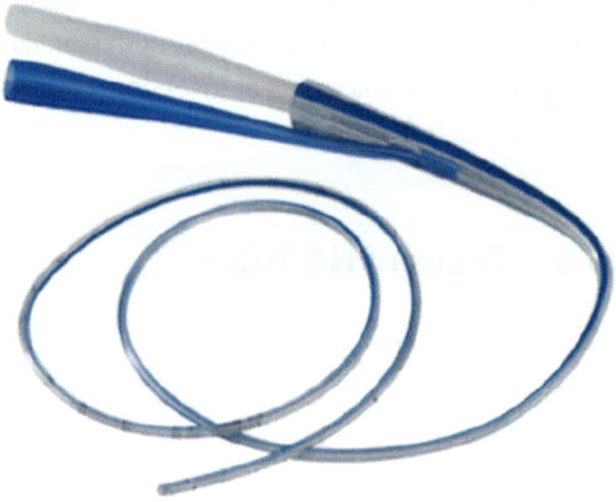

Salem sump tube

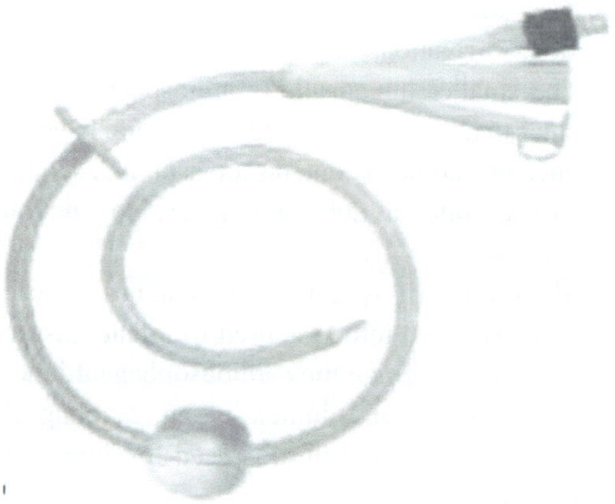

Moss tube

Nasogastric tubes used for feeding are:

- Short term nasogastric feeding tubes: Made of PVC or low-grade polyurethane. They are recommended for use up to 7–10 days.
- Long term nasogastric feeding tubes: Usually made of polyurethane and often have guidewire to help in insertion of tube. These kinds of tubes can usually be used up to 6–8 weeks.

28.4 Indications

28.4.1 Therapeutic Uses

- To administer feed or medication through enteral route in case patient cannot take per orally.
- To relieve ileus or mechanical bowl obstruction.
- For gastric lavage in some centers in case of drug overdose.
- Warm or cold saline can be given through NG tube to aid in aggressive warming (e.g., in hypothermia) or aggressive cooling (e.g., in malignant hyperpyrexia).
- To improve ventilation post-intubation in small children (e.g., incomplete drowning).

28.4.2 Perioperative

- Preoperative decompression of stomach to reduce risk of aspiration
- To facilitate surgery in laparoscopic procedures where stomach decompression is needed
- Intra or post operatively where ileus is expected to occur
- To administer radiopaque dye in stomach or gut when gut resection anastomosis is done to rule out any leak

28.4.3 Diagnostic Uses

- For pH monitoring and to determine motor activity of GI tract
- To obtain specimen of gastric contents for diagnostic purposes in case of intestinal obstruction

- X-ray studies of the upper gastrointestinal tract by administering radio opaque dye
- Diagnosis of upper GI bleeding

28.4.4 Contraindications

- In patients who have history of caustic ingestion or esophageal strictures (risk of perforation)
- Nasogastric tubes should never be inserted in patients with confirmed or suspected base of skull fractures. There is a risk of tube going in to cranial vault.
- Severe mid-face trauma (risk of cribriform plate disruption with NGT entering the brain)
- Coagulopathy (epistaxis risk)
- Choanal atresia
- Unstable cervical spine injuries
- Nasal/pharyngeal/esophageal obstruction
- Tracheoesophageal fistula
- Esophageal/pharyngeal pouch
- Oropharyngeal tumors or have undergone oropharyngeal surgery
- Esophageal tumors or have undergone esophageal surgery
- Post- laryngectomy
- Actively bleeding esophageal or gastric varices
- Patient refusal

In case of nasal bone fracture, base of skull fracture or choanal atresia orogastric tube can be inserted.

28.5 Preparation

28.5.1 Consent

Informed verbal consent explaining purpose of procedure and risk associated with it should be discussed with the patient. After discussion patient should be given some time to take decision. Discussion and patient decision should be documented in relevant patient notes. If procedural consent form is available then that can be filled and signature can be taken. In cases where patient is minor or patient demonstrate a lack of capacity to take decision then informed consent should be taken from family members/parents.

28.5.2 Equipment

- Non sterile gloves and apron
- Appropriate PPE
- Appropriate size NG/OG tube suitable for intended purpose. 14 FG is adequate for general gastric decompression. For long-term feeding fine bore tubes with guidewires are preferred. Refrigerated NG tubes are also used sometimes
- Water soluble lubricating gel or lignocaine 2%
- Tongue depressor
- Vomit bowl
- Appropriate enteral syringe usually 60 ml
- Facial tissues
- pH indicator strips
- Glass of water with straw
- Hypoallergic tape for fixation
- Alcohol swab
- Functioning suction equipment
- Wash cloth with soap and water
- Skin barrier wipes
- Flashlight

28.5.3 In Anesthetized Patient

- Laryngoscope (checked)
- Magill's forceps

28.5.4 Sites

- Nostril

Either right or left nostril should be selected depending on patency or deformity

- Oral

This route is preferred in patients with head injury or trauma to nose or sometimes when tube is required only during surgery

28.5.5 Procedure in Awake Patient

1. Follow proper hand hygiene before putting gloves and apron. Prepare equipment on a clean surface area.
2. Patient should be given a signal so that during procedure they can tell their problem or ask to stop the procedure.
3. Patient should sit in a semi-upright position with the head supported with pillows and tilted neither backwards nor forwards.
4. Each nostril should be examined for any deformity or obstruction and sniff test should be done to check for more patent nostril.
5. Place towel over patient's chest and place vomit bowel within reach.
6. Perform procedure from right side of the patient if right-handed otherwise left side.
7. Nasogastric tube should be opened and lubricated from outside as per manufacturer guidelines.
8. Next the length of nasogastric tube to be inserted is measured. Tube tip is placed from nasal bridge to tragus of ear and from there to xiphisternum. Note down the mark corresponding to xiphisternum. This gives an estimate of the length of the tube to be inserted and might be adjusted.
9. Lubricated tube should be inserted in decided nostril and direction should be parallel to the floor of nasal cavity not upwards. Then further advance the tube towards the back of the nose and along the nasopharynx.
   (a) If resistance is met at any point till tube goes just past the nasopharynx, then apply only gentle pressure to advance the tube. If resistance is met again then try through another nostril.

   For oral insertion: Direct tube to the back of the tongue and then direct tube downwards through the oropharynx
10. Once past the nasopharynx stop tube advancement and allow patient to relax.
11. Now ask the patient to swallow to help in tube advancement and give them glass of water with straw.

    Note: If potential for aspiration, a few ice chips on a spoon may be offered or the patient can be asked to dry swallow
12. Ask the patient to flex head forward and take a small sip of water and swallow to aid in advancement of tube.
13. If patient begins to cough, gag, choke—withdraw the tube slightly and ask the patient to relax and take deep breath and then advance the tube further till the predetermined mark.
14. Once the tube has been inserted to predetermined mark, confirm the position of the tube with the confirmation methods (as discussed later).
15. Secure the nasogastric tube at the nose or cheek with hypoallergic adhesive tape.

28.5.6 Procedure in Anesthetized/Unconscious Patient

- Usually, endotracheal tube is present, sometimes anesthetists put NG tube before intubation in elective surgeries.
- Different methods can be used to insert NG tube either laryngoscopy is done when the tube passes nasopharynx and NG tube is visible in mouth then Magill's forceps is used to hold the tip of tube and tube is passed bit-by-bit in to esophagus.
- **Blind technique**: In this technique as the name suggest, NG is passed through either of the nares (usually right or more patent looking, can be checked pre op in elective surgeries) till the stomach after calculating the length. In this procedure, head is kept in neutral position and if resistance is felt at any point, then tube slightly withdrawn and inserted
- **Trouble shoot in blind technique**: Reverse Sellick's maneuver: in this cricoid cartilage is lifted anteriorly to aid in passage of tube. This helps in opening of the esophageal passage.
- Neck flexion can be done which helps to keep the tube close to the floor of the posterior pharyngeal wall and this helps in smooth passage of the tube in to esophagus.

- Sometimes patient's head is kept in the lateral position or lateral neck pressure is applied to prevent impaction of the tube on the arytenoids and in the piriform fossa
- A cold NG tube prepared by keeping in the freezer can also be used. It has slightly less chances of coiling as it is more stiff. It becomes soft also after some time due to body heat.
- To aid passage through nostril, a nasopharyngeal airway cut along its length can be inserted inside nostril and after inserting NG later can be taken out.
- NGT insertion with angiocath wire/ureteral guidewire are other methods to stiffen the tube.
- Fine bore NGT placement based on Seldinger technique has also been described.
- Inflation with air via a facepiece attached to a self-inflating bag applied firmly with the face while NGT being inserted through the nostril has also been found easy after sedating and paralysing the patient posted for surgery.

28.6 NG Tube Insertion Under Vision

- Conventional laryngoscopy/video laryngoscopy is done when tube passes nasopharynx and NG tube is visible in mouth then Magill's forceps is used to hold the tip of tube and tube is passed bit by bit in to esophagus.
- Fiberoptic scope placement can also be done.

28.6.1 Troubleshoot

- In some intubated patients when it is not possible to pass the NG tube in to esophagus under vision during laryngoscopy, endotracheal tube/tracheostomy tube cuff might be deflated to aid in passage through esophagus.
- Alternatively, digital placement of an NGT can be accomplished in a paralyzed, sedated, and intubated patient. The emergency physician places the second and third fingers in the posterior pharynx of the patient and depresses the tongue. The tube is passed through the nose into the posterior pharynx with the fingers in the pharynx to direct the tube into proper location.

28.6.2 Tips and Advice

- In awake/unconscious patient, NG tube insertion should be tried during expiration as it may avoid tracheal placement.
- Use of excessive force during insertion should be avoided. If resistance is encountered then consider removal and reinsertion otherwise false passages can be created.

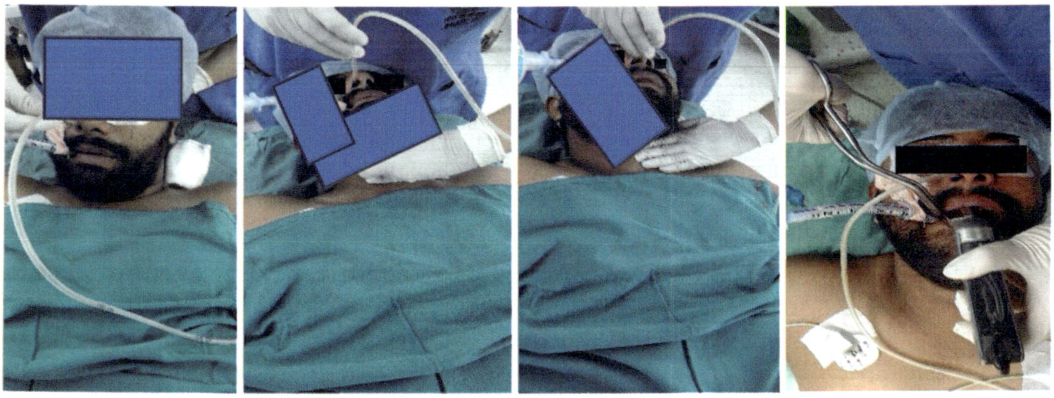

Different maneuvers to aid nasogastric tube insertion

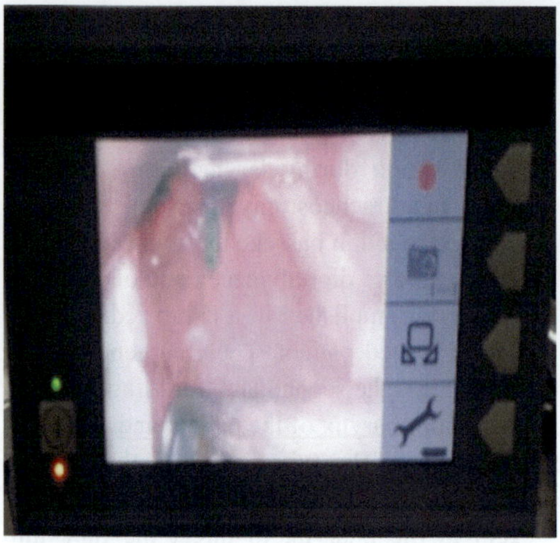

Insertion of nasogastric tube with the help of video laryngoscope and Magill forceps

28.6.3 Confirmation of Correct Placement of NG/OG Tube

1. Patient should be able to speak. There should be no vomiting, retching, or drop in oxygen saturation.
2. Throat should be checked for any coiling.
3. Try to aspirate the gastric contents through 60 ml catheter tip syringe and examine the visual characteristics of aspirate
4. pH of the aspirate should be checked by using pH strips and pH less than 5.5 indicate correct placement. If patient is on antacids, then try to take the sample before taking antacid. With antacids pH may be up to 6.
5. Chest/upper abdominal X-ray may be ordered to confirm tube placement. Tube tip should be visible below diaphragm.
6. Capnography might be attached to NG tube intraoperatively to rule out intratracheal placement.
7. Air can be insufflated through the tube and epigastrium or left upper quadrant of the abdomen can be auscultated for gurgling sound following insufflation of air (unreliable)
8. Abdominal ultrasound can be done though it is better suited for nasogastric tubes with weighted tips.
9. Fluoroscopy can be used.
10. It can be palpated by the surgeon intraoperatively.

28.6.4 Complications

- Trauma to nasal, pharyngeal, esophageal, and gastric mucosa.
- Tracheal or bronchial placement. It is uncommon in awake patient.
- Cranial placement through basal skull fracture.
- NG tube might go in esophagus and it might lead to regurgitation and aspiration of administered substances.
- NGT may induce a hypersalivation response, a depressed cough reflex, or mechanical or physiologic impairment of the glottis which can lead to pulmonary aspiration.
- Rarely pneumothorax can occur.
- Blocked tube also increases the chance of aspiration.
- Gastric or duodenal rupture.
- Gastrothorax and tension gastrothorax

28.6.5 Care of the NG/OG Tube

1. Patient should be nursed with bed elevated at 30°.
2. Secure the NG tube to patient gown also apart from nose or cheek.
3. If patient present with gagging, coughing, and vomiting, check for the coiling of tube.
4. NG placement should be checked at least once per shift for correct external measurement marking at nose/mouth, for fixation, coiling, blockage.
5. If blockage of the tube is suspected, then 15–30 ml of warm water should be pushed with 60 ml enteral syringe. Under no circumstances a guidewire is inserted to remove the blockage.
6. pH testing for gastric placement should be done when there is evidence of tube displacement, e.g., external measurement marking at nose/mouth is different or device used for securing

the tube has become loose or there is unexplained respiratory symptom or desaturation.

Suggested Reading

1. ng-og-verification-clinical-standard-preview-2015.pdf [Internet]. https://www.childrensmn.org/departments/webrn/pdf/ng-og-verification-clinical-standard-preview-2015.pdf.
2. Sigmon DF, An J. Nasogastric tube. In: StatPearls. Treasure Island: StatPearls Publishing; 2022. http://www.ncbi.nlm.nih.gov/books/NBK556063/.
3. 1040.pdf [Internet]. https://www.saskatoonhealthregion.ca/about/NursingManual/1040.pdf.
4. Nasogastric tube [Internet]. http://www.sharinginhealth.ca/procedures/nasogastric_tube.html.
5. https://nnng.org.uk/wp-content/uploads/2016/06/NNNG-Nasogastric-tube-Insertion-and-Ongoing-Care-Practice-Final-Aprill-2016.pdf.
6. Mandal MC, Dolai S, Ghosh S, Mistri PK, Roy R, Basu SR, et al. Comparison of four techniques of nasogastric tube insertion in anaesthetised, intubated patients: a randomized controlled trial. Indian J Anaesth. 2014;58(6):714–8.
7. Appukutty J, Shroff PP. Nasogastric tube insertion using different techniques in anesthetized patients: a prospective, randomized study. Anesth Analg. 2009;109(3):832–5.
8. Mandal M, Karmakar A, Basu SR. Nasogastric tube insertion in anaesthetised, intubated adult patients: a comparison between three techniques. Indian J Anaesth. 2018;62(8):609–15.
9. Kim HJ, Lee HJ, Cho HJ, Kim HK, Cho AR, Oh N. Nasogastric tube insertion using airway tube exchanger in anesthetized and intubated patients. Korean J Anesthesiol. 2016;69(6):568–72.
10. Madhusudhan S, Srinivasaiah B, Pai RK, Gopalaiah VK. Guidewire-assisted nasogastric tube insertion in post stroke patients: a simple bedside trick. Neurology. 2019;67(5):1367.
11. Doshi J, Anari S. Seldinger technique for insertion of a nasogastric tube. Laryngoscope. 2006;116(4):672–3.
12. Gupta D, Agarwal A, Nath SS, Goswami D, Saraswat V, Singh PK. Inflation with air via a facepiece for facilitating insertion of a nasogastric tube: a prospective, randomised, double-blind study. Anaesthesia. 2007;62(2):127–30.
13. Moharari RS, Fallah AH, Khajavi MR, Khashayar P, Lakeh MM, Najafi A. The GlideScope facilitates nasogastric tube insertion: a randomized clinical trial. Anesth Analg. 2010;110(1):115–8.
14. Cureus | role of endotracheal tube cuff deflation in facilitating passage of nasogastric tube [Internet]. https://www.cureus.com/articles/104849-role-of-endotracheal-tube-cuff-deflation-in-facilitating-passage-of-nasogastric-tube.
15. Khair J. Guidelines for testing the placing of nasogastric tubes. Nurs Times. 2005;101(20):26–7.
16. Metheny NA, Stewart BJ, Smith L, Yan H, Diebold M, Clouse RE. pH and concentrations of pepsin and trypsin in feeding tube aspirates as predictors of tube placement. JPEN J Parenter Enteral Nutr. 1997;21(5):279–85.
17. Taylor SJ, Clemente R. Confirmation of nasogastric tube position by pH testing. J Hum Nutr Diet. 2005;18(5):371–5.
18. Xu LC, Huang XJ, Lin BX, Zheng JY, Zhu HH. Clinical nurses' nasogastric feeding practices in adults: a multicenter cross-sectional survey in China. J Int Med Res. 2020;48(4):300060520920051.

29 C-Spine Protection

Gyaninder Pal Singh

Key Points

- C-Spine injuries are frequent, often caused by blunt trauma and have the highest reported mortality of all spine injuries.
- Treat all trauma patients as spine-injured unless otherwise proved.
- Care provider should remain vigilant about preventing secondary injury in patients with C-Spine injury and immobilize head and neck (MILS, rigid cervical collar, sandbags and tapes, or a combination of these).
- Rapid sequence induction and intubation is a safe and acceptable approach in these patients. Use of Cricoid pressure during RSI is controversial and may increase the injury to spinal cord in C-Spine injury patients.
- Neck immobilization may present unique difficulties for tracheal intubation. Remove the anterior portion of the hard collar and perform manual in-line stabilization (MILS).
- Use of a gum elastic bougie as first line approach with direct or video laryngoscopy increase chance of first-pass tracheal intubation (endotracheal tube with stylet is an alternative)
- Awake fiberoptic intubation is an alternative if the necessary expertise and equipment is available, the patient is cooperative and the situation is not a true emergency.
- Timely and adequate measure for C-Spine protection are important to prevent secondary injury to the underlying spinal cord and to improve outcome in patients of cervical spine injury.

29.1 Introduction

Approximately, 1 million people sustain spinal cord injury each year. Spinal Cord Injury (SCI) is a devastating injury, particularly when it involves the cervical region. Nearly 51% of all the spinal injuries are located in C-spine and approximately 10% of the C-Spine injury are associated with injury to cervical cord. The overall prevalence of C-Spine injury among all trauma patients is 3.7%.

SCI can result in partial or complete loss of various functions (motor, sensory and autonomic function) below the level of injury. Higher cervical cord injury may lead to complete quadriplegia, loss of sensation and autonomic dysfunction

G. P. Singh (✉)
Department of Neuroanaesthesiology and Critical Care, Neurosciences Centre, All India Institute of Medical Sciences, New Delhi, India

N. Gupta et al. (eds.), *Techniques in Anesthesia, Intensive Care and Emergency Medicine*,
https://doi.org/10.1007/978-981-96-1202-4_29

below the injury including inability to breath and ventilator dependency. Due to these significant effects of cervical cord injury, all measures should be taken to protect the cervical cord in patients of suspected C-Spine injury. Thus, all patients of trauma must be presumed to have a cervical spine injury unless ruled out.

29.2 Assessment of C-Spine

29.2.1 Clinical Assessment and Predictors of C-Spine Injury

Assessment	Predictors of C-Spine injury
Rule out C-Spine injury while maintaining in-line immobilization • Assess for neck pain and neurological symptoms • Gentle palpation of the neck (posterior midline from the nuchal ridge to the 1st thoracic vertebra and repeat the process lateral to the midline on both sides) • Assess active range of movement of neck (patient is asked to slowly rotate their head 45° to the left and right; stop if this causes pain or abnormal sensations in their arms)	Neck pain, weakness, paralysis or paraesthesia[a] Midline C-Spine tenderness[a] Painful or limited neck movements[a]

If there are no neurological symptoms or midline tenderness and active neck movement is possible without pain or developing any symptom, the C-Spine is cleared and the cervical collar may be removed

[a] In presence of clinical symptoms, radiological investigations (X-rays/CT-scan) are indicated to rule out C-Spine injury

C-Spine protection is indicated in the trauma setting if there is

- Neck pain or neurological symptoms
- Midline C-Spine tenderness
- Significant blunt injury above the clavicle
- Altered level of consciousness (clinical examination not possible)

29.3 Protection of C-Spine

In C-Spine injury patients, neck movements (flexion, extension, rotation) can lead to shift in the alignment of the C-Spine and can cause injury (compression or transection) of the cervical cord. Thus, the neck should be aligned in neutral position to avoid injury and/or aggravation of injury to the underlying cord. Conscious patients should be encouraged to remain still to avoid risk of injury to the spinal cord.

29.3.1 Measures to Prevent Movement of C-Spine

(a) *Manual-in-line stabilization (MILS)*: The C-Spine should be held in neutral position, with the hands of the rescuer on either side of the patient's head either by standing on the head-end of the patient or on the patient's side facing towards the face of the patient (Fig. 29.1a, b). This technique should be used till the cervical collar and/or sandbags and tapes are applied for immobilization of the C-Spine.

(b) *Cervical collar (CC)*: A stiff neck collar (e.g., Philadelphia Collar, Fig. 29.2) should be used in all the trauma patients to reduce the movement of neck till the C-Spine injury is ruled out or it is fixed by surgery. The cervical collars are available in various sizes and should be in place during patient transfer. The neck and head should be supported while shifting the patient (Fig. 29.3) with the neck collar in place.

(c) *Sandbags or blocks and tape*: These can be used either alone or in conjugation with cervical collar to fix the neck in neutral position before transporting the patient (Fig. 29.4). The sandbags or blocks are placed on either side of the patient's head (prevents lateral movements of neck) and are held in place by two tapes one crossing over the forehead and other over the chin. This maintains the neck in neutral position. A hard flat board or Spine

Fig. 29.1 Manual in-line stabilization (MILS) technique for immobilization of C-Spine. (**a**) from the head end and (**b**) from the side of patient

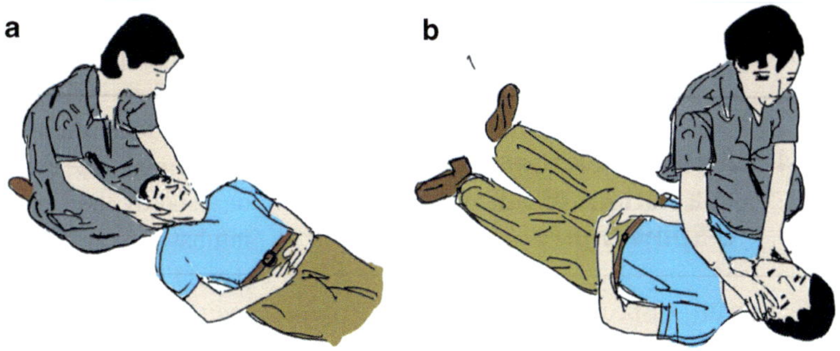

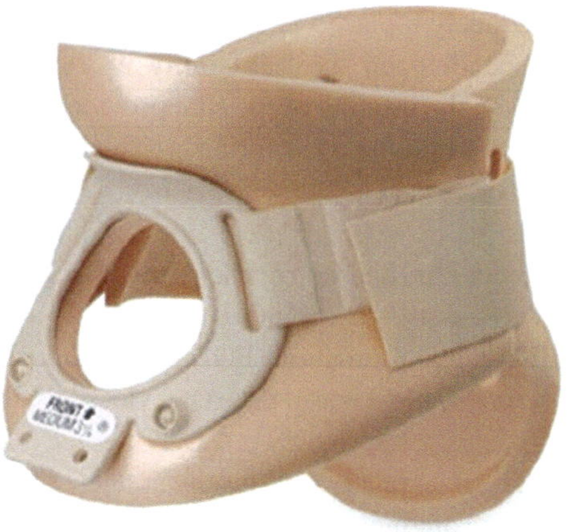

Fig. 29.2 Philadelphia collar (stiff neck collar)

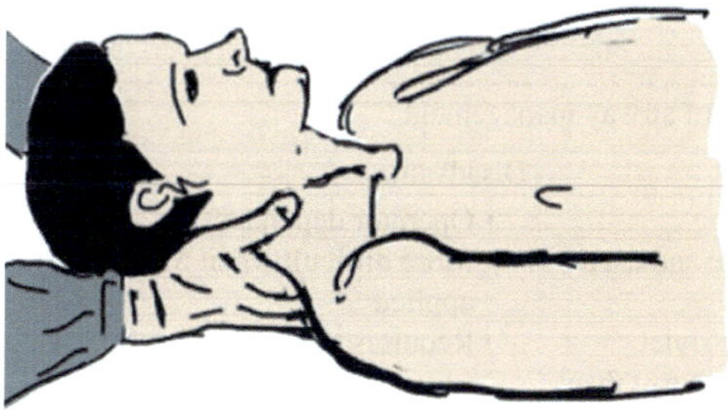

Fig. 29.3 Technique to support head and neck together while shifting the patient

board should be used to transport the patient to prevent spine movement and further injury to underlying spinal cord. The patient should be log-rolled while shifting on to the spine

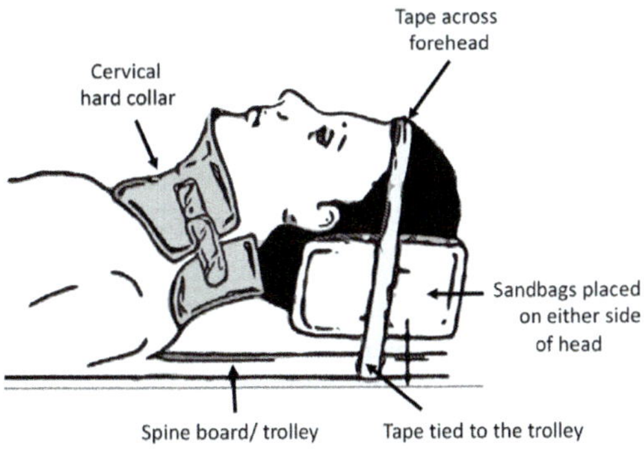

Fig. 29.4 Immobilize the neck using blocks and tape

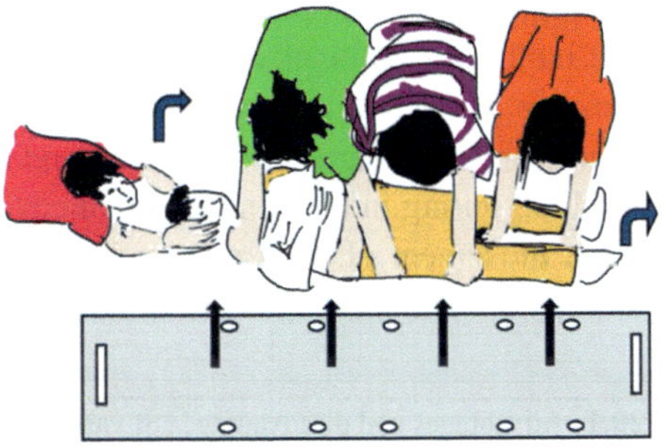

Fig. 29.5 Log-roll the patient to shift on to the

board. During log-roll the patient is turned to one side as a single unit from head to toe (like log of wood) without any movement at the spine. The spine board is placed underneath the patient and the patient is rolled back on to the spine board as a single unit again (Fig. 29.5).

A combination of hard board, cervical collar, sandbags or blocks, and tape or straps is the best method to immobilize the neck which can limit the movement to 5% of the normal range.

29.4 Airway Management in a Patient of Suspected C-Spine Injury

Patient with suspected or confirmed C-Spine injury may require tracheal intubation in emergency for various reasons (like maintenance of the airway, hypoventilation, hypoxia, prevention of aspiration) or electively for a planned surgery. In any case, protection of C-Spine is essential during airway management to prevent or minimize spinal cord injury due to manipulation of head and neck.

The standard of care is to immobilize the neck after trauma until C-spine injury is ruled out or fixed. However, neck immobilization severely limits the mouth opening and laryngoscopic view thereby increasing the difficulty for tracheal intubation. Thus, the care provider should be aware about the implications of various methods of neck immobilization on airway management.

As the presence of stiff cervical collar around the neck limits the mouth opening, the laryngoscopy and intubation becomes more challenging. So, a common practice in such cases is to remove the anterior part of the hard cervical collar and to provide MILS during intubation. This maneuver restrict the movement of head and neck during laryngoscopy and tracheal intubation. It should be applied both during direct- as well as video-laryngoscopy. MILS is applied by an assistant who either stands beside the intubator on the head-end of the patient with both his hands placed over the mastoid processes of the patient or stand by the side of the patient in front of the intubator with hands placed on the sides of the patient's head. The assistant providing MILS maintain the neutral position of neck and prevent movements of the head and neck by counteracting the forces of airway intervention. The anterior part of the cervical collar should be immediately replaced after securing the airway.

Depending on the availability of the equipment and the training of the care provider various technique may be used for airway management. These include:

1. Direct Laryngoscopy (DL) with MILS
2. Video-Laryngoscopy (VL) with MILS
3. Fibreoptic Intubation (FOI)
4. Supraglottic Airway (SGA) devices

The advantages and disadvantages of each technique are mentioned in Table 29.1.

29.4.1 Direct Laryngoscopy

Direct laryngoscopy (DL) is the most familiar technique for tracheal intubation and widely available and thus suitable for emergency situa-

Table 29.1 Advantages and disadvantages of various techniques of airway management

Technique	Advantages	Disadvantages
Direct laryngoscopy	• Fast • Most widely available and used technique • Allows use of bougie/stylet • No evidence that it is worse than other methods in practice	• Operator dependent • More difficult when MILS is applied • Requires training and expertise
Video laryngoscopy	• Better view of larynx and glottic opening • Better for anteriorly placed larynx and difficult airway • Allows use of bougie/stylet • Some devices (e.g., C-MAC) can be used as direct laryngoscopes	• View is hindered by blood and secretions • Requires training for hand coordination with eyes on screen • Equipment not readily available at all places

(continued)

Table 29.1 (continued)

Technique	Advantages	Disadvantages
Awake fiberoptic intubation	• Allows documentation of neurological examination before and after the procedure • Least movement of neck and minimal risk of displacement of C-Spine • Preferred method for elective tracheal intubation	• Not suitable for uncooperative patient • View is hindered by blood and secretions • Requires expertise • Equipment not readily available at all places • Time consuming procedure • Not suitable in emergency
Supraglottic airway	• Fast • More effective ventilation than Bag mask ventilation • May facilitate endotracheal intubation (e.g., intubating LMA, i-Gel, Air-Q) • Useful rescue device if unable to intubate	• Not a definitive airway—risk of aspiration • Uncertainty about degree of cervical spine movement

tion. When used with MILS, it is safe and effective technique for tracheal intubation in C-spine injury patients. Use of adjuncts like stylet or gum elastic bougie may improve the chance of success during intubation.

29.4.2 Video-Laryngoscopy

Video-laryngoscopy (VL) has proved to be an excellent method for tracheal intubation. It gives a better view of larynx because of the camera at the tip of the laryngoscope blade and therefore requiring less force for viewing the glottis/larynx. When used with MILS, it is an effective and safe technique for tracheal intubation in C-spine injury with better laryngoscopic view. However, it gives an indirect view on the screen which require hand eye coordination (as against direct laryngoscopy) and thus person need training to use the scope. Moreover, one should be familiar with use of different types of VL scopes available from various manufacturers. Other limitation is the presence of blood or secretions in the oropharynx that could obscure the view. In spite of these limitation, VL has been shown to have better first-pass success rate compared to DL.

29.4.3 Fibreoptic Intubation (FOI)

This technique causes no or minimal movement of neck during tracheal intubation and is thus the ideal method for tracheal intubation in C-Spine injury patients. It can either be performed with patient in awake state or under general anesthesia. Awake FOI has the advantage of patient self-maintaining the airway during the procedure, cooperate in positioning for surgery, and allows for documentation of neurologic exam before and after intubation and surgical positioning. During FOI, the endotracheal tube (ETT) is loaded over the flexible limb of the fiberoptic scope prior to the procedure. The flexible limb is then directed into the trachea through the glottis via oral or nasal passage (using the lever on the scope) and then the ETT is railroaded into the trachea over the flexible limb. This technique does not require removal of the anterior half of cervical collar and application of MILS. However, this technique of intubation require training to gain competence. For awake FOI, the patient should be cooperative and remain still during the procedure. The non-availability of equipment at all times and expertise required to use it, limits its usefulness during emergency tracheal intubation. Moreover, presence of secretions and blood obscure the view as in VL. Thus, FOI is an excellent choice for elective tracheal intubation in C-Spine injury patients but not generally suited for emergency situations.

29.4.4 Supraglottic Airway Devices

Supraglottic airway (SGA) devices may be used to secure the airway in C-Spine cases. Placement of SGA devices do not require laryngoscopy and can be easily placed blindly to provide ventilation. However, their use in C-Spine injury remains controversial as some studies have shown increased C-Spine displacement (by pressure exerted by inflated cuff) while others have not. Moreover, they do not provide complete protection against aspiration of contents into the lungs.

These are frequently used as a rescue device to provide ventilation in a potentially fatal cannot intubate and cannot ventilate situation. Some of the SGA devices (like Fastrach LMA, I-gel, Air-Q etc) may also act as conduit to facilitate tracheal intubation. SGA devices are an essential component of difficult airway algorithm for all patients including C-Spine injury.

29.5 Rapid Sequence Induction

Rapid sequence induction (RSI) and intubation is a safe and acceptable approach in the trauma patient with suspected or known C-Spine injury. This is especially useful in emergency situation to minimize the risk of aspiration of gastric contents in high risk patients (full stomach). It allows for securing the airway with an oral cuffed ETT after rapid induction of anesthesia and neuromuscular block. Appropriate preparation should be done prior to the procedure (e.g., drugs loaded, adequate size masks, LMAs, stylet, gum elastic bougie, laryngoscopes with different size blades, monitors and other emergency equipment, supply of oxygen and working suction, all should be checked and available at hand). A group of four trained people are required for various roles during the procedure (i.e., administration of drugs, application of MILS, application of cricoid pressure, and tracheal intubation). The anterior portion of the rigid cervical collar is removed and MILS is applied by an assistant to immobilize the head and neck of the patient. The patient is first adequately preoxygenated for 3–5 min and then anesthesia is induced with rapid administration of full dose of intravenous (i.v.) anesthetic agent (Propofol, Thiopentone or Etomidate) and neuromuscular blocking drug (Succinylcholine 1 mg/kg or Rocuronium 1 mg/kg) followed by i.v. flush with normal saline. Cricoid pressure (approximately 30 N vertical pressure over the cricoid cartilage against the C5 cervical vertebrae beneath) is applied as the anesthesia is induced. After 60 s, the laryngoscopy is performed, trachea intubated and cuff of ETT inflated to secure the airway. The proper position of the ETT is confirmed and ETT is secured. Cricoid pressure is released after confirming the correct placement of ETT.

Use of Cricoid pressure during RSI is however controversial. Some studies have shown that cricoid pressure is ineffective in preventing the aspiration of gastric content, and rather worsens the laryngoscopic view and increase the difficulty of tracheal intubation by deforming the airway anatomy [1–5]. Moreover, the pressure exerted by this maneuver may cause movement/displacement of cervical vertebrae and cause injury to cervical cord in C-Spine injured patients. Hence, cricoid pressure is currently not the standard of care and is not routinely advocated in C-spine injury.

Succinylcholine (Sch) may be used for rapid sequence induction in spinal cord injuries less than 24–48 h. In patients with spinal cord injuries beyond 48 h, Sch should not be used because of the risk of extra-junctional receptors and hyperkalemic cardiac arrest. Sch in the dose of 1 mg/kg produce excellent intubating conditions within 60 s. Rocuronium in a dose of 1–1.2 mg/kg rapidly provide adequate relaxation for intubation within 60 s and is safe to use within or after 48 h of spinal cord injury. Both Sch and Rocuronium has been found to produce similar intubation conditions during RSI.

29.6 Do's and Don'ts

29.6.1 Do's

(a) Consider all patients of trauma to have C-spine injury unless proved otherwise.
(b) Prevent secondary injury to spinal cord in all cases of C-Spine injury
(c) Provide protection to C-Spine by neck immobilization techniques (MILS, rigid cervical collar, sandbags and tapes)
(d) Log-roll the patient on to the spine board (hard board) before transporting the patient to prevent spine movement.
(e) Assess the patient to rule out spine injury (clinical examination and investigations)
(f) If required secure the airway while maintaining the head and neck immobilization (using MILS)
(g) Always have all the drugs and equipment ready at hand and use the most familiar technique for securing the airway.
(h) Use rapid sequence induction and intubation in case of emergency to prevent aspiration into the lungs.
(i) Neck immobilization should continue after securing the airway.

29.6.2 Don'ts

(a) Don't shift the patient with suspected spine injury without spine immobilization.
(b) Don't use unfamiliar techniques to secure the airway.
(c) Don't allow movement of cervical spine during tracheal intubation.
(d) Avoid using cricoid pressure during RSI. Its role is controversial.
(e) Avoid hypotension. This may cause ischemia and increase secondary injury to the spinal cord.

Suggested Reading

1. Smith CE, Boyer D. Cricoid pressure decreases ease of tracheal intubation using fibreoptic laryngoscopy (WuScope system). Can J Anaesth. 2002;49:614–9.
2. Hartsilver EL, Vanner RG. Airway obstruction with cricoid pressure. Anaesthesia. 2000;55:208–11.
3. Walker RW, Ravi R, Haylett K. Effect of cricoid force on airway calibre in children: a bronchoscopic assessment. Br J Anaesth. 2010;104:71–4.
4. Snider DD, Clarke D, Finucane BT. The "BURP" maneuver worsens the glottic view when applied in combination with cricoid pressure. Can J Anaesth. 2005;52:100–4.
5. Komasawa N, Kido H, Miyazaki Y, Tatsumi S, Minami T. Cricoid pressure impedes tracheal intubation with the Pentax-AWS Airwayscope®: a prospective randomized trial. Br J Anaesth. 2016;116:413–6.
6. Wiles MD. Airway management in patients with suspected or confirmed traumatic spinal cord injury: a narrative review of current evidence. Anaesthesia. 2022;77:1120–8.
7. Lenehan B, Boran S, Street J, Higgins T, McCormack D, Poynton AR. Demographics of acute admissions to a National Spinal Injuries Unit. Eur Spine J. 2009;18:938–42.
8. Schleicher P, Pingel A, Kandziora F. Safe management of acute cervical spine injuries. EFORT Open Rev. 2018;3:347–57.
9. Fredo HL, Rizvi SA, Lied B, Ronning P, Helseth E. The epidemiology of traumatic cervical spine fractures: a prospective population study from Norway. Scand J Trauma Resusc Emerg Med. 2012;20:85.
10. Milby AH, Halpern CH, Guo W, Stein SC. Prevalence of cervical spinal injury in trauma. Neurosurg Focus. 2008;25:E10.
11. Austin N, Krishnamoorthy V, Dagal A. Airway management in cervical spine injury. Int J Crit Illn Inj Sci. 2014;4:50–6.
12. Podolsky S, Baraff LJ, Simon RR, Hoffman JR, Larmon B, Ablon W. Efficacy of cervical spine immobilization methods. J Trauma. 1983;23:461–5.
13. Heath KJ. The effect of laryngoscopy of different cervical spine immobilisation techniques. Anaesthesia. 1994;49:843–5.
14. Goutcher CM, Lochhead V. Reduction in mouth opening with semi-rigid cervical collars. Br J Anaesth. 2005;95:344–8.
15. Mosier JM, Stolz U, Chiu S, Sakles JC. Difficult airway management in the emergency department: GlideScope videolaryngoscopy compared to direct laryngoscopy. J Emerg Med. 2012;42:629–34.
16. Malcharek MJ, Rogos B, Watzlawek S, Sorge O, Sablotzki A, Gille J, Larson CP Jr. Awake fiberoptic intubation and self-positioning in patients at risk of secondary cervical injury: a pilot study. J Neurosurg Anesthesiol. 2012;24:217–21.
17. Keller C, Brimacombe J, Keller K. Pressures exerted against the cervical vertebrae by the standard and intubating laryngeal mask airways: a randomized, controlled, cross-over study in fresh cadavers. Anesth Analg. 1999;89:1296–300.
18. Talucci RC, Shaikh KA, Schwab CW. Rapid sequence induction with oral endotracheal intubation in the multiply injured patient. Am Surg. 1988;54:185–7.

19. Salem MR, Khorasani A, Zeidan A, Crystal GJ. Cricoid pressure controversies: narrative review. Anesthesiology. 2017;126:738–52.
20. Stewart JC, Bhananker S, Ramaiah R. Rapid-sequence intubation and cricoid pressure. Int J Crit Illn Inj Sci. 2014;4:42–9.
21. Smith KJ, Ladak S, Choi PT, Dobranowski J. The cricoid cartilage and the esophagus are not aligned in close to half of adult patients. Can J Anaesth. 2002;49:503–7.
22. Smith KJ, Dobranowski J, Yip G, Dauphin A. Choi, PT Cricoid pressure displaces the esophagus: an observational study using magnetic resonance imaging. Anesthesiology. 2003;99:60–4.
23. Boet S, Duttchen K, Chan J, Chan AW, Morrish W, Ferland A, Hare GM, Hong AP. Cricoid pressure provides incomplete esophageal occlusion associated with lateral deviation: a magnetic resonance imaging study. J Emerg Med. 2012;42:606–11.
24. Robinson JS, Thompson JM. Fatal aspiration (Mendelson's) syndrome despite antacids and cricoid pressure. Lancet. 1979;2:228–30.
25. Fenton PM, Reynolds F. Life-saving or ineffective? An observational study of the use of cricoid pressure and maternal outcome in an African setting. Int J Obstet Anesth. 2009;18:106–10.
26. Timmermann A, Byhahn C. Cricoid pressure. Protective manoeuvre or established nonsense? Anaesthesist. 2009;58:663–4.
27. Gobindram A, Clarke S. Cricoid pressure: should we lay off the pressure? Anaesthesia. 2008;63:1258–9.
28. Gabbott DA. The effect of single-handed cricoid pressure on neck movement after applying manual in-line stabilisation. Anaesthesia. 1997;52:586–8.
29. Ellis DY, Harris T, Zideman D. Cricoid pressure in emergency department rapid sequence tracheal intubations: a risk-benefit analysis. Ann Emerg Med. 2007;50:653–65.
30. Martyn JA, Richtsfeld M. Succinylcholine-induced hyperkalemia in acquired pathologic states: etiologic factors and molecular mechanisms. Anesthesiology. 2006;104:158–69.
31. Putzu A, Tramèr MR, Giffa M, Czarnetzki C. The optimal dose of succinylcholine for rapid sequence induction: a systematic review and meta-analysis of randomized trials. BMC Anesthesiol. 2020;20:1–9.
32. Herbstritt A, Amarakone K. Towards evidence-based emergency medicine: best BETs from the Manchester Royal Infirmary. BET 3: is rocuronium as effective as succinylcholine at facilitating laryngoscopy during rapid sequence intubation? Emerg Med J. 2012;29:256–8.

Temperature Monitoring

30

Surjyendu Ghosh and Nishkarsh Gupta

30.1 Introduction

Body temperature changes can lead to abnormal functioning of the organs and enzyme systems of the body. Patients receiving anesthesia are prone to temperature changes due to multiple causes and mechanisms. Both hypothermia and hyperthermia, when exceed the physiological limits, can lead to adverse outcomes. Monitoring of body temperature is crucial during anesthesia and is required to detect and correct the changes. This chapter discusses the techniques and methods of temperature monitoring during the perioperative period. Relevant clinical information is also included.

30.1.1 Thermoregulation

Thermoregulation, mediated by hypothalamus, ensures normal body temperature to be maintained within a narrow range (mean core temperature in healthy humans is 36.5–37.3 °C). There is a 1 °C variation in the core temperature from 36.5 °C (usually about 3:00 a.m.) to 37.5 °C (usually about 3:00 p.m.) according to the circadian rhythm. Neonates and elderly are more susceptible to temperature changes. Core temperature represents the temperature in the internal organs of the body and is commonly represented by rectal, tympanic, or nasopharyngeal measurements. Superficial temperature measured in the skin or axilla is marginally lower than core temperature. Liver temperature is approximately 1 °C higher than other core tissue. Core temperature is best represented by pulmonary artery blood temperature. Core temperature is the dominant input to autonomic thermoregulatory control. Mean body temperature (MBT) can be estimated from the combination of mean skin and core temperatures.

30.2 Thermoregulation During General Anesthesia

30.2.1 Responses in Infants and Older Adults

Thermoregulatory vasoconstriction is comparably impaired in infants, children, and adults given isoflurane or halothane. In contrast, the vasoconstriction threshold is approximately 1 °C less in patients 60–80 years old than in those between 30 and 50 years old. Nonshivering thermogenesis does not occur in anesthetized adults. In contrast

S. Ghosh · N. Gupta (✉)
Department Onco-Anesthesiology and Palliative Medicine, DRBRAIRCH, All India Institute of Medical Sciences, New Delhi, Delhi, India
e-mail: drnishkarsh@rediffmial.com

N. Gupta et al. (eds.), *Techniques in Anesthesia, Intensive Care and Emergency Medicine*,
https://doi.org/10.1007/978-981-96-1202-4_30

to adult humans, nonshivering thermogenesis is an important thermoregulatory response in animals and human infants. However, nonshivering thermogenesis in animals is inhibited by volatile anesthetics, and it fails to increase the metabolic rate in infants anesthetized with propofol.

30.3 Development of Hypothermia During General Anesthesia

Incidence of inadvertent hypothermia is much higher than hyperthermia during general anesthesia. Mechanisms include anesthetic-induced impaired thermoregulation that causes vasodilation, inhibit vasoconstriction, and reduce metabolic rate by 20–30% and exposure to cold environment (Table 30.1).

Table 30.1 Causes and mechanisms of intraoperative hypothermia under general anesthesia

Cause of hypothermia	Mechanism
OT environment	Set OT temperature and humidity Exposure of body surface Cold irrigation fluid Skin preparation
Cold IV fluid	1 unit cold Packed red blood cells (PRBC) can decrease body temperature by 0.25–0.35 °C Cold crystalloid
Anesthesia	Anesthesia-induced redistribution of heat from core to periphery Hypothermia-associated (HA)-induced reduction in metabolic rate by 20–30% Dry anesthetic gases Volatiles—impair thermoregulatory vasoconstrictions Muscle relaxants—prevent shivering IV sedatives—increases sweating threshold and significantly lower shivering threshold, impair thermoregulatory threshold Vasodilators—promote heat loss Regional anesthesia—heat loss enhanced by vasodilatation and impaired shivering below the level of the block and cold IV fluids
Surgical techniques	Exposure of body cavity Duration of surgery

30.3.1 Heat Transfer

Heat transfer from the human body occurs in four ways: conduction, convection, radiation, and evaporation. Radiation contributes most to perioperative heat losses.

1. Radiation (Majority of Heat Loss: 40–60%).
   (a) The body loses heat by infrared radiation to cooler surrounding objects, with a proportion to fourth power of the absolute temperature difference between surfaces.
   (b) This occurs even without direct contact.
2. Convection (25–30%).
   (a) Heat is lost when air currents carry warm air away from the body and replace it with cooler air, with a proportion to square root of air speed.
   (b) The larger the exposed skin surface, the greater the convective loss.
3. Evaporation (15–25%).
   (a) Heat is lost when moisture (sweat, respiratory water, or surgical site fluids) evaporates.
4. Conduction (3–5%).
   (a) Heat transfers by direct contact with a cooler object, with proportion to the temperature difference between to surfaces.

30.4 Neuraxial Anesthesia and Hypothermia

Neuraxial anesthesia also impairs behavioral and autonomic thermoregulation. It blocks all thermal input from anesthetized regions and reduces vasoconstriction and shivering thresholds by 0.6 °C above the level of block probably by central action. Reduction in these thresholds is proportional to the number of spinal segments blocked. Supplementation with analgesics, sedatives, or general anesthesia further impairs thermoregulation. Hypothermia during neuraxial anesthesia is as severe as during general anesthesia: core temperature decreases by 0.5–1.0 °C. The decrease may not necessarily plateau since nerve block inhibits peripheral vasoconstriction. So, under regional anesthesia, cold defenses are triggered at a lower temperature than normal, defenses are less effective once triggered, and patients often do not recognize being hypothermic. All these factors often lead to a potentially dangerous clinical paradox: a hypothermic patient who denies feeling cold.

30.5 Consequences of Mild Intraoperative Hypothermia

1. Cardiovascular Effects
   (a) Increased risk of arrhythmias (e.g., atrial fibrillation, ventricular ectopy).
   (b) Altered hemodynamics due to vasoconstriction.
   (c) Increased incidence of myocardial ischemia and infarction due to increased oxygen demand.
2. Coagulopathy and Increased Bleeding
   (a) Impaired platelet function and coagulation enzyme activity, leading to prolonged bleeding.
   (b) Increased surgical blood loss, which may require more transfusions.
3. Delayed Drug Metabolism
   (a) Reduced hepatic and renal metabolism, leading to prolonged effects of anesthetic agents and muscle relaxants resulting in increased risk of postoperative sedation and respiratory depression.
   (b) Higher incidence of postoperative complications, leading to longer hospital stays.
4. Increased Risk of Surgical Site Infections (SSIs)
   (a) Impairs immune function and reduces tissue oxygenation, leading to higher wound infections and delayed healing.
5. Neurological Effects
   (a) Increased risk of postoperative cognitive dysfunction and delirium, especially in elderly patients.
6. Increased Patient Discomfort
   (a) Shivering (which increases oxygen demand and metabolic rate).
   (b) Cold stress and discomfort in the postoperative period.

30.6 Temperature Monitoring

The word thermometer is derived from the Greek *thermos* (meaning hot) and *metron* (meaning measure). Several inventors, most notably Galileo Galilei, developed uncalibrated thermometers at the end of the sixteenth century. While, the first calibrated alcohol-based thermometer was developed by the astronomer Olaus Roemer, which was substantially improved by contemporary physicist Daniel Gabriel Fahrenheit, who enclosed mercury in glass in 1714. Nowadays, most of the world uses the scale developed by astronomer Anders Celsius, which is also referred to as the centigrade scale because it divides temperatures between the freezing and boiling points of water into a hundred degrees. The only other commonly used scale was developed by Lord Kelvin; it sets 0 K at absolute zero but otherwise uses degrees of the same magnitude as the Celsius scale.

Although a variety of technologies are available to measure temperature, none is suitable for all situations. Most modern devices have alarms that can be set if the temperature exceeds high or low limits. Temperature-monitoring capability is available on most physiologic monitors used in the OR and perioperative areas.

30.6.1 Thermistor

A thermistor is composed of a metal (i.e., manganese, nickel, cobalt, iron, or zinc) oxide sintered into a wire or fused into a rod or bead. There must be a source of current and a means to measure that current. As the temperature decreases, resistance of the metal oxide increases and vice versa, so the resistance can be converted to a temperature. Advantages of thermistors include small size, rapid response time, continuous readings, sensitivity to small changes in temperature, inexpensive interchangeable, and disposable probes.

30.6.2 Thermocouple

A thermocouple consists of an electrical circuit that has two different metals welded together at their ends [12]. While one of the two metal junctions remains at a constant temperature, the other one is exposed to the area being measured, producing a voltage difference which is measured and converted to a temperature reading. Advantages of thermocouples include accuracy, small size, rapid response time, continuous readings, stability, and inexpensive interchangeable and disposable probes.

30.6.3 Platinum Wire

The electrical resistance of platinum wire varies almost linearly with temperature. Rapid thermal equilibration is possible by using an extremely small diameter wire. Resistance is measured in a way similar to a thermistor. These thermometers are accurate and give continuous readings. Probes can be made interchangeable. If a probe with a thermocouple, thermistor, or platinum wire is to be used inside the body, it must have an outer sheath. The end of the probe designed to be inserted into the patient is sealed and the electrical connection made at the other end. The connection needs to be kept dry to avoid erroneous readings.

30.6.4 Liquid Crystal

Certain organic compounds during thermal transformation from a solid to a liquid state, pass through an intermediate phase that exhibits anisotropic (optically active) properties, known as liquid crystal. When light shines on such a material, crystals scatter some of the light, producing iridescent colors. The liquid crystals are encapsulated so that the colors form letters and numbers. It consists of a flexible adhesive backing with plastic-encased liquid crystals on a black background that prevents reflection of the transmitted light and enhances the color resolution. The disc or strip is placed on the skin after removing the covering over the adhesive. The liquid crystal thermometer is available in two forms: one displays the skin temperature directly; the other has a built-in correction factor (offset) so that the temperature displayed estimates core temperature.

Although less accurate, liquid crystal thermometers are safe, convenient, noninvasive, easy to apply and read, disposable, nonirritating, and inexpensive. They give fast, continuous readings and involve no electronic circuitry. They can be applied before induction of anesthesia and are easily transferred to the recovery area with the patient. Disadvantages of liquid crystal thermometers include the need for subjective observer interpretation and the inability to interface with a recording system. Extreme ambient temperature, humidity, and air movement may result in inaccuracy. Other disadvantages include difficulties with adhesion secondary to skin secretions, allergic reactions to adhesive backing, inaccuracy, and imprecision. If left in the sun for an extended period, an error indicating hyperthermia can be produced. If the device is frozen, all the numbers can be visible at once. Infrared heating lamps may cause erroneously elevated readings.

30.6.5 Infrared

An infrared thermometer is an electronic instrument with an otoscope-like probe that measures a portion of the infrared radiation from surfaces within its field of view. Electromagnetic radiation is emitted by an object in proportion to its temperature. Because the probe is placed in the outer part of the ear canal and has a relatively wide view angle, it detects infrared emissions from parts of both the ear canal wall and tympanic membrane. The displayed value may be the actual temperature (unadjusted, calibration mode) or with an offset to estimate temperature at another site based on selected study samples (site equivalent mode). The probe should be placed carefully but firmly as far as possible into the ear canal, aiming toward the tympanic membrane. Because it does not contact any surface, patients tolerate infrared thermometry well and

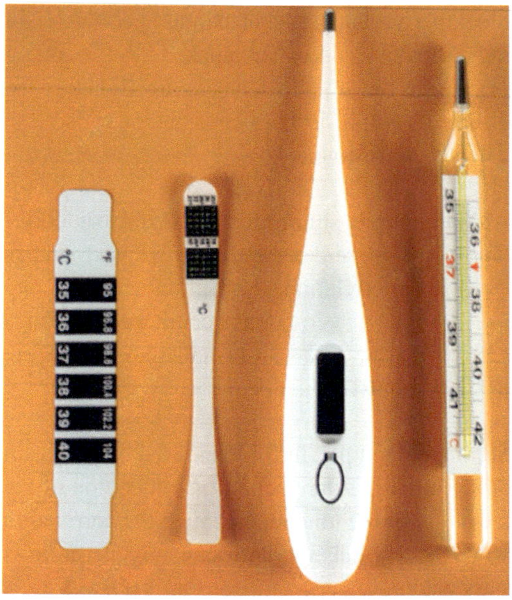

Fig. 30.1 Image of liquid crystal, clinical, electrical, and mercury thermometer

there should be no trauma associated with its use. Although measurements are rapid, improper placement or aiming, and obstructions in view of curvatures of the ear canal, can result in significantly lower temperatures.

30.6.6 Mercury Glass

These thermometers are of limited use during intraoperative anesthesia, as they have a long equilibration period (usually 3–5 min) and cannot be read without being removed from the monitoring site. If a thermometer is broken, the mercury vaporizes and can present a health hazard (Fig. 30.1).

30.7 Temperature Monitoring Sites

Preferred site for temperature monitoring depends on the indication, surgical procedure, duration, access, and availability of equipment. The difference between core and a second site can provide indirect information on blood flow as well.

30.7.1 Pulmonary Artery

Pulmonary artery temperature can be measured in patients who have a Swan-Ganz catheter with a thermistor in place. It is considered to be the best method of measuring core body temperature except during thoracotomy or cardiopulmonary bypass surgery.

30.7.2 Esophagus

Esophageal temperature measurement can be accomplished by using a simple probe, an esophageal stethoscope with thermistor, or a gastric tube with the temperature sensor at a specific distance (located in the lower third or fourth of the esophagus) from the end of the tube. Temperatures in the esophagus may vary up to 4 °C, depending on the temperature probe location within the esophagus. Procedures on the face, oral cavity, nose, airway, or esophagus, and patients who have esophageal disorders are few contraindications for esophageal temperature monitoring. Continuous gastric suctioning will result in inappropriate esophageal temperature also.

30.7.3 Nasopharynx

The temperature of the nasopharynx is measured with a sensor that is in contact with the posterior nasopharyngeal wall posterior to the soft palate (close to the hypothalamus). This site is not useful for patients who are awake. Epistaxis is a known complication.

30.7.4 Urinary Bladder

Urinary bladder temperature monitoring involves inserting an indwelling urinary catheter with a thermistor or thermocouple near the patient end. It generally correlates well with nasopharyngeal, pulmonary artery, and esophageal temperatures [20]. It may be especially useful in the patient with extensive burns. It should be avoided during genitourinary procedures.

30.7.5 Rectum

Rectal temperature is usually somewhat higher than that measured at more central sites during steady-state conditions. It is not influenced by ambient temperature. In spite of easy accessibility, except during gynecologic and urologic procedures and monitoring, it is not usually preferred by the patient or hospital personnel as it is considered esthetically objectionable. Probe with a disposable cover should be inserted to at least 8 cm in adults and 3 cm in children. Bowel perforation is a risk. Pararectal abscess and pneumoperitoneum have been reported with its use.

30.7.6 Tympanic Membrane

Measuring temperature at this site may reflect thermal information at the primary site of thermoregulation. Measurement is done by inserting a thermistor or thermocouple probe into the external auditory canal until it contacts the lower anterior quarter of the tympanic membrane. The external auditory canal should be occluded with cotton wool and covered externally to obliterate free air movement. Contraindications include any ear abnormality that would prevent correct placement, a skull fracture that passes through the osseous meatus, and perforation of the tympanic membrane.

30.7.7 Skin

The forehead is the primary site of choice for skin temperature measurement, as this site has a fairly good blood flow, and devoid of significant underlying fat. Other sites include the back, chest, anterior abdominal wall, fingers, toes, and the antecubital space inside the elbow. Skin surface temperature is typically 2–4 °C less than core temperature. Although in some studies, skin temperature has been found to correlate well with core temperature, most of the investigations could not establish the same. Skin temperature may be used to evaluate the quality of a regional block per se, and a rise in skin temperature is an indication of a successful block.

30.7.8 Axilla

Although a few studies found satisfactory correlation with more central sites [22], most studies show poor correlation.

30.7.9 Mouth

Sublingual temperature is measured by placing a probe in one of the pockets on either side of the frenulum of the tongue. Although the correlation with the central sites varies, in general it is satisfactory.

30.7.10 Trachea

Temperatures in the trachea can be measured by using a tracheal tube with the temperature sensor in the cuff. Studies differ in how well temperatures measured at this site correlate with those at other sites.

30.7.11 Inguinal Area

The inguinal area has also been utilized to measure temperature. Initially the leg is abducted, the femoral pulse palpated, and the sensor is placed just lateral to the femoral artery, then a seal is created by adducting the leg. A significant drawback to this site is the time required to reach equilibrium.

30.7.12 Hypopharynx

A thermocouple can be attached to the cuff of a supraglottic device to measure temperature in the hypopharynx. Temperatures measured in this location have correlated well with those at other sites.

30.8 When Temperature Monitoring Is Required

Core temperature monitoring should be considered during general anesthesia for long duration surgeries, anticipated risks of massive blood loss, malignant hyperthermia by virtue of history or evaluation, deliberate hypothermia, elderly, ASA 3 and 4 physical status, and children. More common than malignant hyperthermia is intraoperative hyperthermia, which has other causes, including excessive external warming, infection, fourth cerebral ventricle hemorrhage, and mismatched blood transfusions. Inadvertent hypothermia is by far the most common perioperative thermal disturbance. Hypothermia results from internal redistribution of heat and a variety of other factors whose effect in different patients is difficult to predict. Core temperature perturbations during the first 30 min of anesthesia thus are difficult to interpret, and measurement is not of great importance. Body temperature should, however, be monitored in patients undergoing general anesthesia exceeding 30 min in duration and in all patients whose surgery lasts longer than 1 h. Local anesthetics (including amides), used during regional blocks, and sedatives, used during monitored anesthesia care, do not trigger malignant hyperthermia. Nonetheless, core hypothermia is as common during epidural and spinal anesthesia as during general anesthesia, and it can be nearly equally severe. Therefore, core temperature should be measured during regional anesthesia in patients likely to become hypothermic, which at the very least includes those undergoing body cavity surgery.

30.9 Temperature Monitoring and Thermal Management Guidelines

Available data suggest the following guidelines:

1. Core body temperature should be measured in most patients given general anesthesia for longer than 30 min.
2. Temperature should also be measured during regional anesthesia when changes in body temperature are intended, anticipated, or suspected.
3. Unless hypothermia is specifically indicated (e.g., for protection against ischemia), efforts should be made to maintain intraoperative core temperature higher than 36 °C.

30.10 Nice Recommends

- Assessment of risk of perioperative hypothermia.
- Maintaining ambient temperature in wards and theatre suites.
- Recording core temperature immediately prior to leaving the ward, every 30 min intraoperatively, and every 15 min in recovery until a temperature of 36 °C is recorded.
- Commencing induction of anesthesia only if the patient's core temperature is above 36 °C.
- Active warming of all patients having anesthesia for longer than 30 min, and warming of IV fluids if >500 mL used.

30.11 Common Problems and Limitation

30.11.1 Damage to the Monitoring Site

Sharp edges of the probe can be traumatic to the tissues which they are in contact with. Trauma to the nose, external auditory canal, rectum, and esophagus have been reported in multiple times in the literature.

30.11.2 Burns

Burns have been reported at the measurement site. Using a battery-operated device is no guarantee of electrical safety, because the chassis may be grounded through a metal support. Temperature probes should be examined carefully before use to detect damage to the insulation. Esophageal burns may be avoided by placing the probe via a small tracheal tube.

30.11.3 Incorrect Information

A faulty probe can cause an incorrect temperature display. Falsely elevated readings may be caused by secretions or fluids in the connection between the probe and reading instrument as well. If the battery in a battery-powered device is discharged, the unit may stop functioning or give incorrect information. Using jacks that fit the receptacle but have internal electronics incompatible with the monitor can give false readings.

30.11.4 Probe Contamination

Reusable temperature probes may be a source of infection even with all precautions.

30.11.5 Faulty Probes

Each probe should be inspected and checked properly before use. A part of the sheath on a probe could break off and be aspirated.

Suggested Reading

1. Bindu B, Bindra A, Rath G. Temperature management under general anesthesia: compulsion or option. J Anaesthesiol Clin Pharmacol. 2017;33(3):306.
2. Rajek A, Lenhardt R, Sessler DI, Grabenwoger M, Kastner J, Mares P, et al. Tissue heat content and distribution during and after cardiopulmonary bypass at 17 degrees C. Anesth Analg. 1999;88(6):1220–5.
3. Sessler DI, Warner DS, Warner MA. Temperature monitoring and perioperative thermoregulation. Anesthesiology. 2008;109(2):318–38.
4. Matsukawa T, Kurz A, Sessler DI, Bjorksten AR, Merrifield B, Cheng C. Propofol linearly reduces the vasoconstriction and shivering thresholds. Anesthesiology. 1995;82(5):1169–80.
5. Lenhardt R, Sessler DI. Estimation of mean body temperature from mean skin and core temperature. Anesthesiology. 2006;105(6):1117–21.
6. Moayeri A, McGuire J, Hynson JM, Sessler DL. Absence of nonshivering thermogenesis in anesthetized adult humans. Anesthesiology. 1993;79(4):695–703.
7. Plattner O, Semsroth M, Sessler DI, Papousek A, Klasen C, Wagner O. Lack of nonshivering thermogenesis in infants anesthetized with fentanyl and propofol. Anesthesiology. 1997;86(4):772–7.
8. Stevens WC, Cromwell TH, Halsey MJ, Eger EI, Shakespeare TF, Bahlman SH. The cardiovascular effects of a new inhalation anesthetic, forane, in human volunteers at constant arterial carbon dioxide tension. Anesthesiology. 1971;35(1):8–15.
9. Hardy JD, Milhorat AT. Basal heat loss and production in women at temperatures from 23°C to 36°C. Exp Biol Med. 1939;41(1):94–8.
10. Ozaki M, Sessler DI, Matsukawa T, Ozaki K, Atarashi K, Negishi C, et al. The threshold for thermoregulatory vasoconstriction during nitrous oxide/sevoflurane anesthesia is reduced in the elderly. Anesth Analg. 1997;84(5):1029–33.
11. Frank SM, Beattie C, Christopherson R, Norris EJ, Rock P, Parker S, et al. Epidural versus general anesthesia, ambient operating room temperature, and patient age as predictors of inadvertent hypothermia. Anesthesiology. 1992;77(2):252–7.
12. Frank SM. Body temperature monitoring. Anesthesiol Clin N Am. 1994;12(3):387–407.
13. Berman MF. The susceptibility of thermistor-based esophageal temperature probes to errors caused by electrically conductive fluids ("artificial saliva"). J Clin Monit. 1992;8(2):107–10.
14. Mackenzie R, Asbury AJ. Clinical evaluation of liquid crystal skin thermometers. Br J Anaesth. 1994;72(2):246–9.
15. Roy RC, Eisenach JE. Clinical monitoring: practical applications for anesthesia and critical care. Anesthesiology. 2003;99(1):243.
16. Weiss ME, Pue AF, Smith J. Laboratory and hospital testing of new infrared tympanic thermometers. J Clin Eng. 1991;16(2):137–44.
17. Sessler DI. A proposal for new temperature monitoring and thermal management guidelines. Anesthesiology. 1998;89(5):1298–300.
18. Lefrant JY, Muller L, de La Coussaye JE, Benbabaali M, Lebris C, Zeitoun N, et al. Temperature measurement in intensive care patients: comparison of urinary bladder, oesophageal, rectal, axillary, and inguinal methods versus pulmonary artery core method. Intensive Care Med. 2003;29(3):414–8.
19. Mitchell S, Brimacombe J, Keller C. Feasibility, accuracy and optimal location for oesophageal core temperature measurements using the proseal laryngeal mask airway drain tube. Anaesth Intensive Care. 2003;31(3):282–5.
20. Shinozaki T, Deane R, Perkins FM. Infrared tympanic thermometer: evaluation of a new clinical thermometer. Crit Care Med. 1988;16(2):148–50.

21. Brinnel H, Cabanac M. Tympanic temperature is a core temperature in humans. J Therm Biol. 1989;14(1):47–53.
22. Kunnel MT, O'Brien C, Munro BH, Medoff-Cooper B. Comparisons of rectal, femoral, axillary, and skin-to-mattress temperatures in stable neonates. Nurs Res. 1988;37(3):162–4, 189.
23. Talo H, Macknin ML, Medendorp SV. Tympanic membrane temperatures compared to rectal and oral temperatures. Clin Pediatr (Phila). 1991;30(4 Suppl):30–3; discussion 34–35.
24. Russell SH, Freeman JW. Comparison of bladder, oesophageal and pulmonary artery temperatures in major abdominal surgery. Anaesthesia. 1996;51(4):338–40.
25. Webb GE. Comparison of esophageal and tympanic temperature monitoring during cardiopulmonary bypass. Anesth Analg. 1973;52(5):729–33.
26. Parker EO. Electrosurgical burn at the site of an esophageal temperature probe. Anesthesiology. 1984;61(1):93–5.
27. Chapin JW, Moravec M. Faulty temperature probe. Anesthesiology. 1980;52(2):187.

Patient Controlled Analgesia 31

M. R. Vishnu Narayanan, Rashmi Ramachandran,
and Vimi Rewari

Key Points

- Patient-controlled analgesia (PCA) technique that allows patients to self-administer analgesic drugs through a pump system by pressing a button in a controlled manner through an IV catheter or epidural catheter.
- PCA is commonly used for acute pain management after surgery or in patients with chronic pain.
- It provides more effective pain relief than traditional methods of pain management and reduces the risk of overdosing.
- PCA requires close monitoring by healthcare professionals to ensure appropriate dosage and avoid adverse effects.
- Patients must be educated on how to properly use the PCA pump and understand the risks and benefits of the medication being administered.
- PCA is not appropriate for all patients and one should be careful in using them in those who are unable to self-administer medication.

31.1 Introduction

Patient-controlled analgesia (PCA) is a modality of pain management where a patient is able to self-administer analgesics in the ward, with the help of a microprocessor-controlled infusion pump. The patient is provided with a demand button which on pushing delivers a predetermined dose of the analgesic. The PCA system also incorporates a data recording system which gives information about the drug usage and patient demands for a given period of time.

Though the most common method of drug administration via PCA has been described with intravenous route (IV PCA), alternative routes like patient-controlled epidural analgesia (PCEA), peripheral nerve block catheter PCA and transdermal PCA has also been described. Sporadic reports also describe a subcutaneous, oral transmucosal, nasal and intrathecal PCA.

31.2 Need for PCA

In 1973, Marks and Sachar published a landmark study suggesting how the misconceptions of pharmacokinetics and addiction potentials of narcotic analgesics among physicians led to the under treatment of pain among hospitalised patients. They had concluded that around 73% of the patients had moderate to severe distress during hospital stay due to inadequate analgesia. This led

M. R. Vishnu Narayanan · R. Ramachandran (✉)
V. Rewari
Department of Anesthesiology, Pain Medicine and Critical Care, AIIMS, New Delhi, India

N. Gupta et al. (eds.), *Techniques in Anesthesia, Intensive Care and Emergency Medicine*,
https://doi.org/10.1007/978-981-96-1202-4_31

to the development of new drugs with improved analgesic properties as well as better modes of drug administration. There was a conversion from the use of intramuscular (IM) analgesics to IV boluses of opioids. Though IV boluses of opioids provide better analgesia than IM, it was observed that each patient had different pain threshold and required different dosing schedule and quantity. A fixed dosing schedule used by nurses to administer opioids lead to frequent periods of dosing above and below the target concentration required for analgesia thus causing sedation or break-through pain, respectively.

Philip H. Sechzer in the year 1971 developed an 'Analgesic-demand system' which delivered IV opioid bolus when the patient pushed the demand button. He described this as an excellent objective method to assess as well as relieve pain with excellent patient satisfaction without causing sedation. A variety of PCA systems have been developed since then with better machine-user interface, accuracy and safety margins.

31.3 Working Principle of PCA

The ideal administration schedule of a drug to cure pain is to provide constant analgesia without breakthrough pain and excessive sedation. PCA aims at maintaining the constant plasma concentration by individualising the dosing intervals according to the patient needs and thereby preventing peaks and troughs. The smallest concentration of an analgesic to do so is termed as 'minimum effective analgesic concentration' (MEAC).

Patient-controlled analgesia maintains a steady state of plasma concentration by a feedback loop mechanism that uses a microprocessor-controlled infusion pump with settings to programme the on-demand bolus does, lockout interval and ability to provide background infusion of the same drug (Fig. 31.1).

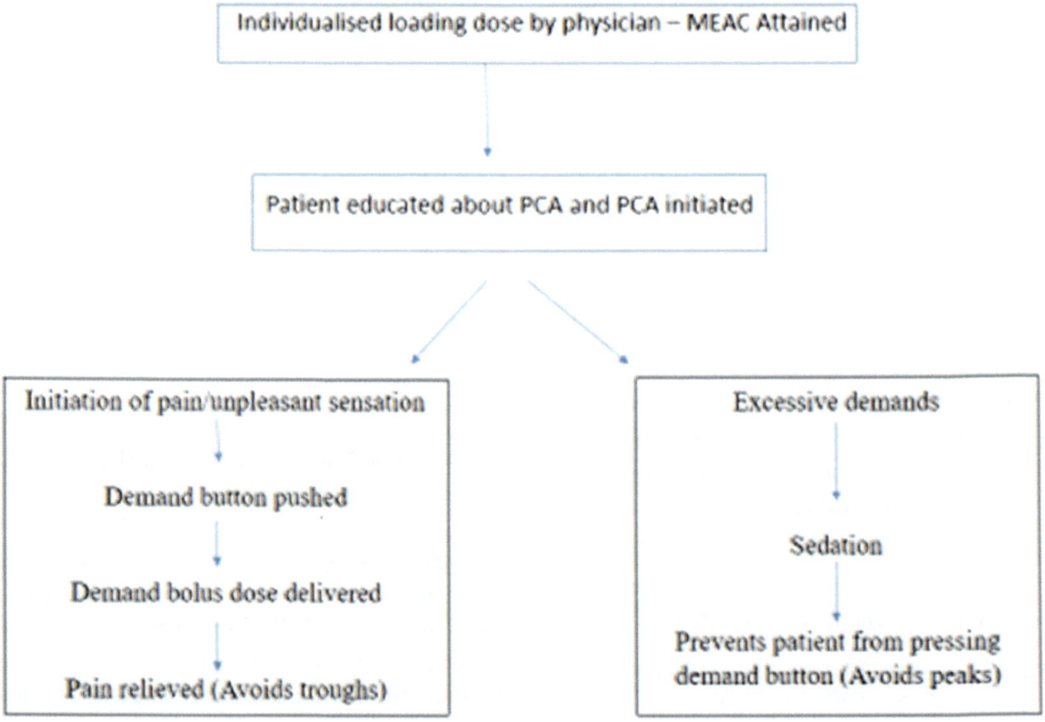

Fig. 31.1 Figure showing feedback loop mechanism of safety with IV PCA

Table 31.1 Terminology associated with PCA

Term	Definition
Initiating loading dose	This bolus dose is given via the pump titrated according to patient need
Demand bolus dose	It is the bolus dose of the analgesic being purged on pressing demand button. It can be entered as ml, mg and mcg. It should be set judiciously to produce appreciable analgesia without adverse effects
Lockout interval	It is the time during which no drug delivery happens even if the patient pushes demand button. It is commonly set at 5–10 min irrespective of the opioid being used. This avoids drug stacking and overdosage
Background infusion	It refers to the continuous delivery of basal infusion of analgesics in addition to the demand bolus. It is more useful in PCEA and peripheral nerve PCA and in opioid tolerant patients
Dose limits	It is the maximum dose of the drug that can be delivered over a period of time. It is a safety feature to prevent overdosing over a period of time

31.4 Terminology Associated with PCA

It is important to know the various terminologies associated with the technique of using PCA (Table 31.1).

31.5 Pre-requisites for Successful and Safe Usage of PCA

PCA, though, simple to use and administer, does have some pre-requisites. An individualised regimen for each patient is then titrated depending upon the opioid tolerance and number of empty and successful demands to provide successful and effective analgesia.

- A co-operative patient with enough comprehension to understand the concept of PCA.
- Educate the patient along with family and the nursing staff involved about the use of PCA.
- A physician titrated loading dose should be given prior to the initiation of PCA.
- Set demand dose according to patient weight, age, and disease profile to provide sufficient analgesia.
- Set the lockout interval to provide maximal effect of the previous demand dose while avoiding break-through pains. The need for a background infusion is assessed and included if needed.
- Separate IV lines dedicated for IV PCA with alarms for blockage of lines and monitoring for side effects, especially sedation and respiratory depression should be used to provide safe analgesia via PCA.

31.6 Benefits and Limitations of PCA

PCA has proven to enhance patients' perception of pain control with decreased breakthrough pain, both of which lead to better patient satisfaction. Certain studies have proven that PCA usage reduces postoperative pulmonary complications in comparison to conventional IV techniques of analgesia.

The major limitation, however, of PCA is the inability to extend its usage to patients who are not understanding enough to use the PCA. Other limitations include restricted postoperative mobilisation, operator errors and opioid related adverse effects. Though it has proven to reduce nursing time for individual patients, PCA usage has been associated with higher maintenance cost due to mechanical malfunctions.

31.7 Techniques of PCA

31.7.1 IV PCA

Opioids are the most common and effective drugs used for IV PCA. Pure mu receptor agonists, such as morphine, hydromorphone, fentanyl and remifentanil, are the first choice of drugs for IV

PCA as they have no analgesic ceiling effect, i.e., a higher dose provides superior analgesia. There is, however, a clinical ceiling due to side effects which are dose dependent, i.e., a higher dose can cause sedation, respiratory depression and psychotomimetic side effects. Morphine is considered as the gold standard drug for IV PCA though recently fentanyl has gained popularity due to its rapid onset of action, high efficacy, intermediate duration of action with minimum accumulation of metabolites. Remifentanil PCA is useful as an alternative to epidural analgesia during labour pain due to its ultra-short action and is thus appropriate for episodic intense pain conditions. The bolus and lockout period regimens of commonly used opioids for IV PCA are given in Table 31.2.

In opioid naïve patients, while using IV PCA, a demand bolus only regimen should be used whereas a background opioid infusion is usually added in opioid tolerant patients and for patients with chronic pain. Infusions should, however, be avoided in elderly, in patients with OSA due to increased risk of respiratory depression. Morphine PCA should be avoided in patients with S. creatinine >2 mg/dl as it can lead to accumulation of its active metabolite—morphine-6-glucuronide (M6G), leading to delayed respiratory depression and sedation. Similarly use of meperidine PCA in patients with impaired renal function can lead to accumulation of its toxic metabolite non-meperidine which can lead to neurotoxic signs and symptoms like, anxiety, tremors and even seizures. Both hydromorphone and fentanyl are good alternatives for patients with renal impairment.

Other IV analgesic drugs like Ketamine have been tried as due to its NMDA antagonism and opioid sparing effect. Morphine and ketamine at a ratio of 1:1 with lockout interval of 8–10 min are commonly used regimen. The use of Ketamine is, however, limited by its adverse effects including nausea, vomiting and psychomimetic effects.

Dexmedetomidine, an alpha 2 agonist, provides opioid sparing analgesia, anxiolysis, sedation without respiratory depression and has a prophylactic role in postoperative nausea and vomiting. A standard combination drug regimen would be a drug mixture of 1 mg/ml morphine with 5 mcg/ml dexmedetomidine. A 1 ml demand bolus of this mixture is delivered with a lockout interval of 5 min.

31.7.2 PCEA

Epidural analgesia with local anaesthetics has proven analgesic benefit over IV opioid administration with decreased adverse effect profile. In PCEA, a background infusion of local anaesthetic is almost always used to maintain a constant sensory blockade. Any breakthrough pain is managed with the demand bolus administered by the patient. The commonly used regimen for PCEA is 0.0625–0.1% bupivacaine/ropivacaine with 2 mcg/ml fentanyl with a background infusion of 4–6 ml/h and a demand bolus of 4 ml with a lockout interval of 10 min.

Several adjuvants have been tried in the local anaesthetic mixture to improve the quality of analgesia. Opioids and when added to the local anaesthetic improves analgesic quality without causing motor blockade. Clonidine an alpha agonist when added to local anaesthetics has shown to decrease the incidence of nausea, vomiting and pruritus at the cost of hemodynamic stability but without any analgesic benefit.

Table 31.2 Opioid regimens for IV PCA

Drug	Demand bolus	Lockout interval (min)
Morphine	0.5–3 mg	5–20
Fentanyl	15–50 mcg	3–10
Hydromorphone	0.1–0.5 mg	5–15
Remifentanil	0.5 mcg/kg	2
Meperidine/pethidine	10–20 mg	6–10
Tramadol	10–20 mg	5–10

Epidurally delivered analgesia is superior to intravenous opioid analgesia because it decreases intraoperative blood loss and the incidence of perioperative thromboembolic events. It is also associated with early restoration of bowel function, enhanced postoperative functional capacity, reduces postoperative cardiopulmonary complications and postulated to decrease the incidence of cancer recurrence.

The use of PCEA like any neuraxial analgesia is associated with side effects like motor blockade, hypotension and potential to cause epidural hematoma, infections and neurological injury. Opioids, if being used as adjuncts, can have their related adverse effects like pruritis, nausea, vomiting and sedation. Caution must be exercised while inserting and removing epidural catheter in patients on anticoagulants and existing guidelines should be strictly followed to avoid complications. Overall, IV PCA might be superior to PCEA in terms of neuraxial blockade related side effects like hypotension, while PCEA is associated with a shorter length of hospital stay due to early mobilisation.

31.7.3 Peripheral Nerve Block Catheter Delivered PCA/ Patient-Controlled Regional Analgesia (PCRA)

In peripheral nerve block catheter delivered PCA aka patient-controlled regional analgesia (PCRA), a catheter is inserted into the perineural space. A continuous infusion of local anaesthetic is usually initiated along with a small on-demand dose delivered via a PCA pump. This technique has been studied with brachial plexus block, femoral nerve blocks and sciatic nerve block.

In upper limb surgeries, interscalene and infraclavicular peripheral nerve catheter has been used with 0.2 % Ropivacaine at 6–8 ml/h background infusion with a demand bolus of 2–4 ml and a lockout interval of 20 min. In lower limb surgeries, sciatic (subgluteal/ popliteal) nerve catheter is used with 0.2% ropivacaine at 5–8 ml/h background infusion with a demand bolus of 3–5 ml and a lockout interval of 20–60 min.

Patient-controlled regional analgesia has shown to provide excellent postoperative analgesia with good patient satisfaction. It also has less interactions with anticoagulants. However, one should always look out for local site infections and neurological complications due to the indwelling catheter.

31.7.4 Transdermal PCA

Transdermal PCA system is a new non-invasive method of drug delivery which provides preprogrammed, self-contained, self-adhesive, on demand drug delivery. Here, the patient has to press the demand button twice, following which, a non-detectable low electric current is generated from the patch, producing an external electric field around the skin. This leads to iontophoresis of the drug and the ionised drug penetrates the skin and is delivered into the target receptors. As the principle involves iontophoresis, only ionisable drugs can be used for transdermal PCA.

Currently, Fentanyl HCl patient-controlled transdermal system is the only available system based on this principle. On pressing the demand button, 40 mcg Fentanyl is delivered over 10 min. The system can deliver six demand doses over 1 h and 80 demand doses over 24 h after which it shuts down and has to be replaced. It is shown to provide equivalent postoperative analgesia as IV PCA with morphine with reduced nursing time and reduced chances of errors. The non-invasive nature of the system allows for greater patient mobility. Breakthrough pain, if present, has to be addressed by an alternative analgesia method as it cannot provide background infusion or additional rescue boluses.

31.8 PCA in Special Population

31.8.1 PCA for Labour Analgesia

PCEA is a very effective method of providing labour analgesia. Here, a demand bolus with background infusion of local anaesthetic–opioid mixture is preferred. The commonly used regimen is Bupivacaine 0.05–0.125% or Ropivacaine 0.08–0.2% with Fentanyl 1.5–3 mcg/ml with a background infusion at 4–8 ml/h with demand bolus of 4–8 ml with lockout interval of 10–15 min. A demand only bolus of 5–12 ml with lockout interval of 10–20 min may also be used.

In comparison to IV PCA, PCEA produces lesser sedation, nausea and vomiting and lesser incidence of neonatal/foetal distress and need of neonatal resuscitation. In comparison to continuous epidural infusion, PCEA requires lesser anaesthetic intervention with lesser breakthrough pain, lesser dose of local anaesthetic usage, lesser motor blockade and hence better patient satisfaction.

Intravenous PCA for labour analgesia is indicated if neuraxial techniques of labour analgesia are not feasible. The pre-requisites for IV PCA for labour analgesia includes one-to-one nursing care, patient, obstetrician and nursing staff education, monitoring for excessive sedation, capnography, respiratory rate, pulse oximetry and hemodynamic monitoring. There should be readily available oxygen delivery devices and ventilation assist devices. Supplemental oxygen should be provided if room air SpO_2 falls below 94%. If SpO_2 falls below 94% despite supplemental oxygen or excess sedation, the anaesthesia provider should be immediately notified.

Compared to intermittent IV bolus /infusion administered by nurses, IV PCA for labour analgesia provides better pain relief with low-drug dosage thereby causing lesser placental transfer of drugs as well as decreasing the incidence of maternal side effects like respiratory depression, nausea and vomiting. However, compared to neuraxial techniques, IV PCA is not effective in providing analgesia to the later stages of labour due to difficulty to co-ordinate the timing of uterine contraction and peak effect of opioid. This can be tackled to some extend by training the parturient to press the demand button on their first perception of uterine contraction. Maternal and foetal side effects of opioids are also a major factor limiting its use as a primary modality for labour analgesia.

Remifentanil is the most commonly used drug for IV PCA in labour analgesia due its short duration of action and rapid titrability. It has a context sensitive half-life of 3.5 min irrespective of the duration of infusion with 50% recovery in minute ventilation following apnoea by 5.4 min. An effective analgesic half-life of 6 min provides excellent analgesia for consecutive uterine contractions in early stages of labour. Though it crosses placenta readily (foetal to maternal blood ratio –0.88), remifentanil is extensively redistributed or metabolised in the foetus leading to decreased incidence of neonatal respiratory depression (umbilical artery to vein ratio –0.29).

The commonly used regimens include a bolus only regimen of 0.2–0.8 mcg/kg with a lockout interval of 2–3 min and a regimen with background infusion of 0.025–0.1 mcg/kg/min with bolus dose 0.25 mcg/kg with a lockout interval of 2–3 min.

The adverse effects of remifentanil in the mother include respiratory depression (decrease in both tidal volume and respiratory rate), apnoea, bradycardia, sedation, dizziness, nausea and vomiting and pruritus. The foetal and neonatal side effects include opioid induced loss of foetal heart rate variability, foetal/neonatal acidosis and need for neonatal resuscitation/naloxone administration.

Other opioids are rarely used for IV PCA due to increased incidence of maternal dizziness and sedation and neonatal respiratory depression. Morphine may be useful for providing analgesia in parturients with intrauterine death.

31.8.2 PCA in Paediatric Population

PCA has been used safely in paediatric age group of more than 7 years who can understand the concept of PCA. A basal infusion is commonly initiated in paediatric cases. All children receiving PCA should be monitored with pulse oximetry and proper education should be given to caretakers.

PCA by proxy/surrogate PCA is a PCA technique useful in children less than 7 years in which a designated surrogate (nurse/parent) pushes the

Table 31.3 PCA and PCEA regimens in paediatrics

	PCA			PCEA
Drug	morphine	Fentanyl	Hydro morphone	Bupivacaine 0.06%/ropivacaine 0.1–0.2%
Demand dose	10–30 mcg/kg	0.2–1 mcg/kg	2–6 mcg/kg	0.1 ml/kg
Background infusion	10–30 mcg/kg/h	0.2–1 mcg/kg/h	2–6 mcg/kg/h	0.1–0.3 ml/kg/h
Lockout interval	7–15 min	7–15 min	15 min	10 min
1 h limit	5 doses/h	4 doses/h	5 doses/h	2.5 mg/kg/h
4 h limit	250–400 mcg/kg	7–10 mcg/kg	50–80 mcg/kg	

demand button when they perceive the child to be in pain. However, it is less safe compared to PCA and has shown to have increased risk of cardio-pulmonary complications and overdose. The commonly used PCA and PCEA regimens in paediatrics are given in Table 31.3.

31.8.3 PCA for Chronic Pain Management

PCA has also found its way in chronic pain management. It has been proven as an effective analgesic option for opioid tolerant patients with moderate to severe cancer pain. Compared to postoperative patients, this population requires a higher dose of opioids and a basal infusion is almost always required. Methadone, an opioid not commonly advocated in perioperative period is useful in this group of patients who are refractory to morphine.

31.9 Recent Advances: Vital Signs Integrated Patient Assisted Intravenous Analgesia (VPIA)

With evolving technology and more complex capabilities of PCA devices and routes, the safety margin for these devices need to be perfect. Vital signs integrated patient assisted intravenous analgesia (VIPA) is a novel intelligent software incorporated in IV PCA system. It has an automated closed loop feedback system with a step up–step down regimen which receives input from vital sign monitoring devices including heart rate and pulse oximeter and regulates drug delivery. The software incorporates a bradycardia and desaturation threshold which can be set, below which the drug won't be delivered even on pressing the demand button. VPIA has been shown to be safe and efficacious in labouring patients receiving IV Remifentanil PCA. Another system of "smart" (computerised) PCA pumps containing dose-error reduction software have been described where the an integrated system would "pause" the PCA pump if either of the predetermined respiratory limits are exceeded (pulse rate <50 beats/min or >120 beats/min; SpO_2 <90%: respiratory rate <10 breaths/min: $EtCO_2$ >60 mmHg: apnoea >30 s).

Suggested Reading

1. Macintyre PE. Safety and efficacy of patient-controlled analgesia. Br J Anaesth. 2001;87(1):36–46.
2. Chumbley GM, Hall GM, Salmon P. Why do patients feel positive about patient-controlled analgesia? Anaesthesia. 1999;54(4):386–9.
3. Walder B, Schafer M, Henzi I, Tramèr MR. Efficacy and safety of patient-controlled opioid analgesia for acute postoperative pain. A quantitative systematic review. Acta Anaesthesiol Scand. 2001;45(7):795–804.
4. Patak LS, Tait AR, Mirafzali L, Morris M, Dasgupta S, Brummett CM. Patient perspectives of patient-controlled analgesia (PCA) and methods for improving pain control and patient satisfaction. Reg Anesth Pain Med. 2013;38(4):326–33.
5. Wu CL, Cohen SR, Richman JM, Rowlingson AJ, Courpas GE, Cheung K, et al. Efficacy of postoperative patient-controlled and continuous infusion epidural analgesia versus intravenous patient-controlled analgesia with opioids: a meta-analysis. Anesthesiology. 2005;103(5):1079–88; quiz 1109–10.

6. Singelyn FJ, Seguy S, Gouverneur JM. Interscalene brachial plexus analgesia after open shoulder surgery: continuous versus patient-controlled infusion. Anesth Analg. 1999;89(5):1216–20.
7. Fentanyl iontophoretic transdermal system for acute-pain management after orthopedic surgery: a comparative study with morphine intravenous patient-controlled analgesia - ScienceDirect [Internet]. [cited 2022 Sep 20]. https://www.sciencedirect.com/science/article/abs/pii/S109873390600530X.
8. Marks RM, Sachar EJ. Undertreatment of medical inpatients with narcotic analgesics. Ann Intern Med. 1973;78(2):173–81.
9. Roe BB. Are postoperative narcotics necessary? Arch Surg. 1960;1963(87):912–5.
10. Sechzer PH. Objective measurement of pain. Anesthesiology. 1968;29(1):209.
11. Sechzer PH. Studies in pain with the analgesic-demand system. Anesth Analg. 1971;50(1):1–10.
12. Evans JM, Rosen M, MacCarthy J, Hogg MI. Apparatus for patient-controlled administration of intravenous narcotics during labour. Lancet. 1976;1(7949):17–8.
13. Keeri-Szanto M. Apparatus for demand analgesia. Can Anaesth Soc J. 1971;18(5):581–2.
14. Austin KL, Stapleton JV, Mather LE. Relationship between blood meperidine concentrations and analgesic response: a preliminary report. Anesthesiology. 1980;53(6):460–6.
15. Gust R, Pecher S, Gust A, Hoffmann V, Böhrer H, Martin E. Effect of patient-controlled analgesia on pulmonary complications after coronary artery bypass grafting. Crit Care Med. 1999;27(10):2218–23.
16. Yan G, Chen J, Yang G, Duan G, Du Z, Yu Z, et al. Effects of patient-controlled analgesia with hydromorphone or sufentanil on postoperative pulmonary complications in patients undergoing thoracic surgery: a quasi-experimental study. BMC Anesthesiol. 2018;18:192.
17. Ashburn MA, Love G, Pace NL. Respiratory-related critical events with intravenous patient-controlled analgesia. Clin J Pain. 1994;10(1):52–6.
18. Tamsen A, Hartvig P, Fagerlund C, Dahlström B, Bondesson U. Patient-controlled analgesic therapy: clinical experience. Acta Anaesthesiol Scand. 1982;26(74):157–60.
19. Jacox A, Carr DB, Mahrenholz DM, Ferrell BM. Cost considerations in patient-controlled analgesia. PharmacoEconomics. 1997;12(2 Pt 1):109–20.
20. Momeni M, Crucitti M, De Kock M. Patient-controlled analgesia in the management of postoperative pain. Drugs. 2006;66(18):2321–37.
21. Trescot AM, Datta S, Lee M, Hansen H. Opioid pharmacology. Pain Physician. 2008;11(2 Suppl):S133–53.
22. Grass JA. Patient-controlled analgesia. Anesth Analg. 2005;101(5 Suppl):S44–61.
23. Soffin EM, Liu SS. Chapter 13 - patient-controlled analgesia. In: Benzon HT, Raja SN, Liu SS, Fishman SM, Cohen SP, editors. Essentials of pain medicine. 4th ed. Elsevier: Amsterdam; 2018. p. 117–22. https://www.sciencedirect.com/science/article/pii/B9780323401968000139.
24. Dal D, Kanbak M, Caglar M, Aypar U. A background infusion of morphine does not enhance postoperative analgesia after cardiac surgery. Can J Anaesth J Can Anesth. 2003;50(5):476–9.
25. Fleming BM, Coombs DW. A survey of complications documented in a quality-control analysis of patient-controlled analgesia in the postoperative patient. J Pain Symptom Manag. 1992;7(8):463–9.
26. Simpson G, Jackson M. Perioperative management of opioid-tolerant patients. BJA Educ. 2017;17(4):124–8.
27. Lam KK, Kunder S, Wong J, Doufas AG, Chung F. Obstructive sleep apnea, pain, and opioids: is the riddle solved? Curr Opin Anesthesiol. 2016;29(1):134–40.
28. Conway BR, Fogarty DG, Nelson WE, Doherty CC. Opiate toxicity in patients with renal failure. BMJ. 2006;332(7537):345–6.
29. Hocking G, Cousins MJ. Ketamine in chronic pain management: an evidence-based review. Anesth Analg. 2003;97(6):1730–9.
30. Petrenko AB, Yamakura T, Baba H, Shimoji K. The role of N-methyl-D-aspartate (NMDA) receptors in pain: a review. Anesth Analg. 2003;97(4):1108–16.
31. Sveticic G, Gentilini A, Eichenberger U, Luginbühl M, Curatolo M. Combinations of morphine with ketamine for patient-controlled analgesia: a new optimization method. Anesthesiology. 2003;98(5):1195–205.
32. Bellon M, Le Bot A, Michelet D, Hilly J, Maesani M, Brasher C, et al. Efficacy of intraoperative dexmedetomidine compared with placebo for postoperative pain management: a meta-analysis of published studies. Pain Ther. 2016;5(1):63–80.
33. Li HJ, Liu S, Geng ZY, Li XY. Adding dexmedetomidine to morphine-based analgesia reduces early postoperative nausea in patients undergoing gynecological laparoscopic surgery: a randomized controlled trial. BMC Anesthesiol. 2020;20(1):11.
34. Nie Y, Tu W, Shen X, Yu W, Yu Y, Song X, et al. Dexmedetomidine added to sufentanil patient-controlled intravenous analgesia relieves the postoperative pain after cesarean delivery: a prospective randomized controlled multicenter study. Sci Rep. 2018;8(1):9952.
35. Lin TF, Yeh YC, Lin FS, Wang YP, Lin CJ, Sun WZ, et al. Effect of combining dexmedetomidine and morphine for intravenous patient-controlled analgesia. Br J Anaesth. 2009;102(1):117–22.
36. Block BM, Liu SS, Rowlingson AJ, Cowan AR, John A, Cowan J, Wu CL. Efficacy of postoperative epidural analgesia: a meta-analysis. JAMA. 2003;290(18):2455–63.
37. Mann C, Pouzeratte Y, Boccara G, Peccoux C, Vergne C, Brunat G, et al. Comparison of intravenous or epidural patient-controlled analgesia in the elderly after major abdominal surgery. Anesthesiology. 2000;92(2):433–41.

38. Epidural anesthesia and analgesia. Their role in postoperative outcome. 2022. https://pubmed.ncbi.nlm.nih.gov/7793661/.
39. Förster JG, Rosenberg PH. Small dose of clonidine mixed with low-dose ropivacaine and fentanyl for epidural analgesia after total knee arthroplasty. Br J Anaesth. 2004;93(5):670–7.
40. Paech MJ, Pavy TJ, Orlikowski CE, Lim W, Evans SF. Postoperative epidural infusion: a randomized, double-blind, dose-finding trial of clonidine in combination with bupivacaine and fentanyl. Anesth Analg. 1997;84(6):1323–8.
41. Rodgers A, Walker N, Schug S, McKee A, Kehlet H, van Zundert A, et al. Reduction of postoperative mortality and morbidity with epidural or spinal anaesthesia: results from overview of randomised trials. BMJ. 2000;321(7275):1493.
42. Carli F, Mayo N, Klubien K, Schricker T, Trudel J, Belliveau P. Epidural analgesia enhances functional exercise capacity and health-related quality of life after colonic surgery: results of a randomized trial. Anesthesiology. 2002;97(3):540–9.
43. Chen WK, Miao CH. The effect of anesthetic technique on survival in human cancers: a meta-analysis of retrospective and prospective studies. PLoS ONE. 2013;8(2):e56540.
44. Practice recommendations on neuraxial anesthesia and peripheral nerve blocks during the COVID-19 pandemic [Internet]. The American Society of Regional Anesthesia and Pain Medicine (ASRA). [cited 2021 Jun 12]. https://www.asra.com/guidelines-articles/original-articles/article-item/legacy-b-blog-posts/2020/04/01/practice-recommendations-on-neuraxial-anesthesia-and-peripheral-nerve-blocks-during-the-covid-19-pandemic.
45. Singelyn FJ, Gouverneur JM. Extended "three-in-one" block after total knee arthroplasty: continuous versus patient-controlled techniques. Anesth Analg. 2000;91(1):176–80.
46. Halpern SH, Carvalho B. Patient-controlled epidural analgesia for labor. Anesth Analg. 2009;108(3):921–8.
47. Lim Y, Ocampo CE, Supandji M, Teoh WHL, Sia AT. A randomized controlled trial of three patient-controlled epidural analgesia regimens for labor. Anesth Analg. 2008;107(6):1968–72.
48. Wilson MJA, MacArthur C, Hewitt CA, Handley K, Gao F, Beeson L, et al. Intravenous remifentanil patient-controlled analgesia versus intramuscular pethidine for pain relief in labour (RESPITE): an open-label, multicentre, randomised controlled trial. Lancet. 2018;392(10148):662–72.
49. Tveit TO, Halvorsen A, Seiler S, Rosland JH. Efficacy and side effects of intravenous remifentanil patient-controlled analgesia used in a stepwise approach for labour: an observational study. Int J Obstet Anesth. 2013;22(1):19–25.
50. Konefał H, Jaskot B, Czeszyńska MB, Pastuszka J. Remifentanil patient-controlled analgesia for labor – monitoring of newborn heart rate, blood pressure and oxygen saturation during the first 24 hours after delivery. Arch Med Sci. 2013;9(4):697–702.
51. Stocki D, Matot I, Einav S, Eventov-Friedman S, Ginosar Y, Weiniger CF. A randomized controlled trial of the efficacy and respiratory effects of patient-controlled intravenous remifentanil analgesia and patient-controlled epidural analgesia in laboring women. Anesth Analg. 2014;118(3):589–97.
52. Das D, Patel N. Management of the woman with an intrauterine fetal death (IUFD). In: Fernando R, Sultan P, Phillips S, editors. Quick hits in obstetric anesthesia. Cham: Springer; 2022. p. 21–4. https://doi.org/10.1007/978-3-030-72487-0_4.
53. Smith LA, Burns E, Cuthbert A. Parenteral opioids for maternal pain management in labour. Cochrane Database Syst Rev. 2018;6:CD007396. https://doi.org/10.1002/14651858.CD007396.pub3.
54. Nelson KL, Yaster M, Kost-Byerly S, Monitto CL. A national survey of American Pediatric Anesthesiologists: patient-controlled analgesia and other intravenous opioid therapies in pediatric acute pain management. Anesth Analg. 2010;110(3):754–60.
55. Berde CB, Sethna NF. Analgesics for the treatment of pain in children. N Engl J Med. 2002;347(14):1094–103.
56. Monitto CL, Greenberg RS, Kost-Byerly S, Wetzel R, Billett C, Lebet RM, et al. The safety and efficacy of parent-/nurse-controlled analgesia in patients less than six years of age. Anesth Analg. 2000;91(3):573–9.
57. Fitzgibbon DR, Ready BL. Intravenous high-dose methadone administered by patient controlled analgesia and continuous infusion for the treatment of cancer pain refractory to high-dose morphine. Pain. 1997;73(2):259–61.
58. Sabatowski R, Kasper SM, Radbruch L. Patient-controlled analgesia with intravenous L-methadone in a child with cancer pain refractory to high-dose morphine. J Pain Symptom Manag. 2002;23(1):3–5.
59. Leong WL, Sng BL, Zhang Q, Han NLR, Sultana R, Sia AT. A case series of vital signs-controlled, patient-assisted intravenous analgesia (VPIA) using remifentanil for labour and delivery. Anaesthesia. 2017;72(7):845–52.
60. Sng BL, Tan DJ, Tan CW, Han NLR, Sultana R, Sia ATH. A preliminary assessment of vital-signs-integrated patient-assisted intravenous opioid analgesia (VPIA) for postsurgical pain. BMC Anesthesiol. 2020;20(1):145.
61. Maddox RR, Oglesby H, Williams CK, et al. Continuous respiratory monitoring and a "smart" infusion system improve safety of patient-controlled analgesia in the postoperative period. In: Henriksen K, Battles JB, Keyes MA, et al., editors. Advances in patient safety: new directions and alternative approaches (vol. 4: technology and medication safety). Rockville: Agency for Healthcare Research and Quality; 2008. https://www.ncbi.nlm.nih.gov/books/NBK43753/.

GPSR Compliance

The European Union's (EU) General Product Safety Regulation (GPSR) is a set of rules that requires consumer products to be safe and our obligations to ensure this.

If you have any concerns about our products, you can contact us on ProductSafety@springernature.com

In case Publisher is established outside the EU, the EU authorized representative is:

Springer Nature Customer Service Center GmbH
Europaplatz 3
69115 Heidelberg, Germany

Batch number: 10731395

Printed by Printforce, the Netherlands